It's that rare thing – a medical book that can be read by lay people and health professionals alike. Dr Barry demystifies subjects that touch so many of our lives and he does so with compassion, wisdom and vast professional knowledge.

Cathy Kelly

Dr Harold Barry, in *Flagging the Problem*, distils impressive amounts of research and practical experience into an accessible and balanced guide to the issues of mental health, depression, addiction, anxiety disorders and suicide. With admirable clarity and compassionate sensitivity, this book offers not just information, but hope, to anyone affected directly or indirectly by these issues.

Breda O'Brien

This is a superb book; it looks at mental-health problems in a fresh and accessible way. The use of an innovative 'flag' method to explain mood disorders offers a unique insight into depression. *Flagging the Problem* could help save lives that might otherwise be lost to suicide.

Dr Muiris Houston, Medical Correspondent, The Irish Times

This is an important book. It provides a new approach to mental health and the intricacy of the variables that influence it. Written with compassion and creativity and informed by decades of General Practice insights, Dr Harry Barry helps the reader to understand the complexity of the normal mood system and the distress of depression, anxiety, addiction and suicide.

Marie Murray, Director of the Student Counselling Services at University College Dublin

Depression is the scourge of the twenty-first century. Dr Barry, in *Flagging the Problem*, offers a unique insight into this illness from a biological/sociological/cognitive perspective, and in this wonderful book has married together all three insights. In particular he defines the hidden dynamic underlying the reluctance of the sufferer to come for help. This is a 'must read' for public and professionals alike.

Enda Murphy, Cognitive Behaviour Therapist and Project Director, ICGP

Dr Barry has produced an innovative, highly readable, challenging text which focuses on the core mental-health disorders associated with suicide. The book will be of major benefit to doctors working in primary care, clinical psychologists and other professionals in the mental-health arena.

Professor Ted Dinan, MD, PhD, DSc, Department of Psychiatry, University College Cork

This outstanding book will be of tremendous help to those who are trying to understand the complexities of mental illness. By integrating a medical and psychological approach, Dr Barry has bridged a gap that has often pitted those espousing either psychological or pharmacological treatments against each other. The book will be of great assistance to everybody who is striving to end the scourge of suicide.

Professor Patricia Casey

Having read *Flagging the Problem*, I now have a much better understanding of why Niall died. This book is written in very simple terms, exploring the complex nature of depression and suicidal tendencies. It is a 'must read' for every parent, informing them of the tell-tale warning signs of depression and suicide.

John, father of Niall, who died by suicide in 2002

First published in 2007 by
Liberties Press
Guinness Enterprise Centre | Taylor's Lane | Dublin 8
www.LibertiesPress.com | info@libertiespress.com
Editorial: +353 (1) 402 0805 | sean@libertiespress.com
Sales and marketing: +353 (1) 453 4363 | peter@libertiespress.com
Liberties Press is a member of Clé, the Irish Book Publishers' Association

Trade enquiries to CMD Distribution
55A Spruce Avenue | Stillorgan Industrial Park | Blackrock | County Dublin
Tel: +353 (1) 294 2560
Fax: +353 (1) 294 2564

ISBN: 978–1–905483–18–1

2 4 6 8 10 9 7 5 3 1

A CIP record for this title is available from the British Library

Cover design by Ros Murphy
Set in Garamond

Printed in Ireland by Colour Books
Baldoyle Industrial Estate | Dublin 13

FLAGGING THE PROBLEM

A NEW APPROACH TO MENTAL HEALTH

DR HARRY BARRY

LIB
ERT
IES

This book is dedicated to Niall, his parents John and Anne, and all his family and friends. It is also dedicated to Jason, his uncle Michael and all those who have lost loved ones to the white flag of suicide. Niall and Jason, you are not forgotten by those who love you in this world, and we pray you are happy in the next.

CONTENTS

Acknowledgements

When I approached an old friend of mine, Dr Tony Bates, for advice on how to get this book published, he gave me the following advice: 'Find an editor who believes in both you and the book.' Tony's advice was as always very wise. I have indeed been very fortunate in finding such an editor in Seán O'Keeffe of Liberties Press. With patience, kindness and a great eye for detail, he has turned my 'ramblings' into a reality. I owe him a debt I can never repay. To Peter O'Connell at Liberties Press I owe a debt for his expertise in the marketing and media side of this book. We are fortunate in Ireland to have such a forward-looking publishing company.

There are so many others who have played a part in this project. To John and Anne, who allowed me to share Niall's story, and to Dr Michael Smurfit for his support and encouragement, and for writing the foreword, I can only say 'thank you'. A special thanks to Kate Kelly for all her help.

To Enda Murphy, the Irish College of General Practice CBT Project Director, I also offer special thanks. He was, and still is, of great assistance in introducing myself and a number of GPs around Ireland into the world of this form of psychotherapy. Many of the clinical and theoretical details about CBT contained in this book were provided by Enda. I hope I have been faithful to his teachings!

To Cathy Kelly, author and UNICEF ambassador, I must offer a special thank you for being of great support and encouragement at a time I needed it most. She is and always will be a real lady.

I would like to send a big thank you to all at Aware, particularly Prof. Patrick McKeown, CEO Geraldine Clare, Annette Byrne, our most able chairman, all the hardworking members of the Board, and the many members around the country, for their support and encouragement. This book is for you all.

To my reviewers, Prof. Patricia Casey, Prof. Ted Dinan, Dr Muiris Houston, Marie Murray, Dr John Connolly (of the Irish Suicidology Association), Mike Watts of GROW, Dr Michael Boland of the ICGP, and Breda O' Brien, along with others mentioned already, another warm appreciation.

To my loyal and devoted staff at 5 Leland Place – Fiona, Carmel, Susan, Anne and my practice nurse Brenda – for all their help and support throughout the period of writing this book. A special thanks also to Darina and Michael for their help with this project.

To my mother Dilly Barry (Thurles) and brothers Gerald and Kevin for their support and encouragement. To my mother-in-law Ciss Lahart (Eyrecourt) for her help and support down through the years, and to all our friends and relatives who have backed this project.

There are a number of people who sadly will not be here to see this published. The first is my brother David (who died recently, following a short illness), and I dedicate this book to him and his family (as well as to Niall and the other people mentioned in the dedication). We will miss you. The second is our great family friend Sister Kieran Saunders MMM. She was by my side during many difficult times in the Developing World and remained close to our little unit over many years till her death. It was she who persuaded me to stay in Ireland rather than return to the Developing World, explaining that there was poverty of a different kind at home. How right she was, for despite our affluence, there are many problems (some of which are dealt with in this book) in modern Ireland. We miss you so much, Kieran, and pray that you will remain our 'spiritual guide' throughout this mysterious journey through life and beyond. We also remember my father Harry and my father-in-law Nicholas, who are sadly not with us to share this moment.

Moving on to my family, I would like to start with my daughter Lara, our 'media expert', who spent a month editing and putting together my initial data into a presentable document. Her expertise, occasionally challenging observations ('Dad, get real!) and support, then and throughout the process of putting the book together will never be forgotten.

I also have to thank my son Daniel, psychology and communications expert, who was my right-hand man throughout this whole project. He was responsible for researching key articles, helping me design and create the diagrams which enrich this book, and also helping with the initial editing. Without his help, this book may never have reached a stage where it could be published.

To my (maths and physics expert) son Joseph, my thanks for his encouragement, support and critical eye during the writing of this book.

Finally, I reserve my greatest thank you to my wife Brenda. She has 'endured' (apart from adventures in the Developing World, mad thousand-mile journeys in a Volkswagen Beetle across the Serengeti Plains, thirty years married to a doctor working within the Irish medical system, and rearing, despite that, three wonderful children) the years of research, writing and editing with patience, love and support.

She is my greatest critic, my best friend, and the love of my life. Without her, all of the rest would be meaningless. *'Mo ghra, mo chroi.'*

FOREWORD

It is a sad fact that many families have experienced the suicide of a relative. We all ask ourselves why it happened and what more could have been done to prevent it.

When that death involves a young person with their whole life ahead of them, the grief that we feel for them is so much greater. We can remember them as happy children and we can see the opportunities that were ahead of them. We wonder how they reached a point when the thought of life became so bleak for them, and whether, no matter how much we tried, we failed them in providing the hope, the help and the encouragement that they needed.

In Ireland we are living through a period when we have more money, and more opportunities for work and leisure, than ever before, yet many of our young people, particularly our young men, find themselves living in a world of despair and drug addiction that ends with their suicide and a legacy of pain for those they leave behind.

Dr Harold Barry's experiences, his research and his findings provide a valuable source of information for the medical profession and for anyone who is trying to help a young person to change their life around, or who, sadly, is trying to come to terms with the suicide of someone they have been close to.

This book could save lives: I believe that it should be dedicated to all those young people whose lives came to such an unhappy and unnecessary end. They have not been forgotten, they are still loved, we still grieve for them and we still treasure memories of the time when they were happy and looking forward to each day with excitement and enthusiasm. They have been the inspiration for Dr Barry's book, which will help us to understand why these lives were lost and what can be done to help prevent other young people from giving up on the glorious journey that is life.

Dr Michael W. J. Smurfit
In memory of my nephew, Jason Smurfit

INTRODUCTION

It is a chilling statistic that as you read this introduction today, at least one person in Ireland will be preparing to end their life by suicide. Even more alarming is the fact that there is an almost 1 in 2 chance that this individual will be under the age of thirty-five. Suicide claims the lives of approximately 450 people each year in Ireland.

Niall, whose story is told in the 'White Flag' section of this book, was one of these people. The main aim of his father John, an inspiration to many because of the way he spoke out publicly about his son's suicide, was that other families could be spared the pain of losing a loved one. Families which have fallen victim to suicide are forever haunted by the question: 'Why?' This book was born out of a search for an answer to this question.

As a family doctor, dealing with the problems of depression, addiction, anxiety and suicide are part of my job. In the past ten years, general practitioners have witnessed a major upheaval in Irish society, brought about by the Celtic Tiger and the increased prosperity that has accompanied this economic boom. Not all the changes have been positive ones, however! 'Stress' and 'fatigue' are words that I hear in my surgery on a daily basis. 'Alcohol misuse' and 'substance abuse' are not far behind. Thankfully, more and more patients are beginning to speak freely about their symptoms of depression and anxiety, particularly men in their late twenties and early thirties. Nonetheless, it is my belief that the numbers presenting are only the tip of the iceberg. Most suffer in silence, hiding behind a mask of normality. This book is aimed at these people in particular, and their friends and families, whose role is often vital in encouraging people to discuss their mental-health problems.

Four things which I have noticed in the course of my professional life over the years are:

1   A lack of awareness or understanding of the ways in which illness can disrupt normal mental health. This includes an inability to accept that the mind is a function of the brain.

2   A misunderstanding of mental illness – that it is a 'weakness' without a biological basis. Just as diabetes is an illness caused by biological abnormalities in our pancreas, depression, anxiety and addiction are illnesses caused, at least in part, by biological abnormalities of the brain.

3   The huge stigma which has been attached to sufferers of these illnesses, and also, by association, to the families of these sufferers.

4   The enduring myth that psychiatrists and psychologists are the only experts who can deal with these illnesses. The family doctor will deal with a large number of such cases on a daily basis, yet this treatment option is often overlooked by both the general public and the media. This is in no way to denigrate the invaluable contribution made by psychiatrists or psychologists. Recent data released by the Irish College of General Practitioners suggests, however, that from the large pool of biological illnesses, which include depression, diabetes and heart disease, very few cases will be treated by a specialist. Meanwhile, although many cases of mental illness are treated by the family doctor, the majority remain undiagnosed.

In the last five years, there has been an explosion of information, based on scientific research, in areas such as neuro-imaging, genetics, neurophysiology and molecular biology. This has led to a transformation in our understanding of how the brain functions, as well as of illnesses such as depression, anxiety and addiction. It marks the beginning of a long and promising journey which may lead to a complete understanding of the brain and the illnesses which affect it. I have attempted to combine these recent findings with my thirty years of clinical experience to produce a book which not only deals with how to stay mentally healthy but also reveals the symptoms of mental illness together with their underlying biological causes.

The book uses a unique system to explain the biology behind these illnesses. During my research, I realised that the first letters of the main components of the biological mood system (the Frontal and Limbic mood departments, the Adrenal gland and the stress hormone Glucocorticsol) make up the word 'FLAG'. Based on this, I have used a colour-coded flag system throughout the book.

The colour coding for the various sections is as follows:

§   *The Green Flag* Normal mood: green indicating normality and balance

§   *The Red Flag* Depression: red as the symbol of warning or danger

§   *The Yellow Flag* Anxiety: yellow as the symbol of fear

§   *The Purple Flag* Addiction: purple as the symbol of pleasure and excess

§   *The White Flag* Suicide: white as the symbol of surrender

This system will, I feel, make it easier for the reader to visualise the illnesses, their symptoms and biology.

The most important part of the book, for me, is the explanation of the symptoms of the Red Flag of depression, and how they are caused. If enough people become aware of the warning signs and symptoms of depression, we will have taken a giant step towards preventing many potential cases of suicide.

The driving force behind this book is hope. For those in Ireland who are suffering from depression, addiction, anxiety and suicidal thoughts, the candle of hope has gone out. This candle needs to be relit, bringing with it the possibility of a new life where the pain and suffering caused by these illnesses can be alleviated. If this book does nothing more than provide a flame of hope to one person whose life seems to them to be so grey, hopeless and empty that ending it appears to be the only solution, and encourages them to come forward for help, then it has been well worth writing.

Let this be Niall's legacy.

A NOTE ON THE TEXT

I am aware that many readers may not want to know all the biological findings relating to the various elements of the flag system. To cater for them, I have given a summary of all the important points at the end of that section. For those who wish to explore the biological findings in greater detail, I include a technical section at the end of the book. Apart from Niall's story, all names, occupations and other details used in the book are allegorical in nature.

I

The Green Flag

The Normal Mood System

1

THE MOOD SYSTEM

Mood is an 'emotional state which lasts for a reasonably long period of time, often hours or days'. It differs from simple emotions like fear, anger, sadness or happiness in that it is of longer duration, is usually less intense, and is less likely to have been triggered by outside events. It is usually positive or negative, i.e. manifests itself in the person feeling 'up' or 'down'. Behaviour, on the other hand, relates to how we act or react to different circumstances in our internal or external environment. It can be conscious or unconscious, and is often strongly influenced by our emotions. These two important functions in our lives, along with our ability to cope with stress, are controlled by a highly organised mood system.

Most of us take normal mood and behaviour (otherwise known as good mental health) for granted. For others who are not so fortunate, disruption of this delicate system through biological illnesses such as depression, anxiety and addiction causes great upset, and sometimes havoc, in their lives.

Many people do not like to discuss issues like depression, anxiety or suicide. Somehow, these words convey an implied weakness or a basic flaw in the personality of those who are suffering from mental illness. Fear lies at the basis of our reluctance to talk about or admit to these conditions. This fear is deeply rooted in a long-standing ignorance and lack of knowledge as to how the brain in particular works.

The majority of mental illnesses arise from a common biological source: problems arising within our 'mood system'. In order to understand these illnesses, it is necessary to understand how the mood system works.

I   WHAT IS THE MOOD SYSTEM?

'Mood system' is a term I have coined to try to simplify for the reader what is, in fact, a highly complex internal biological network within the body. The function of this network is to keep in balance our emotions, behaviour and responses to stress of any kind. So let's take a look at the main components of this system.

Most emotional experiences and behavioural responses are mediated by two departments in the brain – which we'll call our 'mood departments' – one situated at the front of the brain, the other in the centre. These two mood departments are connected by a number of telephone-like cables which are vital for the smooth running of these areas of the brain. Outside of the brain, the mood system is completed by glands situated in our abdomen (perched on top of each of our kidneys), and the hormones this gland produces. This gland and its hormones are key players in our stress response, as we will see later.

So to sum up, these two mood departments, the mood cables connecting them, the adrenal gland in our abdomen and the stress hormones it produces, make up our 'mood system'. The slightest disruption to this delicately balanced system can cause mayhem throughout the body.

The brain is a great integrator of information, so most parts of this organ have an input into every decision we make. It is also extremely adaptable and, like all good computers, is adept at moving information around from one area to another, depending on circumstances. The brain lies at the heart of the mood system because it processes our emotions, creates our thoughts and moods, is the 'biological' source of the mind, and is responsible for instigating our emotional and behavioural responses.

The next section is a discussion of the brain and how it works, and this is followed by an examination of our mood system and how it is organised. I must preface all of this with a caveat. We are only at an early stage in our understanding of the brain: although a large amount of research has been carried out in this area, it remains cloaked in mystery. It is likely to take many years for us to have a complete understanding of the way the brain works – and indeed we may never develop such an understanding. Although functions such as the creation of mood or the control of behaviour will be assigned to different parts of the brain, much of what follows is merely educated guesswork by the world's leading experts in the field.

II   WHAT IS THE BRAIN?

FIGURE 1: THE HUMAN BRAIN

Aptly described as the 'boss organ' of the body, the brain is analogous to the central processor of a computer. It receives, compiles and evaluates information both from within the body and from the external environment, makes the necessary decisions, and issues instructions to every other organ structure in the body.

The brain is composed of around 10 billion cells. These cells are of two basic types:

1   *Neurons* Neurons are the decision-makers. They are individual cells which receive, process and pass on information. Like all other cells in the body, neurons are fluid-filled units surrounded by a fine cell membrane, which helps them to remain distinct from one another. In the centre of each neuron lie the chromosomes which in turn contain our genes. Neurons constitute only 10 percent of adult brain cells.

2   *Glial cells* Glial cells are the support cells. These cells support, protect and nourish the neurons. The glial cells make up the remaining 90 percent of adult brain cells. Many researchers now feel that glial cells may play a much greater role in brain function than was previously thought.

As with any large company, the brain assigns various functions and responsibilities to each department. This organisation mainly involves the neurons; the glial cells are the support staff, servicing all the neurons, regardless of where they are in the organisation.

Within such a large organisational structure, good communication is a prerequisite of efficient operation for the brain. Adjacent neurons must be able to communicate unimpeded, and departments must also be able to exchange important information easily. In order to address this concern, the brain – again like a company – has an excellent 'telephone system' installed, with cables connecting units within a particular department and also linking one department to another. These cables are of great importance in dealing with our mood system.

III   THE BRAIN: IT'S GOOD TO TALK

The brain has an ingenious means of passing on information from one neuron to another. Each cell has the ability to activate itself electrically and to pass this charge on to the next cell, causing it to activate also. As each neuron is an isolated cell, the brain has developed a practical way of sending information from one neuron to another.

Between neurons in the brain are hundreds of small gaps or meeting points, known as synapses (see Figure 2). The neuron which is passing on information produces chemical messengers which it releases in a small bubble into each of these gaps. These chemical messengers are called neurotransmitters, as they are transmitting messages between two neurons. The neurotransmitters cross the gap, attaching to receptors on the surface of the neighbouring neuron, releasing their information and returning to their cell of origin to await further instructions. As soon as this information has been communicated to the next cell, that cell may also decide to fire, based on the information it has received, repeating the process and activating the next neuron. A pathway is formed.

17

A Neurotransmitter (e.g. serotonin) molecule (carrying message from neuron 1) is released and crosses the synapse gap to neuron 2

B Neurotransmitter attaches to receptor on neighbouring neuron 2 and passes message on

C Neurotransmitter is released from this receptor (its job done!) and travels back across the synapse to be reabsorbed into neuron 1

D Peptide neurotransmitters (e.g. endorphins) released from synapse carry messages from neuron 1, which will travel to distant neurons

FIGURE 2: HOW NEURONS TALK TO EACH OTHER

The receptor is like a lock on a door that can only be opened using a key with two notches – the chemical messenger. Receptors are hugely important in our understanding of all illnesses. They are usually generated in the middle of the cell and transported to its outer membranes, where they are positioned to respond to the relevant chemical messengers. Some receptors are designed simply to encourage the cell to fire, others to communicate more detailed messages to the genes at the core of the cell. All this activity shares one key objective: the flow of information. When individual neurons are banded together into long cables, the information can travel long distances to other sections of the brain.

All of these communications between neighbouring cells and departments in the brain take place at lightning speed and occur constantly. Each individual neuron has up to a thousand synapses. A conservative estimate of the number of synapses in our brain is 100 trillion. This fact alone highlights the challenge faced by brain researchers!

IV THE BRAIN: THE MESSENGERS

About two hundred chemical messengers, or neurotransmitters, mediate brain functioning. Of these, the six most influential present in our mood system are:

(i) *Serotonin* Probably the best-known neurotransmitter. It is responsible for mood, memory, sleep, and the control of impulsive behaviour.

(ii) *Noradrenalin* Has an important role to play in the stress response. It is also important in sleep and mood, and is responsible for a person's drive/motivation.

(iii) *Dopamine* Creates a sense of joy and pleasure. It can have an effect on mood and also, when tampered with, addiction.

(iv) *Glutamate* This is present in almost every neuron in the brain. It differs from the first three neurotransmitters in this regard, which, as we will see, are mainly confined to their individual mood cables. Its function is a general 'housekeeping' one and is related to stimulating neurons into action. It is little surprise, therefore, that this transmitter, along with dopamine, is involved in schizophrenia, and, along with serotonin and norodrenaline, in depression.

(v) *GABA* This messenger, which is present in about 40 percent of the cells in our brain, is essential in preventing the brain from over stimulating itself, leading to seizure and death. Its job is to balance out the effect of glutamate by relaxing neurons.

(vi) *Peptides* (see Figure 2) on page 18 These are a group of roaming messengers that are released by neurons. They disperse throughout the brain and attach themselves to cell receptors elsewhere, communicating information to the genes of those cells. They are central to the way in which a person handles stress and anxiety.

Two common examples of peptides are:

1 *Endorphins* Chemicals which induce a state of euphoria, released particularly during exercise.

2 *Stress peptides* Primarily released to help a person cope with stress. Prolonged or excessive release of these messengers (CRH in particular), however, can result in illnesses of the mood system.

V   THE MOOD SYSTEM: MOOD DEPARTMENTS

There are two main mood departments:

1   FRONTAL MOOD DEPARTMENT

FIGURE 3: THE FRONTAL MOOD DEPARTMENT

This department, as its name implies, is situated anatomically at the front of the brain, within the frontal lobe. Most of this part of the brain is taken up by the most important structure we will deal with in this book: the pre-frontal cortex, which we will refer to as the 'behaviour box', because it regulates behaviour. (Both the right and left side of the brain contain individual frontal mood departments with their own behaviour boxes, but for the most part they can be treated as one.) The frontal mood department behaviour box is the thinking (thought-producing), decision-making part of the mood system (the so called 'logical brain'). Its functions, partly related to mood but mostly related to behaviour, are as follows:

(i)   Analysing situations (particularly if they are new to the individual) and making judgements and decisions based on information received. This includes future planning.

(ii)   Managing short-term memory

(iii) Preventing impulsive and destructive behaviour, including self-injurious behaviour and aggressive acts towards others

(iv)   Helping to produce and maintain normal mood and producing positive thinking. This department may also be the source of self-consciousness.

The behaviour boxes (which themselves are composed of different small functioning units) on either side of the brain have different functions. They take up most of the frontal lobes and constitute 29 percent of the total grey matter of the brain; they are therefore of great importance in our lives.

Of primary interest in relation to mental illness is the left-frontal behaviour box. This mediates positive thoughts and impulsive behaviour, and is often called the 'executive decision-maker'. For the most part, when the pre-frontal cortex is discussed, the left behaviour box will be the area that is being referred to. This part of the brain is very influential in both depression and suicide.

2 LIMBIC MOOD DEPARTMENT

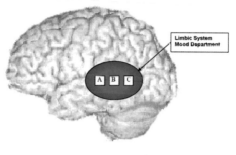

A Memory box
B Stress box
C Pleasure box

FIGURE 4: THE LIMBIC SYSTEM MOOD DEPARTMENT

This department lies in the centre of the brain. It is usually described as the limbic system. It is the part of the mood system that deals with emotion (the so called 'emotional brain'). Composed of different sections with corresponding functions, the limbic system is responsible for:

§ The way in which a person responds to stress

§ The preservation of normal mood

§ Feelings of joy and pleasure

§ Processing of memory

§ Appetite for both food and sex

Within the limbic mood department, there are several sections, which we will call 'boxes', each of which is involved in its own functions:

(i)   *'Memory box' (hippocampus)* This is where memory is generated, filtered and organised before being sent to other parts of the brain for storage. It is also involved in the retrieval of such memories. It plays a key role in putting these recalled memories into context, and in spatial memory. This box becomes very active when we are sleeping, particularly when we are dreaming. It is likely that memories are consolidated at these times.

(ii) *'Stress box' (amygdala)* This unit controls the response to perceived threats both from within the body and from the external environment. Most experts feel that it is also the main processor of the primary emotions of fear, hate, love and anger. It is integral to stress and anxiety and plays a large part in how the brain stores emotions related to unpleasant memories, memories which may or may not be consciously accessible. The negative thinking prevalent in depression probably originates here (or, more accurately, the emotions associated with the negative thinking). This box is larger in males than in females.

(iii) *'Pleasure box' (nucleus accumbens)* This section is activated when we are participating in rewarding activities such as eating food, drinking alcohol, having sex, and so on. In the biological illness of addiction, this box becomes affected by abuse.

These two mood departments, which control emotion and behaviour/logic, are in constant communication. When this communication breaks down – and indeed when communication is disrupted within sections of each mood department – the brain descends into chaos, and illness is a likely consequence.

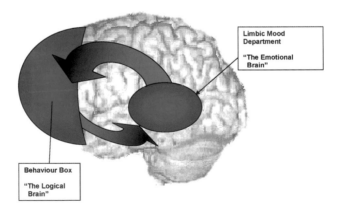

FIGURE 5: THE NORMAL FLOW OF INFORMATION BETWEEN THE LOGICAL AND EMOTIONAL BRAIN

It has been shown that there is a greater flow of information from the stress box to the behaviour box than vice versa (see Figure 5), probably for evolutionary survival reasons. This may explain why our emotions (such as fear) frequently overpower our thoughts and behaviour, but unfortunately we often have difficulty in persuading our thoughts and behaviour to overrule our emotions! As we will see in the section on the Yellow Flag, it is hard for a person in the middle of a panic attack to 'think' their way out of the way they feel.

As a general rule, in the course of normal life, our emotional brain will win out in a battle between the two! If you don't believe me, ask somebody in love to behave in a sensible and rational manner. Thankfully, in this case the 'heart' usually wins out. Another example would be passing a Chinese takeaway and battling between the logical brain (the behaviour box) informing us that getting a takeaway will not help our attempts to keep our weight down, and the emotional mind (the pleasure box) imagining a good tuck-in! Guess which one often wins?

Ideally, in relation to extreme negativity, the behaviour box should exert a large degree of control over the stress box. Not only can the behaviour box produce positive thoughts, it can also switch off, rationalise and overrule overtly negative emotional thoughts that originate in the stress box. For this reason, many experts believe that depression and suicide result in part from a malfunctioning, mainly left-sided behaviour box.

Before leaving the two mood departments, it is worth mentioning the role that both play in memory. We know that the memory box is essential to the formation of all memories and to the ability of the brain to store, retrieve and put in context such memories. It is the destruction of this box that leads to the profound memory loss seen in dementia, and to the memory loss so commonly seen in depression.

The stress box, in comparison, assigns an emotional content (often negative) not only to our thoughts but also to our memories, particularly distressing ones. The stress box, therefore, does not so much store the negative memories we all have (these memories are stored throughout the brain) as assign a negative emotion (such as fear, sadness, anger or anxiety) to the memory.

The stress and memory boxes work very closely together. Both are usually involved in the formation of memories. The latter is felt to be involved in creating, storing and recalling the memory; the former with the emotions associated with it. The inappropriate assignation of excess negativity from this box to both memories and thoughts is the secret to the negative thinking that is so prominent in depression, and to the symptoms of anxiety, both of which we will be dealing with later. Both of these boxes also link in with the pleasure box, so that enjoyable feelings are also stored away in our memories. This, as we will see later, is important in addiction.

VI   THE MOOD SYSTEM: MOOD CABLES

FIGURE 6: THE MOOD CABLES

The two mood departments (and their individual sections) are in constant communication with all other parts of the brain, but in particular are constantly receiving, assimilating and passing on information (through a variety of neural pathways) to each other.

The primary (but by no means only) channels of communication between the two mood departments (and their individual sections) are a series of three long collections of neurons, which will be referred to as mood cables. Each cable will be named after the predominant chemical messenger used by neurons in that particular cable. Because they are so important to the normal health of the mood system, we will be dealing with these cables throughout this book.

Because the information carried by each neuron in these cables has to travel a distance from its source, the brain uses its glial support cells to manufacture, and surround the cells with, a white insulation-type material (similar to that used in electrical wires in our homes) called myelin. This speeds up the passage of information along the neurons. The three main mood cables and their corresponding control boxes are:

(i)   *The dopamine mood cable* The dopamine control box is situated below the limbic mood department at the base of the brain. The dopamine cable travels from this box and continues through the limbic mood department before moving on to the frontal mood department and other structures. It uses the neurotransmitter

24

dopamine, which is produced and mediated by the dopamine control box.

Of the brain's 1 billion neurons, a modest forty thousand make up this cable. The well-being of the entire mood system depends on this small structure, however. This cable produces feelings of joy and pleasure, and its malfunctioning is linked to depression, addiction and schizophrenia.

(ii) *The serotonin mood cable* The serotonin control box is also situated at the base of the brain. The serotonin cable runs from this box through all sections of the limbic mood department, connects with the frontal mood department, and then moves on to pass information to almost every part of the brain. This cable's connections with the memory and behaviour boxes are of particular importance. This cable uses the neurotransmitter serotonin to communicate, which is produced and mediated by the serotonin control box.

Similar to the dopamine cable, the serotonin cable is composed of a relatively small number of neurons. What it lacks in size, it makes up for in significance by virtue of the massive number of connections it makes with all the sections of the mood system, and indeed with the rest of the brain. This is the primary mood cable, which regulates mood, sleep, concentration, memory, appetite, sexual drive, stress and destructive behaviour. Naturally, then, if it malfunctions, this can lead to depression, suicide, anti-social behaviour, addiction and anxiety. Women seem to produce serotonin at a much lower rate than men, which may partially explain the higher rates of anxiety and depression that are present in females.

(iii) *The noradrenalin mood cable* The source of this cable also lies in the brain stem, i.e. the noradrenalin control box. From here it travels up through the limbic and frontal mood departments before dispersing throughout the brain. It has a strong connection with the stress box. The main chemical messenger used by this cable is noradrenalin, the production of which mediated by the noradrenalin control box. It is also composed of a relatively small number of neurons (around 25,000). It keeps us alert, vigilant, driven, sleeping normally, and it also helps us to manage stress. It does not operate properly in patients suffering from depression and anxiety.

The peptide system Alongside the three cables above there is another messenger system. This will be called the 'Peptide System.' Peptides are messengers released by the above cables and mood departments and travel to both local and distant areas of the brain. As mentioned previously, stress peptides and endorphins are two of the most prominent. Peptides (CRH in particular) have a major role to play in depression, anxiety, and suicide.

All three control boxes have a rich supply of glucocortisol receptors and as a result are very vulnerable to excessively high levels of this hormone, as seen in chronic stress and depression.

VII   THE MOOD SYSTEM: THE ADRENAL STRESS GLAND

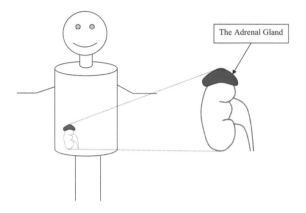

FIGURE 7: THE ADRENAL GLAND

The mood system is completed by the adrenal glands, which are found – in a somewhat unlikely location – a good distance from the brain, on top of the kidneys. The stress box sends messages to these glands, via the bloodstream and the nervous system. Following these instructions, the adrenal glands produce three important hormones: adrenalin, noradrenalin (both of which prepare the body to respond when faced with a sudden threat) and glucocortisol.

VIII   THE MOOD SYSTEM: THE GLUCOCORTISOL STRESS HORMONE

FIGURE 8: GLUCOCORTISOL

The adrenal glands, when instructed by the limbic mood department, produce glucocortisol. This hormone is used to fight stress, illness and infection. It tackles stress by activating pathways which release the energy necessary for the body to cope. The immune system, which fights illness, is very susceptible to fluctuating levels of this hormone. Glucocortisol also affects body fat, sugar levels and bones, is influential in heart disease, and plays a role in the brain's capacity to form memories. This hormone is normally elevated during daytime, and declines at night: this helps keep a person alert during the day and enables them to sleep at night.

When the mood cables and departments are severely disrupted through stress and depression, these normal daily patterns will be destroyed. The system will be bombarded with this hormone day and night, and will travel back to the brain via the bloodstream, where, in a vicious cycle, it will damage the mood cables and departments even more.

Glucocortisol can be described as the body's heavy artillery for dealing with stress. In the case of an over-supply of the hormone, however – where it runs out of its usual targets – this heavy artillery begins to fight the brain itself, resulting in damage to the memory box in particular.

IX   THE MOOD SYSTEM: THE FLAG

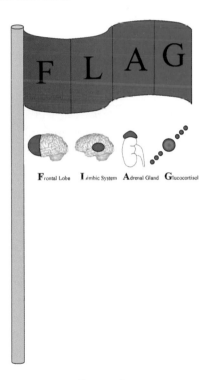

Frontal Lobe   Limbic System   Adrenal Gland   Glucocortisol

FIGURE 9

By now, one can see how interwoven all the parts of the mood system are. Interference with any one section can result in widespread malfunction.

As mentioned in the introduction, a useful way of conceptualising the mood system is to take the first letter of the mood departments, (Frontal and Limbic), the first letter of the stress gland (Adrenal), the first letter of our stress hormone (Glucocortisol), and combine them to form the word 'FLAG' (see Figure 9). In the model seen below, the mood departments are displayed, as is the stress gland and hormone.

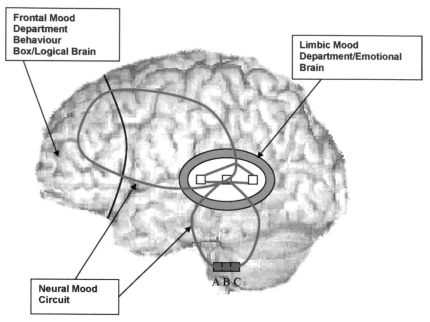

A   Serotonin control box
B   Noradrenalin control box
C   Dopamine control box

FIGURE 10: THE 'MOOD CIRCUIT'

Flags have universal appeal. Beaches during the summertime warrant careful examination of the lifeguard's flags: red warns of danger, yellow encourages vigilance, and green indicates safety. This book deals with normal mood and the various biological illnesses which affect the mood system. These illnesses will be colour-coded using flags. The Green Flag indicates normal mood and behaviour. This is the desirable state, yet for many people is only reached with great difficulty. The Red Flag warns of the inner turmoil and dangerous symptoms that depression can bring. The Yellow Flag of increased vigilance aptly describes the paralysing, cautious, fearful state in which those with anxiety disorders find themselves. The Purple Flag of addiction refers to an infatuation with the pleasures of alcohol, drugs and other addictive substances and activities. Finally, the White Flag of suicide signals acceptance of defeat, and the surrender of the mood system to the illness that has been plaguing it.

An interesting modern approach to the mood system within the brain itself is to consider the brain as a neural 'mood circuit' (see Figure 10) which links the bottom of the brain (which contains the control boxes associated with the main mood cables), the emotional limbic department in the middle of the brain, and the logical frontal mood departments at the top, together. Most mental illnesses are caused by difficulties when this circuit breaks down. If we could shift our understanding of illnesses like depression to encompass this concept of a neural mood circuit, it would revolutionise both our understanding of and our approach to managing this condition.

In attempting to understand the biology of the brain and mood system, it is possible to overlook the unique nature of humanity and individuality. It is important not to see the brain and the individual person as mutually exclusive. It is also important not to see the body or the mind as being somehow distinct from the brain. What affects one will inevitably also impinge on the other. This is why we must look at all illnesses holistically. The mind (both emotional and logical) is a function of the brain, just as blood flow is a function of the heart. So by definition, mental illness – and any approach to dealing with it – must involve the brain itself.

There are those who may worry that, by studying the brain in this way, we are dehumanising or devaluing the human person. Others are concerned that it denigrates the role of religion or spirituality. All these are valid and genuine concerns. But the greatest gift that we have (whatever the origin of this gift) is the ability to observe ourselves and learn about both the universe and our own beings. We can and should be using this gift to ease the sufferings of others.

The family doctor is in a unique position to observe all the highs and lows of human existence – from the joy of the birth of a baby to the mourning of death, with all its unanswered questions. This provides a strong motivation for us to learn as much as possible from current scientific research, in order to alleviate the suffering related to biological illnesses which affect the mood system, particularly in relation to depression and suicide.

Just as the study of coronary heart disease has greatly assisted in the understanding and treatment of this condition, so too have discoveries into the workings of the brain assisted in the understanding and treatment of mental illness. Such study can never diminish the uniqueness of humans beings! The only way to break the taboo of mental illness is to delve into the mystery of how the brain works. Fear of discussing psychiatric conditions is often built on ignorance and a lack of understanding. Human beings are extraordinary organisms! The ability of the brain to examine itself is an extraordinary one, and should be utilised for the benefit of others.

SUMMARY

1   The brain (see Figure 1 on page 16) is composed of 10 billion individual cells. There are two main types of such cells – neurons, which make all the important decisions, and glial cells, which nourish and protect the neurons. Only 10 percent of all cells in the brain are neurons, with glial cells making up the remainder. Neurons and glial cells in the brain are organised into various departments with particular functions.

2   Each neuron stands alone, with lots of small meeting points or gaps (called synapses) present between each cell. Through these synapses, each neuron talks to hundreds of its closest neighbours. It does so by sending messengers from one cell to another across these gaps (see Figure 2 on page 18) in order to communicate information. These messengers are called neurotransmitters, and play a pivotal role in how the brain operates. There are three important neurotransmitters that are crucial to the mood system: serotonin, noradrenalin and dopamine. Another group of neurotransmitters released by neurons into these synapses are called peptides. These roaming messengers 'wander off' to pass important messages to other parts of the brain rather than activating the cells closest to them. Of these messages, the two most important are endorphins (released during exercise) and stress peptides (released during stress).

3   Within the brain, there are two main mood departments: the frontal, situated at the front of the brain, and the limbic system, in the centre of the brain.

4   The frontal mood department (see Figure 3 on page 20) is mainly composed of a section we will refer to as the behaviour box (pre-frontal cortex). This department or box (sometimes called the logical brain) plays a major role in our thinking and behaviour. Its main functions relate to short-term memory, the processing of positive and negative thoughts, analysing and decision-making, future planning, and the control of impulsive thoughts and actions.

5   The limbic mood department (see Figure 4 on page 21) plays a major role in regulating our emotions (and is sometimes called the emotional brain). It has three main sections: the stress box (amygdala), memory box (*Hippocampus*) and pleasure box (*nucleus accumbens*). The primary responsibilities of this department are the regulation of mood, the processing of memory, response to stress, and our experience of joy and pleasure.

6   Our two mood departments are connected by three long telephone-like mood cables (see Figure 6 on page 24). These cables will be named after the main neurotransmitter involved in their operation and are responsible for the smooth running of the mood system. The three cables concerned are the serotonin cable (which deals with mood, sleep, appetite, sex and control of impulsive behaviour), the noradrenalin cable (which deals with energy, drive, concentration, mood, sleep and the stress response) and the dopamine cable (which deals with mood and the sense of joy and pleasure that is extrapolated from positive experiences).

7   The mood system is completed by the adrenal stress gland (situated in the abdomen on top of our kidneys – see Figure 7 on page 26) and the core stress hormone glucocortisol (see Figure 8 on page 26). When under stress for any length of time, the adrenal stress gland helps the system to cope. As we will see later, however, sustained activity in this gland over a prolonged period can give rise to lnumerous problems in our mood system.

8   A useful way of combining all this information to form a unified concept is to take the first letter of the two mood departments, the frontal and limbic system (F and L), the first letter of the adrenal stress gland (A) and the first letter of the stress hormone glucocortisol (G) to form the word FLAG (See Figure 9 on page 27).

Flags have universal significance in our lives. A green flag suggests that all is well, red flags warn of danger, and yellow, purple and white flags can be taken to stand for, respectively, fear, debauchery and surrender. Based on these concepts, the Green Flag represents normal mood, and the Red Flag represents depression. Anxiety is represented by the Yellow Flag, the Purple Flag signals addiction, and suicide will be indicated by the White Flag. All of these illnesses and conditions originate from a widespread dysfunction within the mood system and will be dealt with in subsequent chapters.

9   Although particular functions will be assigned to each of the mood departments and their individual sections, it is important to realise that there is a substantial flow of information between them. These departments also communicate with all other parts of the brain. A modern approach to the mood system is to consider all the above as being part of a neural 'mood circuit' (see Figure 10 on page 28). Interference with this circuit is the basis for many mental illnesses.

When a decision has to be made, there is normally a balanced discussion between the logical, thinking section of our mood system (the frontal department) and the emotional section (the limbic system). Sometimes, emotions prevail, and on other occasions the rational psyche dominates. This balance is a vital and healthy one. When the mood system is functioning properly, decisions that have been reached are balanced and informed. When an illness like depression spreads throughout the brain, this balance is disturbed. A serious consequence of this disruption is suicidal thoughts.

10 Finally, in discussing the workings of the brain and mood system, it must be noted
    that a person is more than simply a conglomeration of neurons and neurotrans-
    mitters! The mystery of consciousness undoubtedly originates from the brain. The
    whole is indeed greater than the sum of its parts, and it will be difficult for any
    study of the brain to capture fully the elusive yet undeniable essence of humanity.
    We are indeed special and unique!

2

The Development of the Brain

and the Mood System

Exciting new research has made a great deal of information on the brain, its mood system, and the illnesses that affect it available to us. The advent of neuro-imaging – the use of scanning to document the development and functioning of the brain – has opened up a new chapter in the understanding and treatment of mental illness.

I   THE DEVELOPMENT OF THE BRAIN

The brain begins it lengthy journey in the womb, around eighteen days after conception. Within three months, hundreds of billions of neurons have been formed, and they are organised rapidly into the different sections which will make up the future adult brain. These cells only survive if they manage to communicate with other neurons within a certain time period via the synapses.

By six months after birth, the brain has developed too many neurons, so it carries out a selective pruning of the neurons. It is a case of survival of the fittest: developing cells must start communicating or die, as those that are unable to form synapses are destroyed. This pruning process is a very important stage in the development of the brain. Illnesses such as autism, bipolar depression and schizophrenia may in part result from abnormal pruning.

At birth, most of the neurons we need for life are already present. It was accepted in the past by the scientific and medical community that, by age twelve, the brain was fully formed and that no new neurons could be formed. It is now known that this is not true and that, in fact, the development of the brain is a dynamic and ongoing process. The memory box is extremely underdeveloped under the age of three: this explains why we have few memories of our existence prior to this age!

Between ages six and twelve, the brain experiences a massive growth in the number of connections between individual neurons. This process reaches its peak just before puberty. Once again, another large pruning process has to occur, or efficiency suffers. Between twelve and twenty-five years of age, a massive reorganisation of the neurons and their synapses occurs. This is probably activated by a combination of our genes working together and the massive release of sex hormones which occurs between ages twelve and eighteen. The neurons themselves do not die during this stage; rather, the connections between them are selectively destroyed. The result is a reduction in the number of synapses but an increase in overall efficiency. Along with this pruning, there is a further increase in the speed of conduction between cells and departments of the brain, due to other cellular changes.

The pruning process begins at the back of the brain, and continues through the limbic system, situated in the centre of the brain, before finally reaching the frontal lobe. Thus, it starts with parts of the brain that are responsible for vision, hearing and coordination, before moving to areas which control emotions, and eventually finishing up in a section of the brain which controls behaviour and decision-making. By the person's early to mid-twenties, most of this work has been completed, and all the brain can do is attempt to improve its speed of conduction and renew dead cells in areas such as the memory box.

From this age onwards, the number of neurons will decline. Over the age of fifty, illnesses such as Alzheimer's and vascular damage to the brain may accelerate this process, resulting in dementia. The three main mood cables also begin to shrink as we age. This, as we will see later, may explain in part the arrival of depression in this group. Alcohol, lack of exercise, and failure to utilise mental faculties also accelerates the loss of neurons. Nonetheless, most of us will retain sufficient neurons to keep us functioning adequately for the duration of our lives.

II   THE DEVELOPMENT OF THE MOOD SYSTEM

New research into brain development has improved our understanding of how the mood system evolves from the womb to full maturity by the mid-twenties. In the last few months in the womb, during the massive pruning process, the frontal mood department seems to become particularly vulnerable to damage. If certain genetic vulnerability or intra-uterine environmental influences are present, a susceptibility to illnesses such as schizophrenia, autism and bipolar depression may become established at this stage; these illnesses will not reveal their presence until later, however. Recently, the frontal mood department has been demonstrated to be of greater importance in unipolar (or simple) depression than was previously believed. Therefore genetic or intra-uterine environmental influences may turn out to be a causal factor in this illness as well.

In childhood, major stress factors such as abuse and loss interact with genetic vulnerability to create a lifelong predisposition for people to react inappropriately to stress.

The behaviour and stress boxes seem to be the most vulnerable targets for the creation of such a lifelong susceptibility. This predisposition may, as will be shown later, explain the emergence of depression, anxiety and addiction in the lives of such people.

The pruning process from the age of twelve to the early to mid-twenties is a vital period in the development of the mood system. The limbic system is dealt with first, before the brain moves on to its final objective, the maturing of the behaviour box in the frontal lobes.

As the limbic system is responsible for how we feel, it is inevitable that feelings will run riot under the massive influence of our sex hormones from the age of twelve to eighteen. If we feel down, the pain will be more intense; and the same applies to positive emotions. As the immature behaviour box can exercise only a weak control over the limbic system at this stage, emotions will influence thoughts and actions more than common sense. This explains the excessive behaviour of many teenagers: their exuberance and great enthusiasm on the one hand, and their apparently complete disregard for the consequences of their actions on the other. Lacking effective control over the behaviour box, teenagers engage in impulsive and often reckless behaviour, including binge drinking, unprotected sex and joyriding. This is why the teenage years are so turbulent for those going through them – and for the parents of teenagers.

By the early to mid-twenties, the brain's 'commander in chief', the behaviour box, has begun to exert its control over the great surge of emotions originating from the limbic mood department. Parents have observed their good-humoured, sociable eight- to ten-year-old undergoing extraordinary behavioural changes and becoming an impossible thirteen- to seventeen-year-old who demonstrates huge swings in mood and behaviour – only for the process to be reversed again as their offspring enter their twenties. This explains why teenagers are reached more easily by appealing to their emotions rather than to reason. Then, finally, out of the caterpillar stage of mood development emerges the butterfly of maturity.

This phased development of the teenage or young-adult mood system has huge implications for how messages relating to smoking, alcohol and drug misuse are communicated to young people. These are an issue because our pleasure box, dopamine cable and limbic system are much more active during this phase of development, due to an inability to exert control on the part of the behaviour box, which is still immature. The pleasure that such activities brings outweighs the inevitable negative consequences of these activities in the mind of the teenager.

There is increasing focus on why most illnesses of the mood system, particularly depression and anxiety, often appear for the first time when a person is between fifteen and twenty-five years of age. It is speculated that the answers lie at earlier stages of development, both in the womb and in early childhood. Abnormalities originating from genetic or early environmental influences, or both, seem to weaken the mood structures, making them prone to breaking down during the emotional stress barrage of the teenage years. The behaviour and stress boxes in particular are very vulnerable during this early stage. A vicious circle can then ensue, with the affected individual becoming prone to further bouts of depression and anxiety in the future.

Schizophrenia also often develops during this phase of development. Scientists are of the opinion that this illness originates from poor development of the frontal lobe behaviour box in the womb. When pruning takes place, from ages twelve to twenty-five, this deficiency is exacerbated, and the illness appears. Of concern recently is the increasing number of cases where abuse of drugs, particularly cocaine and marijuana, is triggering schizophrenia, because the use of these drugs affects the pruning process. This, unfortunately, may delay a diagnosis of schizophrenia, as many of the symptoms of schizophrenia may be attributed to the drug use itself.

If those in the twelve-to-twenty-five age group (particularly the under-fifteens) begin to misuse alcohol, drugs and nicotine from an early stage, the risk of a later, full-blown addiction increases, especially if the person comes from an 'addictive background' (a home where the parents may have been addicted to nicotine, alcohol, gambling or illegal drugs). This explains why so many young people in Ireland are hardened drinkers in many cases by the age of twenty-one. Many have started drinking from an early age, and as a result their dopamine and limbic system becomes hooked on the pleasurable feelings that alcohol can bring, and binge drinking becomes the norm rather than an aberration.

A similar situation exists with regard to smoking: we now know that if we expose the immature brain and mood system to nicotine before the age of eighteen, the chances of members of this group becoming long-term smokers dramatically increases. We live in a culture where alcohol and nicotine are freely available and where many young people (unlike in previous decades) are in a position, both financially and in terms of the freedom they enjoy, to avail of both: the interaction of an immature mood system with modern Irish life is leading to problems.

Lastly, suicide is unfortunately very common in the fifteen-to-twenty-five age group. One could query whether the individual's stage of development is a contributing factor to this situation: common sense dictates that it is. Firstly, at this age emotions are running wild due to the person's over-active limbic system. Secondly, illnesses such as depression and schizophrenia may appear. Thirdly, the dopamine/pleasure box is highly susceptible to the effects of alcohol and other drugs. Lastly, and possibly most importantly, the behaviour box – which controls impulsive and violent behaviour – is slowly maturing from the mid-teens to the early and mid-twenties. When the immaturity of the behaviour box is combined with an illness like depression, impulsive suicidal thoughts and behaviours become more likely.

Before leaving this section, it is worthwhile to reflect briefly on the development of personality (defined as the consistent emotional thought and behaviour patterns of an individual) as opposed to that of the mood system. All of us, from a very early age, begin to show distinct personality traits; as a result, we differ in how we look at life, which consequently determines how we behave. There is a large genetic component to the development of our individual personalities, but positive and negative early child-hood experiences also play a role. Some of us will be extroverted, and others more introverted and cautious. Lots of us have developed set behavioural patterns by adult-hood. Our reactions to most life situations will of course be influenced by the type of person we have become. It is likely that key departments of the brain, like our behav-iour box, play an important role in determining our personality.

This is supported by neuro-imaging research which shows that extroverts have a very active left side of the behaviour box and that those who are more introverted and cautious show more activity in the right side of this box. Since the former have a lower incidence of depression and the latter a higher incidence of anxiety, it is clear that in some areas our mood system and personality intermingle.

One of the difficulties that professionals encounter when dealing with mental-health issues is that many people assume that an illness like depression is simply a weak-ness of personality. This implies that, firstly, it is personality development that is at fault and, secondly, that those with this illness are in some way inferior to others. This think-ing also extends to suicide: many people erroneously believe that those who commit suicide are generally suffering from a major personality problem and should be consid-ered to be weak individuals.

Such perspectives are of course completely misguided. Personality is important in how we cope with many of life's difficulties and stresses, and it is also important in how an illness like depression might express itself. An anxious person by personality might show a lot more anxiety features if they develop depression; an impulsive or aggressive person might display their depression through heavy drinking or by lashing out in bursts of anger, or they may be more likely to self-harm. Men sometimes exhibit all three. Those with perfectionist personalities may become severely self-critical or nega-tive in their thinking if they develop this illness.

It is not a defect in the development of our personality, however, or a weakness in character that leads to depression and suicide, but rather illness infecting the mood sys-tem. Rather, personality is more relevant when it comes to how the illness will manifest itself in a particular person.

The need to make this distinction is one of the driving forces behind this book. All of us need to try to understand that, despite the relationship between personality and mood, the two things are essentially different.

III ENVIRONMENT VERSUS GENES IN THE DEVELOPMENT OF THE MOOD SYSTEM

Whether it is our genes or our environment that controls the healthy development of our mood system is an age-old debate. It is now accepted, however, that there is a dynamic relationship between our genes and the way in which we interact with our environment, and that this relationship continues right through our lives. Everything begins with the genes we inherit. So what are our genes?

Each cell in the brain – like every cell in the body – contains a 'book' of instructions and information called DNA. This book is broken up into chapters and paragraphs which instruct the individual cell to make special proteins to perform particular functions. Each paragraph can be considered to be a gene. It is estimated that each human being has around a hundred thousand genes, which together control all the functions of the body and mind.

In the case of the mood system, a number of these paragraphs, or genes, determine the workings and functions of each cell in the mood cables and departments. If we combine these paragraphs together, a chapter on how each of our individual mood systems function is formed. The problem is that multiple flaws in these instructions – analogous to spelling or grammatical mistakes in a sentence – can lead to a malfunction in the development of our mood system.

Environment also plays a key role in the development of the mood system. From conception to the point when brain maturity is reached, at age twenty-five, a variety of environmental factors can influence our genes, predisposing them to malfunction at a later stage. In the womb, such influences include alcohol, nicotine, drugs and viral illnesses which affect the mother. In childhood, the influences include severe physical or sexual abuse, loss or separation of a parent, or any major trauma.

In adolescence, it is recognised that abuse, severe loss, and alcohol and substance misuse can also affect the genes. One other factor that is often overlooked in this crucial period of development is nutrition. From the womb to age twenty-five, the presence or absence of vital building blocks from our diet may also play a role in the development of the mood system. We will be dealing with this subject in more detail later.

The way in which environmental factors influence the development of the mood system has to be mediated through our genes. This is because everything that happens in the neurons of our mood system is controlled by the genes. In some people, environmental factors may interact with genes which are programmed to malfunction (to a greater or lesser extent) from the beginning.

Some illnesses of the mood system appear in the teenage years, when the limbic system is only maturing. During this phase of development, environmental triggers seem to activate underlying genetic or early-development malfunctions, causing these illnesses to appear. Researchers also speculate that the stress factors noted above in childhood and early adolescence combine with malfunctioning genes to produce a life-long vulnerability to stress in adult life. This may lead to depression and anxiety later.

A useful way of looking at how genes and environmental factors interact in rela-tion to the development of many common illnesses (including those affecting the mood system) is to use the analogy of a profit-and-loss sheet. All of us have genes which predispose us towards illnesses, and other genes which protect us from the same illnesses. In some of us, the genetic balance is tipped in favour of us developing or expressing this illness if environmental factors are favourable.

On the other side of the equation, all of us will experience both positive and neg-ative environmental influences in our lives (both in our past and in our present) which may make it more likely that such illnesses develop. Once again, the overall balance can reduce or increase our chance of developing these illnesses. When we put these two sets of genetic and environmental balances together, we can assess our risks of developing such illnesses. (If the overall balance is tipped in the wrong direction, then it is likely that these illnesses will appear at some stage in our lives.)

Common examples of such conditions are coronary heart disease, diabetes and depression. In coronary heart disease, for example, the genetic predisposition may be towards overproducing cholesterol in the liver, combined with a tendency for the body's immune system to attack this fat within the wall of the coronary arteries; these factors may predispose some towards developing angina and dying from a heart attack. The environmental factors in this case might be poor diet, lack of exercise, smoking and stress. When we put all these factos together, the person's overall risk of developing CHD will be high. In general the stronger the genetic predisposition, the more likely the illness will be expressed, often at a younger age. As we will see later depression is another classical example of this delicate balance.

To conclude, it is the complex interaction between our genes and the environment that lies at the core of the development of the mood system. A proper understanding of the causes of mental illness therefore depends heavily on a comprehensive knowl-edge of this interaction – a knowledge which researchers have so far been unable to develop.

3

THE 'STRESS SYSTEM'

One of the main functions of the mood system is to control the stress system Stress is a universal phenomenon: everyone experiences periods of acute stress (such as exam pressure) and chronic stress (including financial pressures and job difficulties). The body also has to deal with the internal stress of infection and illness. Stress is now felt to be pivotal to the creation and maintenance of certain mental illnesses such as depression and anxiety.

Stress is not always a bad thing, however: it is the way in which the body deals with stress which is crucial. We will also examine how chronic activation of the stress system can lead to many difficulties relating to our general health, even in the absence of mood-system illnesses.

I   THE BIOLOGY OF THE STRESS SYSTEM

The body's stress response is coordinated by the stress box, situated in the limbic mood department. When under attack from any internal or external stress, the frontal mood department behaviour box activates the stress box. The stress box then releases CRH, one of the peptide messengers. This in turn activates two areas in the brain: the hormone control box and the brain stem, both of which send information to the adrenal stress glands, through the bloodstream and the spinal cord respectively (see Figure 11).

The brain stem instructs the adrenal glands to release adrenalin and noradrenalin into the blood stream. This instant response to stress occurs in a period lasting anything from a few seconds to several minutes. The hormones adrenalin and noradrenalin prepare the body for combating the immediate threat. Heart rate increases, blood pressure rises, the mind is vigilant and alert, the mouth becomes dry, and the stomach starts to churn. The body is diverting resources away from non-essential organs towards those which will be used in combat to maximise the person's chances of survival. This is known informally as a 'fight or flight' reaction.

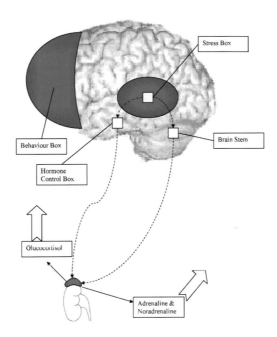

FIGURE 11: THE STRESS SYSTEM

The hormone control box also receives instructions from the stress box, and sends a message via the bloodstream to the adrenal stress glands, instructing them to release glucocortisol. This is a longer process and can last anything from a few minutes to several hours. Glucocortisol is a vital hormone, and is involved in making glucose available to all the cells in the body. Every cell in the body, including the neurons in the brain, has receptors for this hormone. Glucocortisol also helps to break down fats in order for the body to release more energy.

Both adrenalin and glucocortisol feed back to the brain. When the stress or threat has lifted, they encourage the stress box to switch off. Everything then goes back to normal. When stress becomes prolonged or chronic, however, problems begin to arise. Whereas the immediate effects of stimulation of the adrenal gland to produce adrenalin and noradrenalin usually settle, the production of glucocortisol continues, and has the following negative effects on the mood system:

1   EFFECTS ON MOOD CABLES

The three main mood cables originate from their control boxes, situated below the limbic system. Each box is responsible for controlling its own cable, so interference with them will automatically damage the cable in question. Chronic stress forces the stress

41

system to produce too much glucocortisol, and this interferes with the mood control boxes in the following ways (see Figure 12):

FIGURE 12: THE BIOLOGY AND EFFECTS OF CHRONIC STRESS

§   *Serotonin mood control box and cable* Persistently high glucocortisol levels deplete serotonin levels in this box and cable, and have a negative effect on serotonin receptors. This combination of damage to the brain results in mood, memory and sleep difficulties.

§   *Noradrenalin mood control box and cable* Initially, stress encourages this box and cable to be highly active, but continually high glucocortisol levels eventually deplete the noradrenalin reserves. Initial tension and vigilance becomes severe exhaustion. Chronic stress also results in reduced concentration and drive, and sleep disturbance. Overstimulation of the noradrenalin cable results in a 'tired but wired' state.

§   *Dopamine control box and cable* Stress initially activates this system, producing a temporary high. Again, however, it does not take long for the supplies of this neurotransmitter to become depleted, and activities which are normally rewarding then become tiring and laborious. Our normal enjoyment of life becomes impaired.

Those who have been exposed to long periods of sustained stress will be familiar with this lack of energy, drive, concentration, appetite and libido.

2   EFFECTS ON MOOD DEPARTMENTS

The relentless bombardment of stress peptides and glucocortisol due to stress also affects the two mood departments.

§   *Frontal mood department* (see Figure 13) The behaviour box is very sensitive to both stress peptides and glucocortisol, making it vulnerable to an attack. As this box produces positive thoughts and reduces impulsive actions, it is no surprise that, under sustained stress, negativity and impulsiveness begin to manifest themselves.

Some experts believe that the susceptibility of the left-sided of the behaviour box to stress triggers depression. In certain people, this vulnerability may be pre-programmed by genetics and early environmental factors, possibly due to a short-age of glial support cells. For these people, depression is a ticking time bomb, awaiting detonation from a bout of stress.

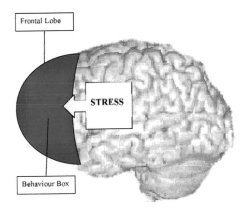

FIGURE 13: STRESS AND THE FRONTAL MOOD DEPARTMENT

§   *Limbic mood department* (see Figure 14) Due to the heightened activity of the stress box, anxiety and negativity will be a likely adjunct to stress. The major casualty in this department during stress, however, is the memory box, which is rich in gluco-cortisol receptors. The memory box requires the presence of this hormone for routine memory formation, but the presence of excessive amounts has a counter-productive effect. The latter interferes with the routine production of memories and also prevents new nerve cells from developing, resulting in memory and con-centration impairment. A similar process occurs, as we will see later, in depression.

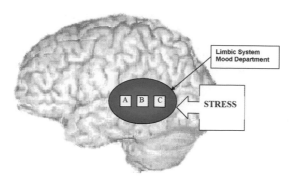

A Memory box
B Stress box
C Pleasure box

FIGURE 14: STRESS AND THE LIMBIC SYSTEM MOOD DEPARTMENT

3   EFFECTS ON GENERAL HEALTH

While it may sound from what we have seen above as though stress is the body's most dangerous adversary, it is in fact a key ally. A healthy stress system is very important to our general physical well-being. Constant bouts of acute and chronic stress can, however, give rise to various problems. For instance, high blood pressure, stroke and cardiac problems result from heightened levels of adrenalin and noradrenalin. Immune-system damage and the clumping together of platelets (an important component of our blood's clotting system) due to an excess of glucocortisol give rise to infection and heart attacks, respectively. The body's ability to defend against a potentially fatal illness like cancer may also be compromised.

SUMMARY

1   The stress box in the limbic mood department is in charge of the whole stress system. During times of stress, this box activates two major pathways. One works via the brain stem (especially in response to acute stress) by sending instructions to the adrenal stress glands to release adrenalin and noradrenalin into the bloodstream (see Figure 11 on page 41). The presence of these hormones gives rise to symptoms such as dry mouth, palpitations, stomach churning, sweating and alertness. These feelings are common before an important exam or job interview.

2   The second pathway works via the hormone control box (especially in response to chronic stress) by sending instructions to the adrenal glands to release the stress hormone glucocortisol (see Figure 11 on page 41). This prepares the body for a longer fight by reorganising its energy reserves to tackle the threat exclusively.

3   When the threat has passed, the body restores levels of these hormones to within normal parameters again.

4   When the person feels under constant threat, however, and stress is prolonged, levels of glucocortisol may remain high. This damages the mood cables (see Figure 12 on page 42) and mood departments (see Figures 13 and 14, on pages 43 and 44, respectively). It also increases the risk of heart attack and damages the immune system, making the body vulnerable to infection.

5   The effects of chronic stress on our mood system are fatigue, poor concentration, reduced drive, sleep problems and an inability to derive any pleasure from life.

II   THE INTERACTION BETWEEN THE MOOD AND STRESS SYSTEMS

The stress system and mood system are intertwined. This intertwining underlies all the illnesses discussed in this book. For most people, periods of chronic stress are inevitable, but normally the mood system is robust enough to survive the onslaught of stress hormones. The body is designed to help the person cope with stress, not force the person to succumb to it. That is not to say that a period of normal stress will be without fatigue, poor concentration, sleep disturbance and a general dissatisfaction in life. These complaints will be temporary ones, however, and will subside when the perceived threat has passed.

Some people do not recover from chronic stress so easily, however, because their mood system becomes dysfunctional when they are faced with stressful situations. Their system does not bounce back from stress in a normal fashion, and is more likely to deteriorate rapidly until the more serious conditions of depression, anxiety and substance abuse (if they are vulnerable to this) seize control of their brains.

Further research may reveal more about the relationship between the stress and mood systems. This will not only foster a better understanding of these illnesses but may also provide radically different and more effective treatments than the ones that are presently available.

4

THE SYSTEMS AND BIOLOGY OF NORMAL MOOD

Having explored the nature and function of the mood system, the Green Flag of normal mood and behaviour will now be discussed. For many people who are unaware that they are suffering from depression, anxiety and addiction, what they consider normal may be a horrendous experience for someone who is free of these illnesses. To understand what it means to be depressed, anxious and dependent on addictive substances, one first has to be aware of the features, biology and course of normal mood.

I   THE GREEN FLAG CHECKLIST

When asked about their mood, people are likely to respond that they feel 'up', 'down', or simply 'fine'. When a doctor is asked to make the same assessment about a person, he or she will apply much more stringent criteria before reaching a conclusion. A doctor is likely to check for the prevalence of a number of key symptoms which will give a better indication of the state of the person's mood. The checklist of symptoms on the next page is designed to identify problems in the mood system (see Figure 15).

How can I tell if my mood system is well?

1   MOOD

This is arguably the easiest to assess. All of us will regularly experience feelings of happiness and sadness in our lives. These emotions originate from our limbic mood department (probably mediated through our serotonin and dopamine systems). It is possible to feel both these emotions within minutes of each other, due to the situation in which one finds oneself; it is also possible to experience more prolonged phases of positivity, and negativity. These variations are normal, and are heavily influenced by normal life events such as relationships.

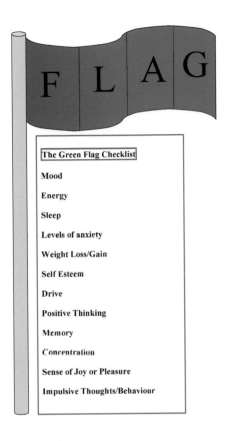

FIGURE 15: THE GREEN FLAG CHECKLIST

If mood drops down to a level where it becomes debilitating, however, there is cause for concern, particularly if low mood lasts for a sustained period (of between two to four weeks). If it continues past this point, the Red Flag of depression may have arrived. The longer this low mood persists, the higher the risk of such a bout deepening. It is important, therefore, for people in this situation to seek help as early as possible; indeed, these early weeks should be seen as a critical warning period.

Sometimes the opposite may occur, and mood may rise to an unnaturally high level. While this may not appear to be cause for complaint, it constitutes an equally vital warning of impending illness. In both cases, help should be sought to assess the cause of the mood changes.

2   ENERGY

Exhaustion is not just a symptom of mental illness; it is a feature of life. It can result from intense physical or mental activity, or from stress, and is usually corrected by an adequate amount of rest and sleep. When stress or illnesses are absent, a person usually has sufficient energy to cope with day-to-day activities. If the mood system is not functioning properly, however, an paralysing fatigue can emerge. This leaves a person physically and emotionally drained. In the absence of any physical ailment, this is an important sign that the mood system is experiencing difficulties.

3   SLEEP

Normal sleeping patterns are a function of the mood system. Sleep allows the brain to rest and provides an opportunity for minor damage inflicted during the brain's day-to-day operation to be repaired. The most notable warning sign of a malfunctioning mood system is a disturbance of these patterns. This can range from difficulty in falling sleep, awakening too early, awakening periodically throughout the night, or feeling exhausted upon waking in the morning.

Depression, anxiety and addiction all create sleep-pattern disturbance. As sleeping patterns are highly individual, a warning sign is a drastic change in the usual pattern. Some people prefer eight to ten hours' sleep, whereas others function well on only four to six hours'. The need for sleep tends to decrease as a person gets older. There is no set 'abnormal' sleeping pattern, but if a person's sleep deviates from its usual pattern, it can be considered abnormal for them – and a possible indicator of mood problems.

4   LEVELS OF ANXIETY

Anxiety, which can be defined as a state of apprehension, fear or worry, is a normal reaction when faced with final exams, a driving test or a first date, for instance. When these feelings are unremitting and evoked by even the most benign of situations, however, to a point where they begin to interfere with a person's day-to-day functioning, it is indicative of illness.

For those suffering from a long-term anxiety disorder, this paralysing anxiety is all they know. Others suffering from depression or addiction may be familiar with this feeling too. The persistent fear that such people experience originates in the mood system.

5   APPETITE

This refers to the satisfaction that is sought from eating and sexual activity. Metabolic rates differ from person to person: some people will struggle to keep their weight at a healthy level, for instance, whereas others will remain slim apparently regardless of what they eat. As with sleep, it is not the appetite itself that is an indicator of illness, but a sudden change in that appetite.

Depression can suppress appetite, resulting in a loss of interest in food, with consequent rapid weight loss. It can also increase appetite, as the mood system attempts to compensate for the declining pleasure derived from eating. A loss of interest in sex is also common. As with eating, however, a small number of those affected will experience increased libido. If the appetite for food and sex remains constant, it is a good sign that the mood system is functioning normally.

6   SELF-ESTEEM

This symptom is often well-concealed, and hidden even from the person affected by it. It concerns our perception of ourselves. In illnesses such as depression, feelings of self-worth are greatly diminished. Questions to ask yourself include: Do you feel uncomfortable in the presence of others? Do you think your ideas and feelings are unimportant? Do you feel useless? Do you constantly evaluate yourself negatively? Do you accept yourself 'unconditionally'?

If you are well, you will feel comfortable with others and confident in yourself. You may doubt yourself in certain situations, but in general you will feel good about yourself. If you answer 'yes' to these questions, and in particular 'no' to the last one, you may be suffering from low self-esteem.

7   DRIVE

Motivation and drive are highly individual. Some people have a strong drive to excel at work, while others focus on their relationships or aim for sporting achievement, and so on. Others may be of a more relaxed disposition, and may be content with their current situation. If your drive has been extremely low for a long time, however, and you do not have much interest in anything, or if you suddenly find yourself not doing activities which you would normally be involved in, because you simply 'can't be bothered', this may be an indication that you are suffering from an illness such as depression.

8   POSITIVE THINKING

Positive thinking involves an interpretation of the world, and our relationship with others, that is optimistic, hopeful and upbeat. Some personalities are prone to pessimism, and see the 'glass' as being half-empty. This common attitude could also be interpreted as cautious, realistic and sensible. When this pessimism becomes almost apocalyptic, however, and the person starts to wonder what the point of the glass existing in the first place is, it is likely that a mood disorder affecting thought processes is present.

9   MEMORY

At first glance, this seems an unlikely symptom, and is often overlooked by those not familiar with mental illness. Memory loss is normally associated in the mind of the layperson with Alzheimer's disease or dementia. Memory disturbance is also a feature of mood disorders, however, as the processing of memory is embedded deep in the mood system. This becomes evident when those suffering from depression and anxiety struggle to remember even the simplest of things, making their life chaotic and confusing. For instance, not being able to remember things at work will impair performance, and can be perceived as incompetence, whereas the cause is in fact a widespread malfunction of the mood system. Students both at school and university will suffer from this condition even more, as their success in examinations depends in large part on their ability to commit information to memory.

10   CONCENTRATION

Concentration – the ability to focus one's attention on a particular task for a length of time, and to process information received efficiently – has a direct effect on memory. Obviously, if concentration cannot be achieved, there is nothing to commit to memory! People suffering from depression of anxiety will find it difficult to read a book or newspaper, watch a film, or finish any task they start. This has serious negative ramifications for those who are at work or in full-time education.

11   SENSE OF JOY OR PLEASURE

Normal sources of pleasure in life include relationships, sex, food and alcohol. Hence the joy and pleasure that is extrapolated from such activities are major incentives to a person's participation in a full and active life. Without such rewards, the world appears an empty and meaningless place.

For those suffering from mental illness, the world is exactly that. As the reward system is a component of the mood system, general malfunction in the latter results in a generalised lack of enjoyment. The negative thinking outlined above can only be confirmed and exacerbated by this absence of positive biological feedback from the environment. Known officially as 'anhedonia', this vacuum of pleasure is a trademark symptom of depression.

12   IMPULSIVE THOUGHTS AND BEHAVIOUR

Some individuals are naturally impulsive, novelty-seeking risk-takers, whereas others are of a more cautious disposition. It is the job of the mood system to regulate impulses that will result in potentially harmful consequences if the person indulges them.

If the mood system is not working, a person's rational inhibitions are often diminished. In such cases, suicide, self-mutilation and violence directed towards others may become acceptable, reasonable and often unavoidable. When a person is going through a difficult period, fleeting and impulsive thoughts of self-harm can emerge. These thoughts are quickly and forcefully eliminated by the mood system when it is working normally. In illnesses such as depression and addiction, however, the ability to control these thoughts is substantially impaired, and the person in some cases may begin to elaborate on such thoughts and plan in detail how they will carry out the violent acts. Recurrent thoughts of self-harm, and how it can be achieved, is an indicator of serious mood-system disturbance.

*

Having read this checklist, you should have a clearer indication of your mood state, and whether it is really 'fine'. As we have seen, mood is not just a feeling of well-being but a cluster of different functions, all of which originate from the same system in the brain. The majority of people reading this list will find their mood system to be in good working order. Others will realise that they may be ill, and require support, empathy and assistance from those around them.

Whether or not you are suffering from, or at risk of, a mood problem is determined by the amount of the aforementioned symptoms you can relate to. Whether you feel you have been having some of these difficulties for a long time, or if you have noticed them appearing only recently, you should contact a health professional for further assessment. Difficulties which have lasted longer than four weeks warrant careful investigation by your doctor.

As a general rule, illness in the mood system results in a 'domino effect': the longer it remains untreated, the more the symptoms appear. For this reason, it is recommended that the Green Flag checklist be consulted on a regular basis. Early detection facilitates early treatment, and the damage to the brain caused by such illness can then be minimised.

One advantage of a healthy mood system is that the immune system will be strong and capable of fighting infection, illness and cancer cells. Other advantages are a decreased risk of osteoporosis and heart attacks. Those who are sceptical about the direct link between mental illness and general illness should note that those who are suffering from a serious bout of depression, for example, are five times more likely to suffer a heart attack than an average person.

The body and the mood system are interdependent. If mood is normal, general health is improved. This is not to say that someone who is free from mental illness will remain immune from other diseases, but they *are* better protected against them.

51

II   BIOLOGY OF THE GREEN FLAG

If the flag is green, then the mood departments, mood cables, glands and hormones are all working smoothly and within normal parameters (see Figure 16). In this case, the various boxes which control memory, stress and behaviour are doing what they were designed to do: promoting homeostasis, or balance within the body. The adrenal stress glands are producing adequate, but not excessive, amounts of its two main hormones, adrenalin and glucocortisol. Responses to stress, illness and disease are not impaired. The immune system is working efficiently, and the heart and bones are not in any immediate danger.

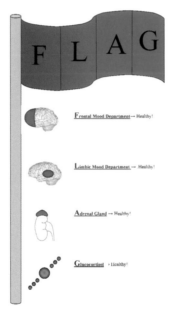

FIGURE 16

III   COURSE OF THE GREEN FLAG

The flag will be green for the majority of a person's life. It is almost inevitable that it will change colour at some stage. Many people go through periods of depression, anxiety or addiction, and some will spend their whole lives dealing with these illnesses. Statistically speaking, between 10 and 15 percent of the population will experience a bout of the Red Flag of depression at some stage. Others will be paralysed by the Yellow Flag of anxiety, or will fall victim to the Purple Flag of addiction.

The Green Flag's most formidable adversary (genes and early environment aside) is stress, for which the fast pace of modern life is a breeding ground. Other challenges to the Green Glag include alcohol abuse, relationship breakdown, and isolation.

Over the last five years, there has been a huge focus on healthy living in Ireland. Diet assessment, cholesterol measurement, prostate checking, breast screening, and cervical smears are seen as critical to the health of the nation. Yet the mood system is not discussed. Such neglect is not only allowing mental illness to remain undetected and run rampant but is also, as has been discussed, increasing the chances of various illnesses, such as heart disease and cancer.

5

How to Keep Your Mood System Healthy

The Top Ten Ways of Keeping Your Mood System Healthy

1   FOLLOW THE GREEN FLAG CHECKLIST

As one should regularly check for the presence of a tumour to protect against testicular and breast cancer, reviewing the Green Flag checklist regularly ensures that you have a good chance of detecting mental illness at an early stage. If significant symptoms are persistent, medical advice should be sought.

2   REDUCE PERSONAL STRESS

The key to fighting stress is identifying its cause. This will be different for each person. For most people, work, commuting, family problems, and relationship and financial difficulties are common sources of stress.

Solutions to work-related stress may include working part-time, reducing commuting times by working closer to home and, as a last resort, removing oneself from stressful working situations. Relationship or family problems should be dealt with as quickly as possible. Financial situations should be constantly reviewed, especially bills and credit cards, to prevent debt-related pressure and stress emerging.

Another important cause of stress in our lives is unrealistic self-expectations. Many of us do not accept ourselves as being genuinely human – that is, 'warts and all'. If we fail – as all of us will regularly do – to reach the often impossibly high goals we set ourselves, we become our own worst critics. We often extend these ideal standards to others and are disappointed when they too fail to reach them. Learning to accept ourselves unconditionally and to look at others in the same way is a vital component of mental health. Examining various areas of our lives with this core concept in mind will help ensure that the Green Flag flies!

3   EXERCISE

Exercise is a powerful stimulant of the mood system. The euphoria-inducing chemicals known as endorphins which are released during exercise provide both energy and relaxation. Exercise also stimulates the dopamine system, alleviating symptoms of mental fatigue. The memory box in particular benefits greatly from exercises like walking and swimming, which encourage the creation of new neurons.

Thirty to forty minutes of exercise per day is ideal for maintaining a healthy mood system. All forms of exercise deliver similar benefits, so it is simply a case of personal preference. Apart from controlling weight and helping the heart, exercise will also help to keep the flag green.

4   GET BACK TO NATURE

Shopping centres and busy department stores drain a person's energy – along with their bank account! Walking in the countryside – or by our lakes, sea shores, or rivers – fishing and swimming are all excellent ways of clearing the mind and providing much-needed relaxation for body, mind and spirit. The emotional part of the brain is particularly affected in a positive manner by interaction with Mother Nature.

5   RELAX AND CONTEMPLATE

For those who live in or near cities, the world is a noisy place. Traffic, television, computer games and mobile phones break the silence which is necessary for relaxation. People often return from work, where they have been staring at a computer screen all day, to stare at a television screen all night.

Our mood system needs periods of calm and silence. Activities such as yoga, meditation or massage, or just going for a walk, fulfil this requirement. Time for quiet contemplation also helps to keep the flag green.

6   IMPROVE YOUR DIET

You are what you eat, and the mood system does not escape this concept. Instant dinners, sugary food, and takeaway treats, although convenient, are damaging to the body. Although it takes time and energy to cook properly, the rewards for mood are great.

Fresh fruit and vegetables, fish, grains, meat and water help the system cope with day-to-day life. Cooking in olive oil, and reducing the intake of meat, dairy products (apart from eggs) and vegetable oils, and increasing the consumption of fish and soya is a good place to start.

Changes like this will reduce the likelihood of obesity and diabetes, and it should also be pointed out that up to a third of the energy derived from food is used by the brain, and that the mood system itself depends on certain vitamins and minerals. These include vitamin C, the B vitamins, zinc and magnesium. Supplements which help to keep the mood system healthy include the whole family of B vitamins, vitamin C, Omega 6 oils like evening primrose, and Omega 3 fish oils (so called because oily fish like mackerel, herring, tuna, salmon and sardines are the best natural source of such oils).

There has been a great deal of interest in these oils in recent years. They contain essential fatty acids which are usually absent from the Western diet. The body cannot manufacture these acids on its own, so it relies on either diet (in the form of oily fish, flax seeds or flax oil, walnuts and some green vegetables) or supplements to ensure the efficient operation of the mood system.

The most important oils are EPA (Eicosapentaenoic Acid) and DHA (Docosahexaenoic Acid). These are essential for the smooth running of our mood cables, helping to build the receptor sites for neurotransmitters and in the day-to-day maintenance of the cell membranes of our neurons. DHA is significant in the formation of the foetal brain in the womb, the neurological development of children under five, and general heart function.

Most brands of Omega 3 oils contain a mixture of EPA and DHA. Some experts believe that capsules containing higher doses of pure EPA (without vitamin E and with smaller amounts of DHA) are of more value when dealing with illnesses of the mood system, like depression. The recommended dose for the average healthy person who does not have such illnesses is probably 250 to 500 milligrammes, or two portions of oily fish a week. (The only exception is for people who are also on anticoagulants (blood thinners).)

Omega 3 oils have also been shown to reduce deaths from heart attacks by 30 percent and sudden death by 45 percent in heart watch prevention trials. (This programme, run by family doctors and practice nurses, monitors the continuing health of those who have either had a heart attack, or who have required a coronary artery bypass or stent to maintain the patency of the blood vessels serving the heart.) Whilst there seems to be a benefit from taking higher doses in such cases, the general view is that two helpings of oily fish (equivalent to 500 milligrammes) per week, or low doses of these essential fatty acids, is generally sufficient.

It is interesting to note that, in parts of the world, such as Japan, where there is a higher consumption of oily fish, there seems to be a lower risk of breast cancer, depression and coronary heart disease. This suggests the importance of diet in general, and possibly fish oils in particular, in preventing these illnesses. Whether this will prove to be of significance, only time and further research will tell.

A diet rich in these essential fats should begin from infancy onwards. Our typical diet in the West often lacks the building blocks necessary for the development of a healthy body and mind. Just observe the contents of the lunchbox or 'deli diet' of the typical school-going child. Some schools are challenging this trend and are at the forefront of encouraging healthy eating habits. This is a very welcome development.

A close examination of the contents of the average supermarket trolley will often reveal a huge dependency on tins and packets, large bottles of high-sugar-content or caffeinated drinks, and a notable absence of fruit and vegetables. Fast-sugar-release foods like white bread and rolls, white rice, confectionery, processed meals and so on have become the norm in a cash-rich, time-poor economy. Are we at risk of becoming an overfed, undernourished generation? Obesity may prove to be one of the major health problems over the next few decades. The obvious medical consequences of this are diabetes and coronary heart disease.

The consequences for the young person's developing mood system are equally alarming. The brain requires proper nutrition for normal growth, development and function. The widespread ignorance of this information could turn out to be one of the casual factors in the increasing prevalence of child behavioural problems and depression in the under-twenty-five age group. Most parents worry about the increasing rates of depression in young men and women, but they rarely consider the role of proper diet, exercise and supplements in the prevention of depression.

It is advisable that young people eat plenty of freshly prepared and cooked healthy food, together with regular portions of fruit and vegetables. Soft drinks should be replaced with milk, water or fruit juices. Growing children, teenagers and young adults should, unless they are eating a proper healthy diet high in fruit, vegetables and oily fish, take B vitamins and fish-oil supplements. Age twelve to twenty-five, in particular, is a period of dramatic brain and mood-system development, and a supply of these essential fatty acids is essential. If we wait until late in the teen years to implement these dietary changes, the benefits are greatly reduced.

7   WATCH YOUR ALCOHOL INTAKE

Alcohol, when taken in moderation, helps a person to relax, especially in social situations. There is no major health risk associated with alcohol if it is used in a sensible manner. Nonetheless, alcohol is classified as a depressive substance, and in genetically vulnerable people its misuse can lead to addiction. Alcohol misuse leaves a person depressed and irritable and can also result in a greater risk of impulsive, violent behaviour.

The international guidelines set arbitrary weekly limits of 21 units for males and 14 units for females (1 unit = 1 glass of beer, or 1 small glass of wine (125 mls) of 8 to 9 percent strength; 2 units = 1 pint of beer, 1 average size (175 mls) glass of wine of 12 percent strength, or 1 large measure of spirits).

Some experts regard 21 to 50 units of alcohol per week as hazardous, and more than 50 units as harmful. In practice, this weekly allowance is sometimes consumed on a single night. When 12 units of more (6 pints of beer, or 6 measures of spirits) are consumed in one sitting, it is classified as a binge. Alcohol is best consumed in small amounts, or with food.

Some useful guidelines to healthy drinking should include the following:

§ Try if at all possible to avoid binge drinking

§ Learn to drink slowly rather than gulping down alcoholic drinks

§ Be aware of what constitutes 'safe' drinking by memorising the limits given above

§ If you feel guilty when approached about your drinking habits, then it is quite likely that you have a problem

§ Avoid drinking as a means of overcoming shyness or boredom, or as a solution to any other problem

§ Have a number of alcohol-free days every week

§ Taking food with alcohol is always preferable to drinking on an empty stomach

§ Avoid buying rounds where possible

§ Avoid using alcohol to self-medicate during times of stress, anxiety and low mood

§ If you are finding Mondays difficult due to excessive alcohol intake over the weekend, you need to review your drinking habits

§ Do not allow friends or workmates to dictate your personal drinking patterns

§ Do not be afraid to say 'no'

Heavy drinking over the age of fifty-five to sixty can be extremely harmful, and results in an increased risk of falls, interaction with medication, impotence, sleep and memory problems, depression and dementia. The older you get, the less alcohol you should consume. Unfortunately, in practice the reverse is often the case.

It is frequently in the aftermath of a binge-drinking session that the underlying symptoms of illnesses such as depression begin to rise to the surface, in the form of decreased mood, anxiety, and suicidal thoughts and actions. Heavy alcohol intake is not compatible with the Green Flag.

8   SPIRITUALITY

Religion and spirituality are commonly misunderstood terms. Religion is a specific system of beliefs; spirituality relates to a more general search for the meaning of existence. This search can bring peace and harmony.

Many rush through life without reflecting on its meaning or relevance. Time spent on such reflection may be beneficial to mental health. Many experts feel that the increased incidence of depression and suicide particularly in the young may lie partially in the absence of such a focus. The religious structures that existed before and are now in dramatic decline may not have been perfect, but their removal has left a vacuum. Whether or not the filling of this vacuum is of any benefit to those at risk of mental illness is for the individual to decide.

9 LIFESTYLE

One of the major causes of stress in modern Ireland is money. The current generation earns far more money than previous ones did, and spends it in an equally excessive manner. Over-spending has led to increased reliance on credit cards and bank loans, which leads to unnecessary worry and stress for the individual concerned.

Advertising gives the impression that if one generates and consumes a great deal of money, life will be perfect. Those who feel as though they cannot reach such lofty materialistic heights may start to feel that they are failures. In short, the pressures on young people to achieve and consume are immense.

As long as this ideology is predominant, the Green Flag is under threat. Consumerism is an empty promise, and its rewards are without substance. While impulse buying is thought to be mediated by dopamine, and people often feel better after a shopping spree, this positive effect on the mood system is short-lived.

10 COMMUNICATION

Just as neurons in the brain only survive the harsh and unforgiving pruning process by communicating with others around them, people can only survive the harsh and unforgiving events in life by doing the same. Loneliness is one of the hidden enemies of normal mood and happiness.

Equally, as a breakdown in communication between neurons results in illness, a breakdown in communication between partners or families results in separation and divorce. This can lead to a major assault on the Green Flag.

In particular, men in such situations find it difficult to admit to feelings of sadness, confusion and loss, as it is often not socially acceptable for them to do so. So instead of reaching out for help, they conceal their emotions. This repression creates problems in the mood system, and increases the risk of depression and suicide. It is important for both men and women to express freely how they feel, without experiencing humiliation or rejection for being honest and open.

An absence of emotional expression makes the Green Flag difficult to maintain. It is advisable to keep lines of communication with significant others open, to set aside time to converse with them without any distractions, and to allow them to express any feelings of unhappiness.

CONCLUSION

For the mood system to remain healthy, proper diet, taking dietary supplements, exercise, meditation, communication, monitoring of stress, and moderating alcohol intake are all important. If these changes are made, improvements to our physical and mental health may not be the only benefits: a feeling of peace and tranquillity is also likely to result. Try it and see. You will be amazed at the results!

II

THE RED FLAG
DEPRESSION

1

SIMPLE DEPRESSION

Depression has been clouded by myth for a long time: it is often believed that it is a weakness, a personal flaw in the sufferer. This myth leads to a fear of discussing the problem. The fear results in silence, which maintains ignorance. Such ignorance compounds the sufferer's misery and effectively seals their fate. It is time to break this myth. Depression is not a weakness: it is a biological illness which damages the body's mood system. It presents with distinct symptoms, operates via well-known biological mechanisms and, most importantly, is in many cases easily treatable.

In order to break this myth, depression must be regarded in the same light as diabetes and heart disease – illnesses resulting from genetic and environmental interaction. The brain is classified as an organ just like the heart, liver and lungs, and is just as vulnerable to malfunction and illness as these organs.

Generally, a diabetic does not ignore their symptoms and view them as a weakness; rather, they seek medical help and treatment that will keep them alive. The chronic suffering, health risks, damage to quality of life, and mortality rates associated with diabetes are also associated with depression, so why should the sufferer not react in the same way as a diabetic?

The symptoms evident in depression (negative thinking, low mood, fatigue, lack of pleasure, suicidal thoughts, and so on) leave the victim ill-equipped to deal with society's ignorance about the condition. Statements like: 'Pull yourself together!' and 'Snap out of it!' are not only naive but counterproductive. Such ultimatums make the sufferer feel responsible for their own condition, and weak for not being able to defend against it. If they could 'snap out of it', they would do so instantly, but they can't, and as this is seen as the only solution by society, they conclude that they are not going to get better. Thus such statements end up making the depression worse.

The time has come to promote an understanding of this illness, and to support those who have suffered in silence for so long. This chapter deals with the symptoms, causes, course and treatment of the biological illness of depression. There is also a question-and-answer section for those who are trying to understand their own illness, or the illness of a person close to them.

I   SYMPTOMS OF THE RED FLAG OF DEPRESSION

Some people reading this chapter will suspect that either they themselves, or someone close to them, are suffering from depression, but need more information on the subject. Others will know that either they, or a person close to them, are definitely suffering from depression, and are seeking to understand the condition. To help such people identify and understand this illness, the following is a list of symptoms that the depressed person may be experiencing, and a description of how these symptoms will manifest themselves to those around them.

1   LOW MOOD

I feel weighed down by hopelessness and sadness. It is a physical pain in my heart, and no one understands how terrible it feels.

John, a nineteen-year-old undergraduate student who has developed depression on moving away from his family for the first time, to live in a flat in Dublin. He is successfully hiding his depression from his family and friends. Alcohol relieves the pain for short periods, but its embrace is fleeting and illusory.

Low mood is an overwhelming feeling of inner sadness, gloom and despair. It is the main warning sign that the mood system is in trouble. Even when the mood system is operating normally, mood swings are inevitable, and are easily influenced by life circumstances.

Low mood, however, is different to 'feeling blue'; those who have not experienced it will not understand the distinction. In depression, these feelings are overpowering and devastating. To people with depression, particularly if the condition is severe, it feels like having fallen down a deep dark well: the individual is alone, hurt, and unable to communicate with others. As they feel that there is no chance of receiving help, or of climbing out on their own, they lie inactive and succumb to their inevitable fate. The feelings of pain they experience may be beyond the comprehension of an outsider.

What John feels:

§   A deep emotional pain so intense he would gladly replace it with any physical pain

§   Enduring despair, sadness and inner turmoil

§   Frustration that no one understands his pain, or cares about it

§   An increasing reliance on alcohol to numb the pain

What those close to John may observe:

- § He may smile less, and his emotional reactions may often be subdued
- § At times he may suddenly lash out in anger at those closest to them
- § He may be drinking excessively
- § He may withdraw into his room, listen to dark angry music, play video games, or use Internet chat rooms

2   FATIGUE

The simplest of tasks drains me of all my energy. I just want to sleep all the time.

Mary, a twenty-seven-year-old mother with two small children, who has started to develop symptoms of depression following a series of stressful events, in particular the death of a close friend from cancer

Exhaustion is an inevitable consequence of intense and stressful physical or mental activity. In depression, however, a more serious form of exhaustion emerges. This form of exhaustion is best described as fatigue: it is a complete lack of energy, resulting in an inability to perform the easiest of tasks.

What Mary feels:

- § Completely sapped of energy
- § Normal functioning becomes a battle: work, shopping and other day-to-day activities all require a level of effort she cannot muster
- § Unrefreshed by sleep
- § Unrelenting exhaustion all the time
- § A further drop in self-esteem and a feeling of uselessness, as she is not able to complete even the most mundane activities

What those close to Mary may observe:

- § She may return to bed frequently in the middle of the day
- § She complains that she is tired all the time, and is prone to yawning and falling asleep
- § She is having difficulties completing normal activities
- § At times she appears listless and apathetic
- § She appears to be acting in a lazy fashion

3   SLEEP DIFFICULTIES

Why can't I sleep when I'm tired all the time? I lie awake all night, or if I do manage to fall asleep, I wake early. It's so frustrating.

Thomas, a thirty-two-year-old successful businessman, who has been suffering from un-diagnosed bouts of depression for more than a decade

Sleep disturbance can refer to a sudden change in a person's normal sleeping pattern, or a long-standing pattern of sleeping which is broken, fitful and unsatisfactory. It presents most commonly in depression as pure insomnia.

What Thomas experiences:

§   Difficulties falling sleep despite the fact that he is exhausted

§   Early-morning waking

§   Waking intermittently throughout the night

§   Unpleasant nightmares

§   Somnolence during the day

§   An increased reliance on alcohol to induce sleep

What those close to Thomas will observe:

§   He walks around the house at night looking for things to do

§   He lies awake for a long time before falling asleep

§   He is exhausted in the morning

§   He may return to bed during the day when the opportunity presents itself

§   He regularly drinks alcohol before going to bed

4   ANXIETY

I am constantly on a high state of alertness, and I always feel under pressure. I cannot cope when something goes wrong. I sometimes feel panicky for no obvious reason.

Peter, aged twenty-two, who for the previous three years has successfully hidden how he feels

66

Anxiety often occurs alongside depression, and can be described as constant panic, tension and worry about things going wrong. It is a vicious circle because anxiety uses up so much energy that the person is too tired to deal with the situations of which they are afraid. This results in further anxiety when other situations arise, as the first ones have not been tackled.

What Peter feels:

§   Agitated and irritable

§   Worried about not being able to perform simple tasks properly

§   Excessively fatigued

§   Episodes of panic

§   A reluctance to start new tasks or take on new responsibilities

What those close to Peter will observe:

§   He appears tense and often 'snaps' when asked a simple question

§   Restlessness

§   Sensitivity to criticism

§   Regular alcohol intake, often drinking alone or at odd times

§   Persistent inability to make decisions

§   He may complain of physical irregularities such as headaches, palpitations and stomach pains

5   WEIGHT LOSS OR WEIGHT GAIN

I'm just not hungry any more. Food does not look appetising and it's too much energy to eat. Hopefully I will waste away into nothing.

Catherine, a single parent aged twenty-four. The stress of coping with a small child on social welfare, living in a small, poorly equipped flat, and with a partner who abuses alcohol (and her), has triggered a bout of depression. She has lost more than a stone in weight. Her diet (already poor due to lack of money and knowledge about nutrition) has been reduced to coffee and cigarettes.

Or:

> Eating has become a habit for me. It distracts me from how I feel for a while. Then I feel worse as I get fatter and uglier, but who is going to look twice at me anyway?

Michael, who, although presenting an outer image of seeming normality, has suffered for years with poor self-esteem. Now, at the age of thirty, he is grossly obese from years of using food as a coping mechanism for his bouts of low mood.

Usually in depression, a sudden and complete loss of interest in food ensues. The weight loss prevalent in depression does not usually result from a person's negative self-image and dissatisfaction with their appearance, however: it occurs because eating becomes a laborious chore that yields no enjoyment. Sometimes, although not as often, the depressed person will eat excessively because it makes them feel better, and weight gain becomes the symptom to look out for.

What Catherine experiences:

§ A sudden and absolute lack of interest in food

§ Difficulty in finishing a meal

§ A tendency to regard food as one area of life that she can control

§ Decreased energy

§ Weight loss

What those close to Catherine will observe:

§ A rejection of food when it is offered

§ A seeming loss of any interest in food

§ Visible weight loss

§ Irritation when friends try to encourage her to eat

§ That she seems to be withdrawing 'into herself'

What Michael experiences:

§ A desire to hide his true feelings behind his large girth and a mask of seeming good humour

§ An increasing craving for food to numb his emotional pain

§ A complete lack of interest in his personal appearance

§ A feeling that food is the one area of his life that he can control

§ A deep seated lack of self worth: 'I'm just a fat, useless nobody'

§ A denial of the consequences of his obesity: 'After all, who will notice if I was gone anyway'

What those close to Michael may observe:

§ He takes no interest in his appearance

§ He rejects any offers of help or advice

§ He has complete disregard for the consequences of his obesity

§ He seems to binge-eat at every opportunity

§ Although he is always smiling, it seems to be 'skin deep'

6   LOSS OF SELF-ESTEEM

I am ashamed of the weak, useless, boring, incompetent failure that I am. People hate spending time with me.

Carl, a twenty-four-year-old mechanic whose quiet disposition and painful shyness has disguised his inner torment from those close to him. Depression visited him first at the age of seventeen and has been an unwelcome but frequent visitor ever since.

Self-esteem refers to whether we love and value ourselves unconditionally. Depressed people feel unloved, unworthy, and of no value. It is a common and distressing set of symptoms.

How Carl feels:

§ Of no value or use to society

§ An unnecessary burden on others

§ That his opinions are irrelevant

§ Completely non-accepting of himself

What those close to Carl will observe:

§ He has become self-absorbed

§ He avoids and withdraws from social interaction

§ He makes negative comments about himself

§ He is reluctant to express his opinions

7   LOSS OF DRIVE

I don't enjoy any of the activities that I used to. It all seems like so much effort now, and I don't see the point.

> *Maura, a twenty-four-year-old working mother who developed depression*
> *three months after the birth of her first child*

Drive refers to a person's willingness to participate in an activity. This is usually absent in depression, and results in idleness. Loss of drive is compounded by fatigue, as the person lacks either the will or the means to do anything.

What Maura feels:

§   Apathy, an inability to see the point of any activity

§   A lack of purpose

§   A pervasive boredom with regard to life

What those close to Maura will observe:

§   Avoidance of tasks and situations

§   Unwillingness to become involved in normal activities

§   A dissolving of ambition and goals

8   NEGATIVE THINKING

I cannot wait till I am dead. Then I will be at peace, the loneliness and hurt will be gone. I cannot go on, not like this. I have often thought of trying to explain how I feel to those closest to me: to share the pain. But what would be the point. After all, there's nothing they or anyone else can do to help, and I would only be burdening them with my troubles.

> *Andrew, a twenty-six-year-old postgraduate student, suffering from his second major bout of depres-*
> *sion. Andrew, like many others with this illness, is having relationship difficulties with his girlfriend,*
> *blaming her for not seeing his pain, and using alcohol in large amounts. This does little, however, to*
> *silence his negative thoughts that he does not deserve to live: he reasons that no one, including her, would*
> *notice if he was gone.*

Negative thinking is a distorted and often false interpretation of the world (sometimes called 'rumination') which focuses exclusively on unpleasant events and results in pessimistic predictions. Although to others this thinking seems odd and irrational, to the depressed person it is an important explanation as to why they feel the way they do. Because they view the world and their own existence as being empty and futile, there is no point in seeking help: they feel that it is unlikely that anything can be done. This fosters a sense of predestined and unavoidable suffering, and explains why they isolate themselves, and in certain cases rationalise suicide.

What Andrew feels:

§ An inability to see the positive aspects of anything or anyone (including his girlfriend, who cares deeply for him), particularly himself

§ A sense of futility about existence in general

§ Pessimism about the prospects of treatment

§ A conviction that his life is not salvageable

§ That he deserves the pain he is feeling

§ That the hidden cigarette burns he occasionally inflicts on himself to ease the emotional pain are 'all he deserves'

What those close to Andrew will observe:

§ A predominantly negative verbal assessment of health, family, friends and themselves that seems to bear no relation to reality

§ A decline in goal-oriented behaviour, as he is not working towards anything

§ A refusal of help from anyone

§ Occasional bursts of anger (particularly after drinking alcohol) that nobody can understand the world (of negativity) he lives in

9   POOR MEMORY

I have become increasingly forgetful, and have difficulty remembering the simplest of things, like what I did yesterday.

Noreen, a single, very busy twenty-seven-year-old manager who is struggling to cope with her day-to-day duties due to depression triggered by a prolonged period of sustained stress

Depression reduces short-term memory – the ability to retain information concerning recent events. Naturally, if this continues, the capacity to form, store and retrieve long-term information is also adversely affected. This, combined with damage to the part of the brain which filters and organises the storage and retrieval of long-term memories, leads to chaos in the life of the person.

What Noreen experiences:

§   Difficulties remembering exceptionally simple things, e.g. repeating what she has just read in a newspaper

§   A reduction in the effectiveness of studying and memorising data, regardless of the amount of time she spends on it

§   Difficulty performing in a job in which memory is an important component

What those close to Noreen will observe:

§   Noticeable and often bizarre forgetfulness, bordering on eccentricity

§   Exasperation when trying to remember data

§   Slowed performance in the workplace

10   REDUCED CONCENTRATION

I don't read any more, it is too much effort to make sense out of the words, and it is becoming difficult to pay attention to anything.

George, a seventeen-year-old Leaving Cert student, struggling to study as he battles internally with a bout of unrecognised depression

Concentration is the ability to focus exclusively on a task for its duration, from start to completion. Concentration is a prerequisite for learning to occur. One cannot commit to memory what one is not paying attention to. Furthermore, the initial performance of a task in work, for example, demands concentration. Subsequent improved performance depends on memory. Without the initial concentration, this cannot be achieved, and new skills cannot be learnt.

What George experiences:

§   Easily distracted when performing any task, particularly in relation to the upcoming exam

§   An inability to focus on individual words when reading a newspaper or a book

§   Study that is unproductive and constantly broken up by his mind wandering

§   A pile-up of projects and tasks, all of which are unfinished

§ An increasing sense of panic as the exam looms and his ability to prepare seems to diminish

What those close to George will observe:

§ Unfinished projects and tasks, or projects that have been completed taking an extremely long time

§ What seems like laziness in relation to his studies

§ Impaired performance at school, university or work

§ He will read much less, if at all

11 LACK OF PLEASURE (ANHEDONIA)

I can barely manage a smile any more. I'm sick of people telling me to 'cheer up' or 'it can't be that bad', but it is, and much worse than they can imagine.

Paula, aged twenty-eight, who was sexually abused at the age of nine and has had bouts of depression for the previous five years

An inability to enjoy anything that life has to offer is one of the trademark symptoms of depression.

How Paula feels:

§ Complete indifference to activities which would normally be considered enjoyable

§ Dejected, wondering what the point is of going anywhere or doing anything

§ Curious and confused as to why people enjoy and participate in activities like sport, socialising and eating out

What those close to Paula will observe:

§ Her face may seem blank and emotionless

§ She rarely smiles or laughs

§ She seems to avoid social situations

§ It takes a lot to persuade her to take part in any optional activity

12   SUICIDAL THOUGHTS

The world will be a much better place without me. I am a burden on everyone and they won't miss me at all.

Jack, who is twenty-nine, has already quietly planned in great detail how he will end the pain he is experiencing. If his depression is not recognised and remains untreated, he may soon put these thoughts into action. This is made more likely by a dramatic increase in alcohol consumption to numb the pain of the recent breakup with his girlfriend.

Suicidal thoughts are the most perilous symptom of depression. Sometimes a healthy mind will experience impulsive thoughts of self-harm, but such thoughts will be fleeting due to the brain's ability to control them. In depression, however, this control is lacking, and urges to self-harm may become habitual. The suicidal thoughts are bolstered and rationalised by low self-esteem, low mood, and a generally negative outlook on life. If these impulses become too strong, the person may feel compelled to cut themselves or attempt suicide. Death becomes something to look forward to, and is seen as a favour to those around them. The combination of alcohol and suicidal thoughts should be avoided: alcohol makes it easier for the depressed person to act on their suicidal thoughts.

How Jack feels:

§   The only way to end this intense emotional pain is to kill himself

§   A feeling of helplessness and hopelessness

§   A burden on everyone around him

§   A craving for the peace and quiet that death will bring

§   A compulsion to do anything that will result in self-injury

§   An inability to see any future for himself

§   That his girlfriend was right to leave him, as he is worthless and deserves to be left on his own

§   A sense of isolation

§   A sense of relief in working out in detail how he will end it all

What those close to the Jack may observe:

§   Gradual physical and emotional withdrawal from loved ones

§   Spending increased time on his own

§ An increased amount of time spent in front of computer games or in Internet chat rooms

§ Increased dependence on alcohol

§ Throwaway statements such as 'Wouldn't it be a lot easier if I just killed myself'

THE RED FLAG CHECKLIST

The above symptoms are summarised in the Red Flag checklist (see Figure 1). This is a useful tool for assessing the health of our mood system. These symptoms can be summarised as a combination of 'physical' symptoms such as fatigue and sleep difficulties and 'psychological' ones such as low mood and negative thinking. This physical and emotional cocktail makes the condition difficult both to recognise and to treat. The mystery and secrecy that cloud and maintain depression can only be lifted by a frank and open discussion of these symptoms.

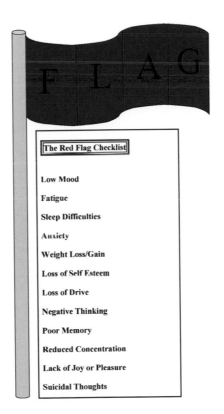

The Red Flag Checklist

Low Mood

Fatigue

Sleep Difficulties

Anxiety

Weight Loss/Gain

Loss of Self Esteem

Loss of Drive

Negative Thinking

Poor Memory

Reduced Concentration

Lack of Joy or Pleasure

Suicidal Thoughts

FIGURE 1: THE RED FLAG CHECKLIST

How many of the above symptoms does a person need to have in order to conclude that he or she is depressed? Technically, the doctor will diagnose 'major depression'(the commonest form) as depressed mood for more than two weeks, combined with at least four of the above additional symptoms, particularly difficulties with sleep, appetite, fatigue, feelings of worthlessness, and anhedonia.

Most people with the Red Flag will usually experience the majority of these symptoms, of which low mood, negative thinking, reduced self-esteem and sleep or appetite disturbance are the most common. Reduced energy and concentration are not as obvious, but are usually just as prevalent. The crux of the issue is that, if these symptoms are consistently present for a period of two to four weeks or longer, it is likely that the person is suffering from a mood disorder and needs to get help.

The longer an episode of depression continues, the more of these symptoms appear. As a result, early detection and treatment is vital before the person's life is completely disrupted, or even in some cases destroyed. References to suicide should be regarded as the most alarming symptom of depression because they are often a quiet cry for help, and warrant immediate referral to a specialist.

Lastly, as many of these symptoms reflect internal states, and not overt behaviour, it can be difficult for those around the depressed person to notice that anything is wrong. Fatigue, low mood, anxiety, anhedonia, reduced self-esteem, and thoughts of suicide are not readily observable, especially to a person who is not looking for them. This is why it is crucial to encourage people to talk about how they feel.

The illnesses of depression, anxiety and addiction all revolve around and are sustained by emotional disturbance. The mood system is responsible for these emotions; illness affecting this system leads to such disturbances.

If you have read through the above section and are experiencing many of the symptoms of depression, your mood system is in trouble, and you need to seek help. Depression is an illness, and is eminently treatable. The symptoms that are causing such misery in your life can be successfully eliminated.

If you suspect that you are living with somebody who may be depressed, sit them down in a quiet room, and ask them to talk to you about how they are feeling. Let them know that you care, and that they are worth a lot to you. Remember, they will probably think that you hate even spending time with them, and that they cannot be helped, so it is important to reassure them that this is not the case.

If major suicidal thoughts are present, the mood system is in real trouble. It is an indication that the depression is taking over complete control of the brain. If you or anyone close to you is feeling suicidal, help must be sought and alcohol avoided till the situation is brought under control.

II   THE BIOLOGY OF THE RED FLAG

Of all the illnesses that can affect the mood system, depression causes the greatest disruption. The symptoms outlined above cover every aspect of the mood system. The causes of this illness and its exact neurological mechanisms will take some time for researchers to understand fully. Science is only beginning to explain the workings of the brain, and how an illness like depression operates. New research continues to lift the veil from that mystery. Taking this into consideration, we will look at what is known to date about the biological causes of depression.

There may be many people reading this chapter who are not particularly interested in the biological underpinnings of depression. To cater for them, following this section is a summary of the main biological findings relating to depression. Others may be curious about the specifics of how the condition operates.

*

The whole 'flag system' is in chaos, but why? This is the question that modern researchers are struggling to answer. At the moment, it seems likely that some of us are programmed (by virtue of genes and our early environment) to be particularly vulnerable to stress. In such people, once the stress response has been activated, particularly in a chronic fashion, the mood departments and cables come under sustained attack, and the whole neural mood circuit starts to malfunction.

This, in turn, impairs the ability of the mood system to shut down the stress response. So a vicious circle ensues, and the mood system deteriorates, until the symptoms of depression increase and take over the person's life.

In chronic depression, there may not be any trigger: the mood system can just break down. This may be due to previous structural damage to various departments, such as the behaviour box in particular, and also the memory box, from earlier episodes. Therefore, the more episodes of depression the brain has to deal with, the more likely it is that depression will occur again in the future. This is why detection and treatment of initial episodes is crucial.

The genetic vulnerability of the mood system to stress varies widely from person to person. The greater the vulnerability, the less stress that will be required to kick-start the depressive process. What follows is a detailed look at the damage caused by depression in the brain.

(A)   MOOD DEPARTMENTS

Depression causes mayhem in both mood departments, especially to the key sections that regulate memory, stress, behaviour and pleasure.

1   FRONTAL MOOD DEPARTMENT

FIGURE 2: THE FRONTAL MOOD DEPARTMENT

Malfunctioning of this department usually involves the behaviour box. In depression, this leads to the following problems:

§   Decreased short-term memory and concentration

§   Slowed thought processes

§   Fatigue

§   Low mood

§   Pessimism

§   Impulsive thoughts of self-harm

§   Ruminating or negative thinking

Reduced activity in most sections of the behaviour box, combined with increased activity in others, seems to play a vital role in the arrival of many of the symptoms of depression. The behaviour box in particular plays a major role in negative thinking. Reduced functioning of one section of this department (and the serotonin cable supplying it) also increases the prevalence of suicidal thoughts.

This dysfunction in the behaviour box promotes negative thinking for two reasons:

1   Positive, logical thinking depends on activation of the behaviour box in particular

2   Negative emotional thoughts originating from the stress box are not overruled. This is because some parts of this box have the function of dampening down such

thoughts. In depression, the normal functioning of these parts of the box is impaired. This allows the stress box to pour out these negative emotional thoughts.

One prominent theory of depression is that it begins in the frontal behaviour box (particularly on the left side). Neuro-imaging and post-mortem studies have demonstrated increased activity in those sections at the base of this box (involved in the creation of mood) and reduced activity in those at the apex (involved in the cognitive control of mood).

A key section of the behaviour box involved in depression is one called 'Area 25' (see Figure 3). This area, along with other sections of the behaviour box, seems to play a major role in the creation of mood. Area 25 appears to be over-active in all forms of major depression, and at the heart of the breakdown of information between the emotional and logical mood departments. Structurally, it is positioned at the junction between these two departments. For this reason, some experts call it a 'gateway'. It is activated (or opened) under normal conditions when we are sad, but in depression this activation becomes chronic. This seems to allow a torrent of negative emotions from the stress box to overwhelm the logical brain, creating the negative thinking that is so prevalent in depression.

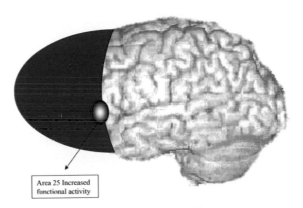

Area 25 Increased functional activity

FIGURE 3: THE ROLE OF AREA 25 IN DEPRESSION

At present, doubt exists as to whether this is the actual biological source of depression (which would be a major breakthrough), or, more likely, a consequence of it. A great deal of research into this question is under way. Whatever the role of Area 25, it is obviously well placed on the neural mood circuit to influence, for better or worse, the pain that the illness brings into people's lives. We will be examining its role both later in the treatment of depression and in Appendix 1.

It has also been shown that, in chronic depression, reductions in actual physical size and structure of the box itself can affect various parts of the behaviour box. In one study (involving familial depression and bipolar mood disorder), for example, a segment of Area 24 (bordering on Area 25) (see Figure 4) was shown to be reduced in size by 20 to 40 percent. (Subsequent research has suggested that these structural changes are due to a decrease in the number of glial support cells and a reduction in the number of connections between the neurons in this box.) Why this occurs remains uncertain.

FIGURE 4: AREAS 24 AND 25

Other research into depression has shown varying shortages of neurons, connections between neurons, and in particular glial support cells in various other sections of the behaviour box, particularly Areas 9, 10, 24 and 47. Many researchers wonder whether the shortage of glial cells might lie at the heart of this illness.

This hypothesis is born out by research which showed a reduction of up to 19 percent in Area 24 of these support glial cells in a group of young women following an initial bout of adolescent-onset depression. The same study found the same changes in a group of middle-aged women who had suffered repeated episodes of depression. This suggests that these changes may be present in the individual from the beginning of their life.

Some scientists are of the opinion that genetic and early environmental factors increase the vulnerability of the behaviour box, perhaps by creating an initial shortage of vital glial cells, but more likely by increasing their vulnerability to stress, thus beginning the depressive cycle. How the latter might occur is uncertain: it may be due to an attack on these glial cells by high glucocortisol/stress peptides released by the stress system. This process could destroy the glial cells, resulting in some of the deficits in brain matter that are observed in depression. As the neurons depend on these glial cells to function, a reduction in their activity, and indeed in the possibility of them being destroyed, is inevitable. At present, all of this is speculative, but a great deal of research is pointing in this direction.

If depression does begin its journey in this section of the brain, it may explain why a bout of depression makes further episodes of depression more likely. When depression damages the behaviour box, the box's ability (through structural and possibly glial-cell deficits) to cope with stress in the future is compromised. A benign stress trigger (having to deal with simple work problems, for instance) in forthcoming years, which would not have been a problem before the first bout of depression, may be too much for the damaged behaviour box to cope with, and the dysfunctional stress response which precipitates depression will be set in motion.

2   LIMBIC MOOD DEPARTMENT

FIGURE 5: THE LIMBIC MOOD DEPARTMENT

When it comes to the majority of depressive symptoms, this department has the finger of blame pointed squarely at it. When the limbic mood department is not operating properly, the following disabling results may ensue:

§   Low mood

§   Anxiety

§   Sleep difficulties

§   Poor memory and concentration

§   Reduced self-esteem

§   Anhedonia (lack of feelings of joy or pleasure)

§   Fatigue

§   Reduced motivation

§   Reduced sexual drive

§   Appetite and weight changes

§ Disturbance in normal biological rhythms

§ Negative thinking

KEY DEPARTMENTS

THE MEMORY BOX, THE STRESS BOX AND THE PLEASURE BOX

1 *The memory box* Damage to cells in this box interferes with memory. This occurs due to a combination of prevention of new cells being formed and interference with the efficiency of those already present.

2 *The stress box* Over-activity causes anxiety, a common symptom of depression. It is also responsible for a pessimistic outlook on life, negative thinking, and a reduction in self-esteem. Over-activity also contributes to excessively negative emotional responses to many common everyday occurrences, as seen in many people with depression. The stress box is also the chief organiser of the stress system, which in turn leads to too much glucocortisol being produced. Post-mortem and neuro-imaging studies have revealed once again a shortage of glial cells and an increase in activity of this box, respectively.

3 *The pleasure box* The lack of responsiveness of this box results in an inability to derive pleasure from activities which would normally provide pleasure.

(B)   MOOD CABLES

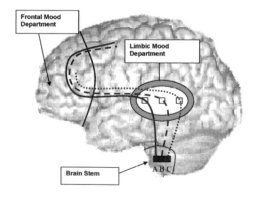

	A: Serotonin Box/ Cable → Reduced Activity
- - - - -	B: Noradrenalin Box/ Cable → Reduced Activity
....	C: Dopamine Box/ Cable → Reduced Activity

FIGURE 6: THE MOOD CABLES IN DEPRESSION

The three mood cables, which communicate using serotonin, noradrenalin and dopamine, are normally depleted in varying degrees during depression. This is due to a decrease in both the production of the transmitters and the sensitivity of the receptors they target. The extent of this damage varies from person to person. As these cables connect the mood departments and their individual sections together, it is clear that any disruption to their normal functioning will contribute to difficulties relating to mood. Such disruption causes the following problems:

1   SEROTONIN CABLE

This is the primary mood cable. Decreased activity results in low mood, anxiety, sleep difficulties, appetite problems and reduced self-esteem. It also leads to suicidal impulses and actions.

2   NORADRENALIN CABLE

Damage to this cable results in fatigue, low mood and lack of motivation. It also interferes with concentration.

3   DOPAMINE CABLE

Dopamine creates a feeling of pleasure. If this cable is not responding appropriately to life events, a person will not enjoy any activities and will not see the point in taking part in them. In some cases, this contributes to fatigue.

4   PEPTIDE SYSTEM

This system is highly activated in depression. It helps to perpetuate the vicious cycle of the stress response and depressive episodes.

(C)   ADRENAL STRESS GLAND

FIGURE 7: THE ADRENAL STRESS GLAND

In depression, the activation of the stress response is often so prolonged and extreme that the adrenal glands in some cases actually increase in size. This results in further extensive production of glucocortisol, which is unnaturally constant, day and night. It is now clear that these glands are one of the long-sought links between stress and depression.

(D)   GLUCOCORTISOL STRESS HORMONE

FIGURE 8: THE GLUCOCORTISOL STRESS HORMONE

This hormone is depression's closest comrade. As depression worsens, the level of glucocortisol rises in unison, launching a vicious assault on the mood departments and cables. This causes continuous damage, day and night.

In depression, this hormone is to blame for the following problems:

§   *Damage to the memory box*, interfering with the creation and organisation of memory and reducing the ability to concentrate. It prevents new cells from growing in this box.

§   *A 200 to 500 percent increase in the risk of heart disease* (depending on the severity of depression), by causing blood platelets to stick together. Prof. Ted Dinan (professor of psychiatry at University College Cork) has done a great deal of work on the effects of glucocortisol in this area (see Appendix 1 and Bibliography)

§   *Reduced defences against illness*, by interfering with the white blood cell receptors and their ability to respond to infection. This includes the ability to fight cancerous cells.

§   *Poor bone formation*, leading to osteoporosis (thinning of the bones).

§   *May increase the chances of developing abdominal obesity and Type 2 diabetes*

§   *Fatigue*

§   *May play a role in suicide* due to the damage it causes to the serotonin cable and behaviour box

It is now clear how the Green Flag of normal mood is turned into the Red Flag of depression (Figure 9).

FIGURE 9

Another useful, indeed revolutionary, way of looking at depression 'within the brain itself' is to view the mood system as a neural 'mood circuit', as discussed in the Green Flag section. Information flows to and fro along this mood circuit between the frontal and limbic mood departments and the mood cable control centres in the brain stem. When this flow is disrupted through malfunctions to any part of this circuit, depression may emerge.

At present, it is felt that the most likely source of such a short-circuit within this loop is a malfunctioning left-sided behaviour box. This allows the emotional limbic mood department to flood the logical brain with negativity and low mood, and sets off the chain of biological effects noted above. Once this neural mood circuit breaks down (see Figure 11), all of the symptoms and signs of depression appear.

This mood-circuit-breakdown model is also very useful in explaining depression in the elderly. For completely different reasons (such as vascular damage to circuits leading into the left-sided behaviour box, or Parkinson's disease damaging the dopamine control boxes), the same neural mood circuit is disrupted, and once again the signs and

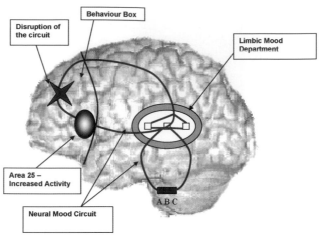

A   Serotonin control box
B   Noradrenalin control box
C   Dopamine control box

FIGURE 10: THE DYSFUNCTIONAL MOOD CIRCUIT

symptoms of depression appear. We can now see that this model of depression allows us, for the first time, to explain how this illness can give rise to the same symptoms in both young and old people.

If we were to theorise on the most likely chronology of a bout of depression, it would probably go like this:

1   A period of stress in our lives causes the stress box to kick-start the body's stress system into action by producing stress peptides and glucocortisol in abundance.

2   These substances begin to attack the already vulnerable frontal behaviour box. This in some cases may already have structural changes in place due to glial-cell shortages.

3   The ability of the behaviour box to switch off the stress box is now compromised. Area 25, a key part of the mood circuit, becomes over-active. Negativity pouring out of the emotional limbic brain's stress box begins to overpower the logical brain. Low mood, anxiety, negative thinking and poor self-esteem move in.

4   Another consequence of the stress box being out of control is that more stress peptides and glucocortisol continue to pour out. As the mood-cable control boxes (which are rich in glucocortisol receptors) are very sensitive to this barrage, the mood cables begin to become under-active, starting with the serotonin cable and then later the noradrenalin and dopamine cables.

5   Gradual involvement of these cables due to their huge importance in linking the two mood departments and their individual sections together leads to the appearance of many of the vegetative symptoms of depression, such as sleep disturbance, increased or decreased appetite, poor drive, fatigue and poor concentration. These symptoms also consolidate some of the psychological symptoms noted above.

6   Now the whole mood circuit, from the mood control boxes and cables to the emotional limbic brain and the logical frontal brain, is dysfunctional. All the symptoms of depression, both physical and psychological, are present.

7   Due to the constant glucocortisol barrage, the body's platelets, bones and white blood cells may become affected, with the appearance of heart disease, osteoporosis and infections.

Why label depression 'the Red Flag'? Red is a warning colour. Depression does not just affect the mood system, it also warns of damage to many other parts of the body. This includes heart disease, infection, osteoporosis and death by suicide. (Up to 15 percent of those who have suffered recurrent bouts of depression commit suicide.) It is a warning to the depressed person and those around them that trouble may be looming.

The behaviour box (particularly one key section which we will be examining later in the White Flag) and the serotonin cable that connects with it are extremely influential in suicide. Thoughts of suicide, and the successful completion of the act, are more likely to occur in those who display marked inactivity in the serotonin cable which feeds a particular section of their behaviour box. Identifying these people is a difficult task. In the future, neuro-imaging of this cable, and possibly genetic screening of high-risk families and individuals, may be the most effective non-clinical means of picking out those who are most at risk.

SUMMARY

Depression can have the following adverse effects on the mood system:

1   *Damage to the frontal and limbic mood departments* (See Figures 2 and 5, on pages 78 and 81, respectively) This damage will be most extensive in the memory, behaviour, stress and pleasure boxes. Such damage results in low mood, negative thinking, poor memory, anxiety, poor self-esteem, anhedonia (absence of joy) and urges to inflict self-harm

2   *Damage to the three main mood cables* (the serotonin, noradrenalin and dopamine cables) (see Figure 6 on page 82) This results in reduced motivation, poor concentration, eating problems, sleep difficulties, fatigue and low mood, and the disappearance of pleasure from the person's life.

3   *Overstimulation of the adrenal glands*, producing too much of the stress hormone glucocortisol (see Figures 4 and 5, on pages 80 and 81, respectively). This will increase the risk of heart attacks, osteoporosis and general infection.

4   A useful way of looking at depression in the brain itself is to view it as *a dysfunction of the mood circuit* (see Figure 10 on page 86)

III   CAUSES OF THE RED FLAG OF DEPRESSION

The cause of depression has been the subject of intense and acrimonious debate for decades. Many researchers previously attributed it to genetic inheritance. Others emphasised the contribution of family upbringing, social problems and general environment. Modern research has deepened our understanding of the condition. The cause is primarily genetic, with outside environmental triggers also influencing the onset of the illness. A similar example would be type II diabetes, where the underlying malfunction is genetic, with environmental influences such as poor diet and obesity also contributing.

A genetic predisposition towards a malfunctioning of the mood system may, in many cases, be the root cause of depression. As we discussed in the Green Flag section, however, the presence of both positive and negative environmental influences in our lives may hasten or reduce the emergence of depression in our lives. The primary environmental trigger is most likely stress, but poor diet, misuse of alcohol and drugs, and lack of exercise all play an important auxiliary role. As is the case with all diseases, a strong genetic susceptibility means that fewer environmental influences (in this case stress) are required to send the system into difficulty. Where this predisposition is not so strong, a major trigger (or triggers) is needed to start the process.

(A)   GENETIC INFLUENCES

The genes that are present in every cell control the activity of that cell and the brain structure they belong to; the mood departments and cables are no exception to this rule. As previously mentioned, genes form part of a book of instructions, inherited from parents and grandparents, and present from birth.

Exactly what mistakes in this 'book of instructions' result in depression is still the subject of speculation. One gene, called Creb1, has recently been implicated in women from families with a history of recurrent early-onset depression. But in general, depression is polygenetic in nature: that is, many genes are probably involved. For those who are interested, five chromosomes – 4, 5, 11, 18 and 21 – and the X chromosome are under particular scrutiny! Also, environmental influence from the womb to adult life determines how such genes express themselves, complicating the situation further.

People vary in the number of malfunctioning genes they have which predispose them to developing depression (as noted earlier, genetic vulnerability increases when the malfunctioning genes outnumber the protective ones). These malfunctioning genes make the mood system more sensitive to stressful situations. The greater the number of malfunctioning genes, the more likely it is that the Red Flag of depression will present earlier and will have a more chronic course. The smaller the number of malfunctioning genes, the more stress is needed to trigger depression, and the higher the likelihood of fewer episodes of depression occurring. In both cases, however, the same biological malfunctions take place, and the same symptoms manifest themselves. The episodes and symptoms will differ only in terms of severity.

In future, scientists are likely to uncover a complete explanation of the complex blueprint that makes up our brain. This should help to isolate the genes involved in the design of the mood system. Although this may only be science fiction at present, one day it should be possible to generate a 'printout' of our own individual genetic blueprint; this printout will reveal an individual's 'potential genetic risk' of developing this illness. This may lead to various ethical dilemmas, with the increasing invasion of patient rights by large insurance companies and employers to elicit such information posing particular problems. Statutory protections may need to be built in when this day finally arrives.

(B)   THE STRESS TRIGGERS (ENVIRONMENTAL INFLUENCES)

Research has suggested that stress is the most common environmental trigger of a depressive episode. The most likely explanation for this is that the cells of the mood system are pre-programmed (by genes and early environment) to malfunction when subjected to stress. Possible stress triggers include:

1   LOSS

Loss is a potent initiator of stress. Loss of a mother, father, child, partner, close friend, or even a beloved pet can be a very traumatic experience. For most people, their ability to cope and recover (due to a mixture of their genes and upbringing) via the natural grief process is adequate. This involves going through various stages of grief, from denial to anger, realisation and, finally, acceptance.

Those with a genetic predisposition towards problems in their mood system may, in such cases, develop the Red Flag of depression. If the loss is of a particularly powerful nature, however, such as a mother losing her child, or a spouse losing a long-time partner, even those who do not have this genetic predisposition may find their defences overrun. The overwhelming stress response that this type of loss produces internally may be enough to trigger a mood disorder.

Loneliness results from a lack of any fulfilling relationship and can be extremely stressful for some people. It can be just as much a feature of isolated rural areas as large anonymous cities. Loneliness may be one driving force behind the growing epidemic of suicide evident in young men. A key risk period is where a young person leaves the security of their family either to begin their studies at college or to take up a new job away from home. Many become isolated in flats or campuses and may find it hard to forge new relationships. If susceptible to depression, some may become quite down.

Loneliness, if it develops, aggravates depression, as there is no one for the sufferer to confide in, and it acts to confirm their thoughts that no one cares about them – or even should do!

The end of a relationship will result in similar problems. Young people are particularly vulnerable when a relationship breaks down, due to their immature mood system's inability to cope with the situation. Loss of a job will be equally devastating for many people. It lowers self-esteem, and there is often a subsequent drop in mood. This is possible in all age groups, but particularly in those aged between forty-five and sixty years old.

2   CHRONIC STRESS

Modern life is fast-paced, and rarely without its troubles. Pressures that almost all of us experience on a regular basis include those relating to housing, commuting, relationships and finances. The time available for family and relationships is limited and, due to stress, is more likely to involve quarrelling than quality time spent together.

When one or more of the above pressures turns into an impasse, stress can become chronic. An average couple, commuting long distances, trying to cope with childminders and under pressure at work, often struggle to find the time to talk to each other. This lifestyle is in large part a result of excessively high housing prices and the demands of a growing economy. Many couples in this situation feel trapped. If either partner is genetically susceptible to the Red Flag, depression may ensue. Unrealistic self-expectations, as dealt with earlier, are another common stressor. Alcohol, when used to relieve such stress, will accelerate the process.

Bullying, a powerful environmental trigger which can occur at work, at home or at school and can be physical, sexual or emotional in nature, will in very many cases result in chronic stress. The chronic stress, and low self-esteem, it produces can combine, in those who are already at risk, to kick-start a bout of depression. In vulnerable young teenagers, it creates the added risk of potential suicide. In Northern Ireland, many young people have been terrorised by paramilitary groups. This extreme form of bullying has led to many developing depression, and in some tragic cases has resulted in suicide.

3   CHRONIC ILLNESS

Long-term illness can often feel like a prison sentence. The lives of many are plagued by pain and immobility. Parkinson's disease, rheumatoid arthritis, stroke, multiple sclerosis and cancer all create huge strain on a person's ability to cope and thereby increase the likelihood of depression – in addition to their direct biological effects on the mood system. Fifty percent of Parkinson's sufferers develop depression, a fact which is often not recognised. Parkinson's causes depression by damaging parts of the mood system, in particular the dopamine cable.

Another important cause of depression among the elderly is dementia. A substantial number of peopl with dementia will develop depression for biological reasons. Alcoholics and drug addicts will also present on some occasions with depression because these illnesses damage sections of the mood system. Finally, illnesses involving an under-active thyroid or over-active adrenal gland can also lead to the Red Flag.

It is worth mentioning in particular the trauma experienced by those who have gone through the ordeal of surgery, chemotherapy or radiotherapy for cancer, and those who are recovering from cardiac surgery. A good example of the former would be women who have treatment for breast cancer. Many become emotionally and physically exhausted – mainly due to prolonged high glucocortisol levels (which attack all three mood cables), which develop as the body tries to deal with the stress of the various treatments used. If the person is genetically susceptible to depression, he or she is at higher risk of developing depression. In my experience, this is one of the most hidden consequences of the battle fought by women who are recovering from breast cancer. Cancer specialists need to be aware of the role of the mood system in this battle, often describing symptoms like fatigue and low mood as a 'normal response'. In reality, the prolonged glucocortisol barrage often overpowers the mood system, and the symptoms of depression appear. The problem is often missed by both the spouse and the medical team looking after the patient, and as a result the condition often remains untreated. Apart from the distress this causes to the patient, who may already be deeply traumatised, it may reduce the body's ability to prevent a recurrence of the disease.

There is also a well-documented link between heart surgery and the potential to develop depression, for the same reasons. So we end up with the unusual scenario where depression increases the risk of developing coronary heart disease, and the treatment for severe cases of the latter increases the risk of developing the Red Flag. The biological machinery of the mood system and the other parts of the body are indeed intimately interwoven.

Those who care for people suffering from chronic illness – dementia being a typical example – are also living under difficult conditions, and can feel trapped. Over a prolonged period of time, their ability to cope with the situation may deteriorate and result in depression – particularly for elderly spouses. Finally, certain drugs used for other medical illnesses, such as high blood pressure and heart disease, and the long-term use of steroids to treat conditions like rheumatoid arthritis and asthma can themselves put stress on the mood system, leading to depression.

4 CHRONIC ANXIETY

Anxiety (which we will deal with in more detail in the Yellow Flag section) can be a chronic condition, and those who suffer from it are extremely vulnerable to bouts of depression. Sometimes such people, when questioned, may reveal a long history of hidden, underlying anxiety, often going back to their teenage years. This anxiety wears down their biological coping mechanisms, resulting in depression. Some therapists feel that many people with depression, who started with anxiety, end up in a vicious circle of anxiety–depression–anxiety, and so on. Breaking this circle is vital in such cases.

5 SEXUAL IDENTITY

For some people (particularly in the fifteen-to-twenty-five age group), confusion about their sexual identity can be a major source of stress. If people have difficulties in forming and maintaining relationships, they may begin to question their own sexual identity. Homosexuals may experience the following problems:

1   If they are openly gay, they may suffer harassment, bullying and rejection from their families, friends or workmates

2   If they are hiding their sexual orientation from their family, friends and workmates, they feel trapped in a world of deceit and lies, unable to be honest with themselves and others. This can lead to feelings of loneliness and isolation.

The above problems can place a continuous strain on the person's stress system, leaving them vulnerable to depression and suicide.

6 OUR PAST

Our present is forged by our past experiences and decisions, both good and bad. There has been much emphasis on the role that upbringing has on the development of depression. In practice, many people with happy upbringings still go on to develop the Red Flag of depression. Genes and present environmental difficulties are more influential in this group.

A certain percentage of people grow up in particularly difficult situations, and are less able to cope with stress as a result. Members of this group are more likely to develop depression. Such examples include those who:

§ grow up in extreme poverty and neglect

§ experience severe physical, sexual or emotional abuse. This can haunt the victim for a lifetime, unless they receive help and counselling

§ lose a parent at a particularly vulnerable stage of their development

§ grow up in a house where addiction was present

§ lose a sibling to suicide

Apart from the above exceptions, our past is often not as important as the present: it is in the present where most of our stress triggers arise.

7   SEX-HORMONE TRIGGERS

It has been suggested that sex hormones act as a depressive trigger. Hormones such as oestrogen, progesterone and testosterone play a huge role in development from twelve to eighteen. Hormones are also important in pregnancy and the months following the birth of a baby. Although such hormones do not control the mood apparatus, they are able to interfere with it. In the past, this was assumed to be the cause of post-natal depression, but many experts now believe that the stress of the post-natal period itself may be a more likely origin of such depression.

8   ALCOHOL AND SUBSTANCE ABUSE

Addiction is extremely destructive. Those suffering from addiction often end up losing everyone and everything close to them, and for this reason alone it is no surprise that depression is a close comrade of addiction. Once again, the greater the genetic predisposition, the more likely an alcoholic is to slide into a bout of depression.

A great deal of interest is emerging in the strong link between alcohol, in particular, and the Red Flag of depression. Many who start by misusing alcohol to 'numb' the symptoms of low mood end up getting 'hooked' on this substance, which in itself is a depressant. The more they abuse it, the more their mood drops. Others who start with alcohol abuse may later develop secondary depression.

In both cases, it is vital to recognise the depression that is lurking under the stormy seas of alcohol abuse. If this does not happen, then the treatment of both conditions may prove to be an impossible challenge. Those who abuse alcohol or drugs, particularly in their teenage years, may also alter the neurochemistry of their brain, predisposing them to subsequent depression. We will deal with this in more detail in the Purple Flag section.

9   POOR NUTRITION

One rarely-discussed environmental trigger is poor diet. It is widely accepted that poor nutrition (along with a lack of physical exercise) lies at the heart of the current

obesity, diabetic and coronary-heart-disease epidemics. Some experts are now beginning to wonder whether depression should be included in this list.

From early childhood, many children are fed a diet in which many of the important ingredients necessary for the smooth running of the developing brain and body
are sadly lacking. This puts great internal pressure on the mood system in particular. We
need a regular supply of vitamins, essential proteins and fats in our diet to keep it functioning properly. Often, poor dietary habits learned in the home are carried into adulthood, and the vicious circle continues.

Some experts wonder whether poor diet actually causes depression. I prefer to
regard it as an important environmental influence which may, when combined with
other genetic and environmental factors, help trigger a bout of the Red Flag.

Before leaving the causes of the Red Flag, it is important to examine the stress–mood
cycle. The Green Flag/Red Flag models are highly influenced by these stress triggers.
As stated previously, the greater the genetic predisposition for the mood cables and
departments to malfunction, the less stress is required to turn the Green Flag red
(Figure 12).

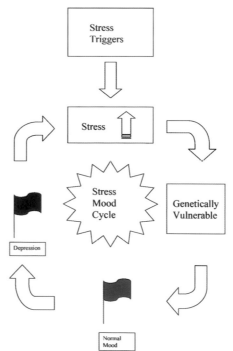

FIGURE 12: THE STRESS MOOD CYCLE

94

IV   SOME COMMONLY ASKED QUESTIONS ABOUT THE RED FLAG
     OF DEPRESSION

So far, we have dealt with what depression is, how it presents itself, and how it is caused. Now let's try and answer some common queries about this condition:

How common is depression?

At least ten to fifteen percent of the population will experience depression at some stage. In Ireland at any one time, 5 percent of men and 10 percent of women will be experiencing a bout of the Red Flag. Women up to the age of thirty are diagnosed with this illness twice as often as men. It is possible, however, that the number of men suffering from this condition is much higher, and that they do not come forward for help.

The true number of people in Ireland suffering from this illness is unknown, but probably lies between 300,000 and 400,000! What concerns many is the frightening reality that probably only 50 to 60 percent of sufferers will seek professional help – and many of these reluctantly. (Prof. Patrick McKeown of Aware estimates that for every four people in Ireland suffering from depression, only two will seek help, and of these, only one will receive adequate treatment.) The rest suffer in pain and silence. The episodic nature of this illness, combined with the confusion created in the media in relation to treatments and the 'stigma' attached to the condition, encourage many to try and 'stick it out'.

The great work being done by Aware in highlighting the issue of mental health, in particular depression, and supporting those who come forward for help should be strongly supported by us all. It is time to break the stigma and misinformation surrounding this illness once and for all.

Of particular concern is the increasing prevalence of depression in young people. Lack of recognition of the symptoms of depression in society is leading to many tragically avoidable deaths. There is a growing concern in Ireland, and indeed worldwide, about the increasing incidence of young males suffering from depression who subsequently go on to take their own lives. The Red Flag is by no means limited to this group, however: depression affects both men and women of all ages.

When does depression appear?

Depression can appear at any stage of a person's life, but often occurs for the first time before the age of thirty, and is more likely following periods of great stress. Twenty-five percent of sufferers will first show signs of the illness during their teens. This group is more likely to become chronically depressed and prone to relapse. Others will develop depression later, either post-natally or in response to stress. The elderly are also vulnerable to depression, although it is often misdiagnosed and dismissed as 'old age'.

How long will a period of depression last?

Most episodes of untreated depression will last between six and twelve months. This may seem like a short period of time, but it is a very long time for the person who is depressed. The brain and the body will desperately try to bring the malfunctioning mood apparatus back into balance before this. Frequently, however, the body's defences are fighting a losing battle with both the illness itself and external stress triggers.

If they are successfully treated, most sufferers will make an early improvement in six weeks, and will experience a remission of most symptoms within eight weeks and full recovery within nine to twelve months.

How often will an individual suffer a bout of depression?

It is estimated that 75 percent of those who suffer from a significant bout of depression will undergo between one and four depressive episodes in their lifetime. In 75 percent of cases, there will be another episode of this illness within five years of the first one.

It is also felt (probably for biological as well as psychological reasons) that each episode makes further ones more likely, particularly if the condition is not treated. These bouts usually occur after a period of immense stress. This is why it is important for people with depression to develop coping mechanisms to deal with stress.

The remaining 25 percent will experience constant bouts of low mood, which will alternate with periods of feeling relatively 'normal'. In this group, the depression is likely to start in the teenage years, and often needs only the most benign of stress triggers to reactivate it.

Why treat depression at all?

This may seem a ridiculously rhetorical question, given what we know of the devastation that depression brings. However, many argue that, if these episodes of low mood are left alone, they will be corrected by the body after six to twelve months, and that therefore there is no need to intervene. Some even argue that depression is a 'normal' life experience.

This solution, although partially correct, is wholly unsatisfactory, because the sufferer is often experiencing intense pain. They feel miserable all the time, cannot remember things, are unable to concentrate enough to read, are constantly tired and anxious, have sleep difficulties, are not eating, have no interest in sex, and cannot derive any pleasure from life. It seems barbaric to suggest that they stay as they are. Such an approach will only confirm in their minds that there is nothing that can be done; in some cases, this makes thoughts of suicide more likely.

The symptoms caused by depression result in mayhem in a person's life. If lifestyle changes, drug therapy or psychotherapy can help to alleviate this emotional pain, there seems to me to be no good reason why the person should be left to suffer alone till it subsides. It has also been shown that each episode can increase the chances of a further episode, particularly if the condition is left untreated.

The second factor that highlights the importance of treating depression is that it sometimes results in suicide. As we have seen, for those who suffer from recurrent bouts of depression, the lifetime suicide rate is 15 percent. Last, but by no means least, depression can cause very serious damage to other organs in the body. Depression, particularly if it is severe, can increase the likelihood of a heart attack by up to five times. This is due to increased levels of glucocortisol; this affects the body's clotting mechanism, making it easier for clotting to occur inside the coronary arteries, eventually blocking them and leading to a heart attack.

Other physical side effects of depression include osteoporosis (thinning of the bones) and an increased risk of infection. There is even the possibility of an increased risk of cancer, as the normal defences which pick up cancer cells in the body may not work as efficiently. Recent research has even linked depression to the later development of Parkinson's disease.

How do I know if I am stressed or depressed?

Stress and depression often present in a similar fashion, due to the overlap of symptoms that exists between them. The stress system (as we saw in the Green Flag section) is intricately interwoven biologically into the mood system, often making the two conditions difficult to separate during diagnosis. Stress also seems to be the catalyst for many of the illnesses which affect the mood system.

The following are the most common warning signs that someone is under prolonged stress:

§ *Fatigue* This is not as extreme as that found in depression, but is usually the first symptom experienced by the person, as they claim to feel 'run down'

§ *Apathy or lack of drive* This is linked to fatigue, as the benefits of a task are outweighed by the effort expended in completing it

§ *Loss of pleasure* Every activity becomes a laborious chore, and it is difficult to relax

§ *Sleep difficulties* Difficulties getting to sleep or staying asleep ('tired but wired')

§ *Anxiety* People who are stressed are more tense, irritable and impulsive

§ *Memory and concentration* These can be impaired by chronic stress

What differentiates stress from depression is the absence of low mood, poor self-esteem, gross negative thinking and suicidal thoughts. The above symptoms of stress are also prevalent in depression, but usually in a more severe form.

Stress symptoms should be a warning to someone that their mood system is getting into trouble. Stress increases levels of glucocortisol, which feed back to damage the behaviour box and mood-control boxes and cables. If prolonged stress continues, particularly in those who are vulnerable to the condition, there is a risk of the mood system breaking down, and full-blown depression emerging. There are also the potential risks of chronic stress detailed in the Green Flag section.

If you are suffering from any of the above symptoms, and feel under major stress, it is advisable to visit your doctor and get help.

Of concern to many is whether strict diagnostic scales (which I have purposefully avoided in this book) should be applied by all family doctors to help them distinguish between stress and depression in their patients. Whilst there is merit in this, I personally am uneasy about rigid assessments in primary care (while being in total agreement with their use in the specialist fields).

I would, however, love to see the availability of personal self-assessment mood and stress questionnaires in all doctor surgeries and possibly in the workplace and in schools, colleges and so on. The person could bring them home and do their own assessment in private. If they felt that they had a problem with either stress or mood, they could then have a chat with their family doctor. For some, this might in itself act as a useful vehicle for expressing how they feel!

Is depression a dietary illness?

Some experts wonder whether a lack of important proteins, fats and vitamins in our daily lives is enough to explain fully the mystery of depression. While I feel that the absence of such things from a person's diet may possibly play a role in the expression and severity of depression, it is highly unlikely that this is the full story: genetic predispositions and other environmental influences play a larger part in this illness. As we have already seen, depression is more to do with structural and functional difficulties within the mood departments and mood circuit. I do feel, however, that diet must play an important part in our journey to recovery from bouts of the Red Flag.

One interesting recent experiment took a group of people recovering from depression who were being treated with modern SSRIs (which, as we will see later, are drugs which boost our serotonin cable) and gave them a diet depleted of a vital vitamin that was necessary to make serotonin. Those who were getting better subsequently relapsed. So clearly, a healthy diet and possibly supplements are vital in the treatment of this illness.

Is depression caused by a chemical imbalance in the brain?

One of the concepts relating to mental health that is most firmly embedded in the mind of the layperson (but which is being increasingly challenged in the media) is that depression is basically caused by a shortage of certain brain chemicals, with serotonin being identified as the main culprit.

In reality, this view of depression is extremely limited. Although a reduction in serotonin, noradrenalin and dopamine play a role in some of the symptoms associated with the illness, this is only part of a much more complex picture. The involvement of the chemical neurotransmitters mentioned above should firstly be seen as having more to do with the mood cables they service than with any individual chemical. It is the malfunctioning of these cables which gives rise to many of the symptoms of depression. The mood cables themselves become dysfunctional, more as a result of difficulties within the departments they serve than because of problems within the two main mood departments.

As noted earlier, the two big mood departments, together with the adrenal gland and glucocortisol, play equally important roles in the onset of depression. Involvement of the former gives rise to many of the physical and psychological symptoms of depression, and the latter explains many of the associated risks of osteoporosis, heart disease and infections.

Also as noted above, the mood cables and boxes, together with the two mood departments, are part of a neural mood circuit, and it is difficulties within this circuit rather than shortages of brain chemicals per se that lies at the heart of this illness. We are also now aware that there are structural difficulties within the mood departments which remain even when depression has been treated and the functioning of the mood circuit has returned to normal. It is most likely these structural deficits which predispose those at risk to further bouts of depression if stress arrives again in their lives.

So depression should be seen as a multifaceted illness rather than as a simple chemical imbalance. It is also important to note that the real underlying cause of this condition lies in the interaction between genetic and environmental (both past and present) factors and the mood system as a whole, which creates the cascade of symptoms seen in this illness.

This distinction is crucial. For example, if a person with depression feels that all their problems are coming from a simple shortage of serotonin over which they have no control, they may feel that they have no role to play in the management of their own illness. In practice, nothing should be further from the truth.

Depression, like most biological conditions, requires the person to be very much involved in all aspects of their treatment, whether that be in the areas of diet, exercise, counselling, drug therapy or CBT (cognitive behaviour therapy, which, as we will see later, is a psychological therapy aimed at reducing negative thoughts and anxiety in depression), and other psychological therapies.

Another problem with this erroneous view of the Red Flag is that it suggests that only drugs which elevate brain chemicals can solve the problem! We now know that psychological therapies like CBT work more on the frontal mood department than directly on chemical neurotransmitters. In fact, both therapies work on the neural mood circuit, with CBT working from the top down, and drugs from the brain stem up, via the mood cables.

Some feel that the emphasis on chemical imbalance has led to an over-emphasis on the importance of drug therapy. Although this has an extremely important place in the treatment of depression, so too do all the other therapies discussed above. Psychotherapists in particular argue, with some justification, that this preoccupation with chemical imbalances has stopped some people from getting the psychological help they may require.

Is depression an inflammatory illness (i.e. an attack by the body's immune system)?

Depression is seen by many researchers as having many similarities to heart disease, and numerous other common illnesses. The common denominator in many illnesses, including multiple sclerosis, rheumatoid arthritis and coronary heart, is clear evidence that the body's immune system is attacking its own structures. Because of this, a great deal of interest is being generated in the possibility that something similar might be going on in depression.

In favour of this theory is the presence of inflammatory markers (called cytokinines) in close proximity to the structures involved in depression. Other indicators are the evidence of excess activity of the stress system, the increased presence of inflammatory markers in the blood of some people with this illness, and, in some cases of depression, an unexplained reduction in the number of glial support cells in various parts of the frontal mood department.

One could ask whether this is evidence of the body attacking itself. For the time being, we can only speculate that the link between stress in our lives and problems within our mood system is probably mediated through the body's stress system. The final answer to this question lies in the future.

Is depression a physical, psychological or biological illness, or a combination of all three?

A common statement made by many laypeople is that depression is a mental or psychological illness alone. This denies the possibility that it may also have a physical or biological basis. So what is the true situation?

In support of the physical-illness argument, it is clear that symptoms such as fatigue, sleep, appetite and drive difficulties, problems with memory and concentration, and increased risks of heart disease and osteoporosis all have a physical basis. The obvious fact that the brain itself is a physical organ and that, as we have already seen, it plays a key role in depression also supports the view that this illness has a physical basis. The presence of structural and functional changes in various parts of the mood system also supports this supposition. Supporting the psychological (i.e. of the mind) basis of depression are the symptoms of low mood, anxiety, poor self-esteem, negative thinking, reduced enjoyment of life, and suicidal thoughts.

As both the physical and psychological symptoms mentioned above have a biological basis, it becomes clear that this illness is due to a combination of all the above. This is crucial in our understanding of the Red Flag. If all of us could grasp this reality, the stigma associated with depression would quickly become ancient history!

Is there a unified theory of the cause of depression?

Albert Einstein spent his life trying to develop a unified theory of all the laws of physics. So far, like Einstein, those working in the field of mental health have failed to bring together all the genetic, chemical, biological, hormonal and environmental influences into one cohesive model. Each group researching the area stakes a claim to the truth – whether it is the psychologist, the psychiatrist, the geneticist, the neurobiologist, the psychotherapist or the nutritionist! In practice, all are helping to provide parts of the jigsaw puzzle. It is useful, however, to put together what we know to date.

It seems likely that most people who develop depression have a genetic potential to develop this illness. This may involve various genes which, apart from having a key role in the development of our personality, also control or retard the following:

§ The manufacture of the crucial neurotransmitters dopamine, noradrenalin and serotonin, and their receptors

§ The healthy development of the mood system, particularly the development of the neurons, and in particular of glial support cells in various parts of the pre-frontal cortex behaviour box and the stress box. The latter may turn out to be the key to this illness.

§ The response of the mood departments (particularly the behaviour, stress and memory boxes) to stress

§ The likelihood of the body's defence system inadvertently attacking the glial support cells

From birth to twenty-five, the expression of these genes is dependent in varying degrees on the environmental influences the person experiences. This is where the psychologist comes in to flesh out many of the potential negative or positive factors, including family upbringing, abuse and addiction. Such influences may affect a person's capability of handling future stresses in life. This is probably mediated through the genes, as discussed above.

In terms of biology, all of the above may create initial structural changes within the mood departments, usually due to a decrease in glial support cells and connections between neurons. This may create a potential for the future functional disruption of the mood circuits when they are exposed to stress.

Whether depression will appear or not in the teenager and adult then becomes dependent on other environmental factors, such as the stresses of life:

§ The difficulties of developing from a teenager to a young adult physically, sexually, emotionally and financially

§ The difficulties of moving from the security of home to the isolation of college or working away from home

§ The joy and pain of relationships

§ Learning to cope with loss, particularly of those close to us

§ Learning to cope with all the stresses of modern civilisation, from commuting to work difficulties, exam pressures, the arrival of a new baby, relationship breakdowns, and so on

§ Learning to cope with loss of a job or severe illness

What is important is that what might seem to be a stress to one person may be seen as a challenge to another, depending on their personality. People who are more anxious or perfectionist by nature seem to be more at risk of depression. It is also worth noting that, in some cases, genetic influences are so strong that it may take only a small amount of stress to trigger an attack. If we add in some other environmental influences, like diet, alcohol and drugs, and exercise, the picture becomes more complete.

The role of nutrition may be more important than researchers originally thought. Suppose that one of the genetic predispositions is to under-manufacture serotonin or dopamine; in this case, a diet lacking in the protein building blocks of these transmitters, and in key vitamins involved in the process, will certainly not help. Maybe this potential weakness is only exposed when the person begins to suffer from a bout of prolonged stress. If the nutritional state of the person was better. the appearance of the symptoms might possibly be delayed, or even in some cases avoided.

So, too, essential fatty acids like Omega 3s are frequently missing in our diet. As these are important for running repairs to the mood system's neurons, a lack of these substances from the diet may help to speed up the appearance of a potential bout of depression. A well-nourished brain cannot but benefit our general mental heath. Only research, however, can confirm or deny the importance of diet in the maintenance of good mental health and the prevention of mental illness.

Lack of physical exercise is another negative environmental influence. Our brain, and in particular our mood system, craves the buzz that exercise brings. If we are not fulfilling this need, maybe we are making the arrival of latent depression more likely. Could this, along with poor diet and alcohol misuse, be the reason why we are seeing such an epidemic of depression in the under-thirty age group?

Lastly, the misuse and abuse of alcohol, and of illegal drugs like cocaine and marijuana (in all age groups, but particularly among the under-twenty-fives, where the mood system is only maturing) is another environmental influence that has a strongly negative impact. These substances exert pressure on the mood system, encouraging the appearance of latent depression and worsening episodes of active depression.

We will be dealing later with the arrival of depression in the elderly, where a different set of factors (particularly a reduction in blood supplies to vital parts of the mood system combined with a natural reduction in the neurons supplying our mood cables) becomes involved.

The key to all of the factors discussed above is that they end up disrupting the neural mood circuit: this seems to be the final common pathway in this illness. So we can see that the arrival (or not) of depression in our lives depends on many different but intermingled factors – genetic, biological, social, nutritional and psychological – coming together. It will take many years of research before we know the whole story!

V   TREATMENT OF THE RED FLAG OF DEPRESSION

One of the most ingrained beliefs held by those with depression (particularly if it is severe) is that nothing can be done to help them and that they are likely to remain in this state indefinitely. The basis for this belief lies in the symptom of negative thinking that is so common in this illness. They come to believe that depression is part of who they are. These beliefs allow the illness to worsen, as the sufferer is reluctant to come forward for treatment; even when they do, they doubt that they will ever feel well again.

A person with depression must first of all grasp the fact that their family doctor, specialist or therapist wants to help them. If they develop this trust, they are already on the road to recovery. Doctors and those close to the person must make a special effort to empathise with and listen to them. This provides a safe and supportive environment that allows them to talk about their illness – which is the first step to recovery.

Because depression is a disease, like diabetes and coronary heart disease, for example, common sense dictates that all forms of treatment that act on the illness have an effect on the body's physiology. Many illnesses are managed with a combination of diet, exercise, drug treatment and counselling, and depression is no different.

These are the treatment options that are available for treating depression:

1   EXERCISE

The first, and most basic, treatment recommended to those with depression is simply to spend thirty to sixty minutes each day exercising. This alone has a hugely beneficial affect on depression by increasing levels of both dopamine and endorphins in the brain; this eases stress, lifts mood and improves the functioning of the memory box.

Many with this illness find themselves in a catch-22 situation when advised of this treatment. The symptoms the treatment will cure prohibit the treatment itself. They are suffering from fatigue, which makes it difficult for them to do anything which requires effort. They are also suffering from a lack of motivation, and do not want to do any exercise. They must overcome these stumbling blocks, however, as exercise elevates mood, improves the sleep and appetite disturbances associated with depression, and increases energy levels, memory and concentration. They should choose an activity that suits their lifestyle. Any form of exercise – be it walking, swimming, dancing, tennis or football – will provide similar benefits.

2   DIET

Another catch-22 situation in which someone with depression may find themselves in is poor diet. A healthy diet is important in the prevention and treatment of depression. In some cases, poor diet may have been one of the environmental factors triggering an attack. In many cases during an episode of depression, those with the Red Flag will lose interest in food. This in turn leads to the mood system running short of vital nutrients, with the risk that the depression may worsen. A good diet rich in essential proteins, fats and slow-release carbohydrates, along with B and C vitamins, fits the bill. This helps the mood system to recover and repair itself. Regular meals of fresh meat, fish, vegetables, grains, nuts and fruit will usually supply most of the above list.

It is also advisable to reduce the intake of caffeine and other drinks that have a stimulant effect. Caffeine produces an immediate yet artificial energy – which is desirable for those who are suffering from unrelenting fatigue. It stimulates the stress box, increasing alertness but also anxiety, and leads to a drop in mood when the effects of the drug have worn off. It also interferes with sleep patterns – which may already be disturbed.

Research has revealed the importance of fish in particular in our diet. Fish oils, which are present in fish like mackerel, salmon, tuna, herring and sardines, help to build, maintain and repair the mood system.

3   SUPPLEMENTS

Alongside a healthy diet, it is advisable that people with low mood take vitamin supplements (especially of vitamin C and the B vitamins) to ensure complete nutrition. Other supplements that are helpful as part of a treatment plan include Omega 3 fish oils. These help the neurons and mood cables to function.

The general consensus is that all adults need around 500 milligrammes of EPA (Eicosapentaenoic Acid) in particular for normal brain health, but that those with illnesses like depression may need up to 1 gramme of it. This can be provided by two to three portions of oily fish, but in my experience many people who are already struggling with a lack of interest in food will be unable to reach this target. I personally recommend supplements in such cases.

This is particularly important if the diet of the person with depression has been very poor, as is often the case. Several studies have shown that patients taking these supplements experience a reduction in anxiety, sleep difficulties and suicidal thoughts.

Fish oils work in a similar way to many antidepressants. Sections of the mood department reduce in size during severe depression. This is in part due to decline in the number of connections between neurons. Brain scans have shown that the essential fatty acids found in fish oils encourage the re-growth of these connections. This effect has been displayed in depression, bipolar depression and schizophrenia. Fish oils have also been shown to exhibit anti-inflammatory properties, and this may also be of relevance to depression.

For the initial management of depression, some experts recommend a starting dose of 1 to 2 grammes of Omega 3 oils containing a high EPA content, with 500 milligrammes to 1 gramme being adequate as a continuous daily dose. Some may prefer to take these oils in the form of seeds (sesame or sunflower) or seed oils. They must be used with caution if the person is on anticoagulants. You should always check first with your family doctor if taking these oils in large quantities.

The importance of these oils is questioned by some experts, and we probably need much more research in order to prove that they have an important effect in combating depression. My own opinion is that there is insufficient proof that they are enough on their own to treat this illness, but it makes sense at least to replace the basic daily requirement of 500 milligrammes of EPA necessary for the running of the adult brain. I therefore always recommend them as part of an overall package of treatment.

Some experts have also looked at the role of essential amino-acid supplements in the treatment of depression. Amino acids are produced as a byproduct when the body breaks down the proteins we consume. These acids are transported through the blood to all parts of the body, including the brain. Many of the key neurotransmitters are derived from amino acids.

A good example is a neurotransmitter called tyrosine. In the neuron, it is broken down to form dopamine and subsequently noradrenalin. It makes sense that a good supply of this essential amino acid (as of many other amino acids) will help us to manufacture the extra amounts of EPA we need if we are suffering from depression.

A detailed discussion of this whole area is not possible in this book, and I would recommend Patrick Holford's interesting book on the subject (see Bibliography).

Certain neurotransmitters (e.g. dopamine, serotonin and noradrenalin) are manufactured with the help of B vitamins. These vitamins have many other important functions in the brain and mood system, so it is wise to keep their level high, especially when the person's mood is down. (A B-complex supplement, a daily combination of all the B vitamins needed by the body, is recommended.

If it can be shown that a person with depression has a healthy diet, there may be no need to add such vitamins, but in my experience this is not usually the case; I often suggest that these vitamins be added to the person's diet in the form of supplements. Finally, it is important to note that supplements like the ones dealt with above can never replace a healthy diet, but they are useful as an adjunct to help the body's defences, particularly in combating depression.

4   COUNSELLING

The simple act of talking about one's depression helps ease the emotional pain associated with the condition. Some people with this illness may have experienced abuse, bereavement, addiction and stormy relationships in their past. They may also have difficulties coping with stress, which may be domestic or work-related.

The aim of counselling is to help the person identify their problem areas and to look at possible solutions that will help them cope. Counselling can be non-directive, where the person is encouraged to articulate their problems and work through them, with minimal interference from the counsellor. It may also be confrontational, either on a personal or group level. This is particularly effective in dealing with addiction. Reality therapy targets the specific areas that are causing difficulty and concentrates on specific methods for dealing with them. This approach is used by family doctors on a daily basis.

All these forms of counselling have their value. When carried out by professionally trained counsellors, they are of great assistance. Counselling should be the first choice for those who are suffering from stress and initial mild depression where obvious stress triggers are present. I do worry, however, about the proliferation of 'counsellors' with little formal training around the country, and feel that it is very important that the proper supervisory structures are in place, to ensure that people in trouble receive help from properly trained personnel.

How can counselling help fight depression? It probably works biologically in a similar way to psychotherapy – by activating the logical behaviour box, which in turn calms down the emotional stress box. In mild cases of depression, this may be sufficient to improve the mood-circuit dysfunction and lift mood.

In moderate to severe cases of depression, the role of counselling becomes complementary to the use of drug therapy. This approach may prove more successful if it takes place four to six weeks after the person has started drug treatment, as he or she will then feel well enough to talk about their problems.

5 PSYCHOLOGICAL TREATMENTS

There is often confusion between the role of the counsellor and that of the psychologist. The counsellor helps a person to deal with life's problems; the psychologist changes a person's dysfunctional thought processes and uses the individual's self-perception to modify their behaviour and help transform negative thoughts into positive ones.

There are many ways in which the psychologist can help when a person's mood system is in trouble:

(A) RELAXATION THERAPY

Exercises to calm the mind and body can help a person to become more relaxed and peaceful within, reducing the over-activity of their stress system and thereby easing the pressure on the body's mood system. This is particularly effective in anxiety disorders, and in depression with associated anxiety.

(B) PSYCHOTHERAPY

There are a number of forms of psychotherapy that are commonly used in treating depression:

1   *Psychoanalysis*, the oldest type of psychotherapy, works on the principle that the source of the person's depression may in some cases lie buried deep in their unconscious. This usually involves unresolved conflicts from childhood. Sometimes these conflicts may relate back to periods of physical or sexual abuse, or other very traumatic experiences. By bringing these back to the surface, the person can deal with them explicitly, and this in turn will eliminate their depression by neutralising the cause.

Although this form of (usually non-directional) therapy has its place, it has generally fallen out of favour. There are many potential dangers in opening up peoples past lives to such an extent, and this approach has been shown to be less effective than the other psychological therapies mentioned below.

2   *'Interpersonal therapy' (IPT)* This form of psychotherapy, which has proved to be of great help to many, is based on the concept that those suffering from depression may be experiencing difficulties with key relationships from either the past or, more often, the present. This can be a catch-22 situation, where depression itself

can cause difficulties in important relationships, often due to lack of understanding of the condition, and the stress of such conflicts may exacerbate the depression itself.

It has been shown that helping a person to learn new ways of handling such relationships, and in some cases to come to terms with previous relationships, can help to lift mood. This approach is used daily by GPs, but more formal work with a psychologist may be necessary. In the case of the latter, a set number (generally between ten and fifteen) of directed sessions is the ideal.

Biologically, IPT probably works by putting the frontal behaviour box (the thinking part of the mood system) back in control over the stress box, where most of the negative memories reside. Recent neuro-imaging studies suggest that IPT and CBT stimulate the same brain areas.

This form of therapy, when utilised properly, reduces the risk of future episodes of depression. It will not suit, and may not be necessary for, everyone, however.

3   *Cognitive Behaviour Therapy (CBT)* This is currently the most popular choice for treating depression, anxiety and addiction. The theory behind CBT is based on the concept that, over time, many people with anxiety and depression develop persistent negative thoughts, and that this in turn leads to destructive behaviour patterns.

In CBT, the psychologist or therapist highlights the negative and dysfunctional thoughts the person experiences (with concomitant negative behaviour patterns) when feeling depressed or anxious. By challenging these erroneous attitudes and explanations, and rationalising them, the person's thoughts (and behaviour) become more logical and positive.

This technique owes much to the pioneering work of Aaron Beck, whose book on the subject (see Bibliography) was a major breakthrough in how to deal with the negative thinking associated with depression. He noted that, while many people with depression who were treated with drugs improved in relation to their physical symptoms, they continued to struggle with the psychological symptoms. In particular, their view of themselves, their present and the future was overshadowed by a black cloud of negative thought and perceptions. Beck felt that this barrage of negative thoughts fostered and maintained the person's depression.

Beck worked out a system of training therapists to work with people whose thoughts had been distorted by the Red Flag of depression. The end result in many cases was an improvement in the thinking and behaviour of those who worked with such counsellors. This concept was also found to be of help in challenging the hopelessness found in those at higher risk of suicide. It has proved to be a very useful tool in the treatment of depression.

Another parallel form of CBT was created by the psychologist Albert Ellis. This was called Rational Emotional Behaviour Therapy (REBT), and in many ways it superseded Beck's approach. Instead of challenging the erroneous negative thought, this form of therapy encouraged the person to look at the emotions these thoughts evoked. This in turn helped them to alter their behaviour.

The best way to explain the difference between the two approaches is to examine the following example. Imagine that Peter, on his way home from work, is passed by a friend, John, who is late, and is rushing home to attend a birthday party for his partner, Mary. Under normal circumstances, Peter would chuckle to himself 'I must pull John's leg at a later date that he is either too busy, or too much in love, to notice his friends.'

But let's assume that Peter is suffering from the Red Flag of depression. His reaction to the same event produces the following response: 'John just ignored me on purpose. He obviously feels that I am not worth stopping to talk to. I must be a boring, useless person if that is the case.'

He then goes home, where the negative thoughts run riot. 'I must really be an awful person if even close friends avoid me. I must avoid John in future, as this encounter made me feel so bad. But maybe John is right and I am really not worth spending time with. The world would be a better place without me.'

Beck's approach to the above case would be to encourage Peter to challenge the initial negative thought, the emotions it provoked, and the subsequent conclusions: 'Did John really choose to pass you by or is that just your perception? What emotions did the event provoke? Were those emotional feelings uncomfortable? Is your decision to avoid John a way of avoiding such emotions?'

Ellis's approach would be to encourage Peter to examine why this encounter bothered him at all. He would help him to rationalise his emotional responses to the situation: 'Why does it bother you at whether John stopped to talk? How and why did you feel so upset that John didn't notice you? Are you really such an awful person as you think you are? Can you give concrete examples to prove conclusively that you are so awful? Is the root of the problem that you don't fully accept yourself unconditionally as a human person without demanding impossible standards from yourself? Once you accept the latter, it won't matter whether or not John bothers to greet you in the street.'

By rationalising Peter's responses to the event, this approach challenges him to alter both his behaviour and his future interpretation of similar situations. The REBT approach (the core of which is unconditional self acceptance) would also help him to understand the difference between the logical and the emotional brain.

Both approaches are extremely useful in many cases, with the latter more commonly being used to treat depression and anxiety, and the former to treat panic attacks.

A recent adjunct to the above CBT therapies, which have been the mainstay of therapeutic approaches to depression for more than thirty years is dialectical behaviour therapy (DBT). This was created by the American psychologist Marsha Linehan as an approach to dealing with people with borderline personality disorders (which we will deal with later in the White Flag section) who were involved in self-harm behaviour. Over the last ten years, this approach is being increasingly used to treat a number of other illnesses, such as addiction and depression.

The core of this form of therapy is the recognition that some patients are so distressed that the usual forms of CBT are not going to be effective unless the distress is both accepted and dealt with first. DBT is often associated with the term 'mindfulness', which is one of the main planks (along with learning new ways of dealing with interpersonal difficulties, coping with life's crises and managing distressing emotional states) of this form of therapy.

Mindfulness, developed from Buddhist meditation, involves developing techniques to stay with experiences (both feelings and actions) in the present moment (sometimes called 'self-soothing'). If ever there was a generation that needs to become more aware of the present moment, it is the current one!

This form of therapy is felt to be of particular help to those suffering from mental (and indeed physical) pain. Instead of trying to run away or avoid these moments, those in this state are taught, with the help of meditation and breathing exercises, to absorb and live with them. In Ireland, a key proponent of this approach is Dr Tony Bates, a leading psychologist who is well known for his writings on depression. At the 3TS conference on suicide in 2004, he explained that: 'Mindfulness encourages an attitude of acceptance and kindness towards your experience instead of one of self-criticism. It offers you a way to be with your bodily sensations, your feelings and thoughts without being overwhelmed by them.' He went on to add: 'Mindfulness meditation is essentially about taking time to be in touch with yourself, so you may feel embodied and grounded, instead of disconnected and alienated.' For those who would like to read Tony's beautifully written lecture on this subject, I refer them to the Bibliography.

In the past, most therapists belonged to either the Beck or Ellis (and more recently the Linehan) 'camp' in terms of how they treated patients. Nowadays, most have a much more fluid approach, switching comfortably from one form of CBT to another, depending on the illness and personality of the person.

A useful way of explaining how CBT and IPT work on a physiological level in depression is to return to the concept of the mood system being composed of an emotional (controlled by the limbic mood department) and a rational, controlling department (the frontal mood department). CBT, through its effects on the mood circuit, helps the person utilise their frontal behaviour box (probably by strengthening inter-neuron connections) to overrule the negative and irrational emotional thoughts originating from the limbic system, particularly the stress box. This fosters a sense of control in the person with depression, which is huge step on the road in their recovery and helps them develop effective long-term coping mechanisms. In eliminating negative thinking and low self-esteem, it reduces the relapse rate among those with chronic depression

Some neuro-imaging studies have shown that, in cases where CBT is successful, activity in the behaviour box initially increases but then, as the person improves, reduces. The memory box was shown to become more active. This suggests that a great deal of intensive cognitive activity occurs as the patient tries to address their negative thoughts. The memory box works harder to consolidate the memories of these cognitive changes. As the person improves, they don't have to use their logical behaviour box as much, and activity there reduces. This is the opposite of what happens during drug treatment!

Needless to say, given the seriousness of the conditions being dealt with, these therapies should only be carried out by trained professionals (psychologists, psychiatric nurses, counsellors, or family doctors trained in CBT).

It is felt that CBT is best suited to those with mild to moderate depression, those who do not want or are unable to take drug therapy, those who are prepared to become fully involved in their own treatment, those with a history of recurrent bouts of depression (to try and reduce relapses), and those who are combating suicidal and impulsive thoughts.

The disadvantage of CBT is the amount of time it can take to produce lasting changes in the mood system compared to drug treatment. It is also not available to most patients in Ireland, due to the great shortage of psychologists and trained CBT therapists within the public-health system, and the high cost of treatment within the private sector. It also involves a time (and motivation) commitment from the patient which is often not possible. Without the latter, CBT will be doomed to failure.

While some GPs (with the help of dedicated Irish College of General Practice CBT tutor Enda Murphy) are starting to study and apply CBT, it can be difficult for them to find the time in a busy practice to deal with the large number of patients who require it. The system needs more therapists who are trained in this area. This would reduce the need for drug therapy, speed up the treatment of depression, and reduce relapses.

The advantages of CBT are the absence of the side effects that are associated with drug treatment, the practicality of the approach in dealing with the person's present state rather than an in-depth analysis of the past (with the former often being more acceptable to patients), its effectiveness in reducing relapse rates of depression, and the clearly defined nature of the course of treatment.

My personal opinion is that CBT concepts would be of use to many with depression and that we need to look at new ways of reaching these people. I feel from experience that a combination of drug therapy and CBT is the ideal approach, as it tackles the mood-circuit dysfunctions at two different levels in the brain and both speeds up recovery and reduces relapses. In the absence of proper health funding, the best way to achieve this ideal may be through a combination of training GPs and possibly working through self-help groups.

4   *Other psychological therapies* There are a number of other approaches that have also been found to be helpful. Of these, 'problem-solving' is one of the most useful. Problem-solving has been shown to be a major difficulty for many with depression, and in particular is very common amongst those who self-harm. Improving these skills has been shown greatly to assist those with the Red Flag and to be a valuable preventative measure in those identified as being at risk of suicide. As always, getting such help (apart from useful advice from the more experienced family doctor) is the problem.

6   DRUG TREATMENT

The most common – and most controversial – form of treatment for depression involves medication. Some maintain that antidepressants are simply placebos, and work by tricking the mind into believing it is getting better. Others compare their use to that of taking paracetamol for a headache: it deals with the symptoms but not the causes. Some believe that they are addictive. Users of antidepressants often complain that the drugs make them feel numb, eliminating some of the symptoms of depression but also leaving them unable to experience happiness. Another common argument against the drugs is that they are having no discernible impact on suicide rates, and that in some cases they may be increasing the risks of a suicidal act.

With such controversy surrounding their use, should these drugs be prescribed at all? Most experts would reply that they are simply one of a number of useful tools available in the management of this illness. Many of the actual users of these drugs (who should know better than anyone!) value antidepressants, but also understand the limits of these drugs. They are not a miracle cure on their own, but they do often enable the person to function and, when used with the above therapies, frequently yield positive results. They do have their disadvantages, but their ability to help a person 'get back to normal' is often invaluable.

Interesting trials have been carried out to compare and contrast psychological (CBT) and drug therapies, using them both individually and together. These trials have shown that both forms of treatment offer advantages and disadvantages. Drug treatment was shown to work faster but, after four months, both approaches were shown to be effective. On finishing individual courses of both, those that had used CBT, in particular, seemed to have a lower relapse rate.

The conclusion was that the use of both, in many cases, maximised the patient's chances of recovery. This view is shared by many modern CBT therapists and is supported by the neuro-imaging data. If symptoms like fatigue and concentration are improved, it is easier for the latter to help the person to change their negative thoughts and behaviour.

In chronic depression, CBT should be utilised to reduce the need for long-term drug treatment. In severe depression, it is often necessary to combine drug treatment with CBT to keep the person well.

How do antidepressants work?

All current prescribed antidepressant drugs operate in a similar manner. Neurons communicate by releasing chemical messengers (neurotransmitters) into the gaps (synapses) between the adjoining cells (see the Green Flag). These messengers cross the gap, activate receptors in the adjacent cell, and are then re-absorbed back into the original cell. Much of what we think, feel and do is partially mediated by these neurotransmitters.

Low levels of serotonin, noradrenalin and dopamine have been implicated in depression. Scientists discovered that drugs which blocked the absorption of these transmitters back into the original cell increased these low levels, and subsequently helped alleviate the depression. They also found that drugs that affected the re-uptake of serotonin and noradrenalin were the most effective.

What has baffled researchers since then is that, although these drugs initially increased the levels of these neurotransmitters in the synapses, within twenty-four hours this effect seemed to stop, and relieving the symptoms of depression then took between two and four weeks. This latter delay suggested that other mechanisms had to be involved. A great deal of research has been done to try to clarify this process, and we still do not know the full story. Here, however, are the possible explanations that have been put forward:

§   Antidepressants block the re-uptake of the serotonin/noradrenalin back into the neuron which released them in the first place.

§   The level of the neurotransmitter tries to rise, but is initially held in check by a normal feedback mechanism which stops this neuron from releasing more into the synapse.

§   This delay lasts about two weeks, but eventually the feedback mechanism weakens and levels of the neurotransmitter increase.

§   The gradual rise in the neurotransmitter within the synapse then instructs serotonin/noradrenalin receptors to pass information into the nucleus of the cells, where the DNA/genes reside.

§   The DNA/genes then issue instructions to encourage neurons to re-grow connections between them. This is particularly beneficial in depression, because it repairs the behaviour and memory boxes. The most likely mechanism for this is encouraging the manufacture of a crucial enzyme within the neuron called BDNF, which encouragesthe neuron to improve its connections with other neurons. This effect is probably mediated through the neurotransmitter glutamate.

§   The DNA/genes also alters receptor function and other key neuron activities.

§   The final result is that the neurons of the mood system are now interacting much more efficiently, and the mood cables and departments start to function better.

§   It is also likely that the growth of new connections takes much longer to consolidate, which may explain why those who stop treatment before this process is completed are more likely to relapse.

§   In this scenario, a neuron would need at least two to four weeks to begin these alterations, and much longer to 'bed in' these changes.

What happens within the mood system when these drugs are taken?

The most likely sequence is as follows:

§   The mood cables (serotonin/noradrenalin cables in particular) are stimulated, initially (within two weeks) by the increased amounts of noradrenalin and serotonin that have become available within synapses. When these cables activate, they calm down the stress box and Area 25, leading to many of the symptoms of depression – such as fatigue, lack of concentration, and eating/sleeping disturbances – gradually disappearing.

§   The mood departments (particularly the frontal behaviour box) start to heal, at a gradual rate, due to neuronal changes directly caused by the antidepressant, and stimulation of the mood cables/circuit. This leads to an increase in positive thinking, self-esteem and memory, and a reduction in suicidal impulses and anxiety.

§   The above changes help to calm the stress box further, and this box sends messengers to the adrenal glands instructing them to produce less glucocortisol. When the normal daytime and nighttime levels of glucocortisol are restored, blood platelets, bones and the immune system start to recover. This reduces the risk of heart disease, osteoporosis and infection.

§   The vicious biological circle of the Red Flag is reversed, and the Green Flag reappears.

It is also worth examining what happens with regard to neuroimaging when this process occurs. The key findings are: an increase in activity of the mood control boxes/cables, a reduction in activity of the stress box, a dampening down of activity in Area 25, a gradual rise in activity of some key sections of the behaviour box (and a reduction in others), and an increase in activity in the memory box .

An interesting way of comparing the neurobiological effects of both drug therapy and CBT is to regard the former as working from the bottom of the brain upwards, and the latter from the top downwards (see Figure 13). Because the two mood departments are, as we have seen, really part of a two-way loop/neural mood circuit, both therapies often end up with similar results. This is the beauty of understanding the flag model of the mood system. It also suggests that combining both may be the ideal way of treating this illness.

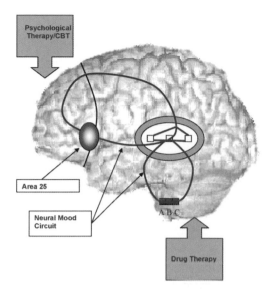

A   Serotonin control box

B   Noradrenalin control box

C   Dopamine control box

FIGURE 13: MECHANISMS OF ACTION OF PSYCHOLOGICAL AND DRUG THERAPY ON THE MOOD CIRCUIT IN DEPRESSION

It is also interesting to reflect on the reasons why there is a difference in the speed at which drug therapy lifts many of the symptoms of depression when compared with CBT and interpersonal therapy. The former acts initially on the mood cable/boxes and, through them, on the stress box. Since, as we have already discussed, many of the vegetative symptoms, such as fatigue and problems relating to sleep, appetite, mood, concentration, drive and so on stem from problems within these cables, it makes sense that a therapy that activates them leads to an early lifting of these negative effects.

It has also been shown that Area 25 normalises much faster with this form of therapy. The effect of drug therapy on psychological symptomsof depression, like negative thinking, comes later. This is due to the normalising of the mood circuit finally improving these symptoms.

In comparison, CBT/IPT works by activating the logical behaviour box. This in turn begins slowly to calm down the circuits leading to the stress box and, by gradually normalising them, leads to a secondary improvement in the vegetative symptoms noted above. This takes much longer. People with symptoms like fatigue and poor concentration often find it difficult to engage with this form of therapy.

TYPES OF ANTIDEPRESSANTS

Antidepressants can be separated into two groups, old and new:

I   OLDER ANTIDEPRESSANTS

These drugs, which were introduced in the 1950s, revolutionised the treatment of depression. The most renowned group are the tricyclics, so called because there are three circles within their chemical structure. They act primarily on the serotonin, dopamine and noradrenalin mood cables.

They prove effective in most cases of depression but can have undesirable side-effects, including sedation, dry mouth, blurred vision, difficulty passing urine, and impotence. Furthermore, some are extremely toxic, and often fatal, when taken in overdose.

This is obviously a serious problem because, although they are effective in severe depression, the person who is unwell may be suicidal: prescribing them a drug like this in effect gives them a means to kill themselves. Side effects like sedation can often simply replace the depressive symptoms, making it difficult for them to function normally. Many have to stop taking these drugs due to the side effects, despite the fact that the medication is working. Nevertheless, they were the drug of choice for decades in treating depression, and have cured millions of patients. To this day, I have patients who respond much better to these older drugs than to more modern ones – although this is the exception.

Two common tricyclics are:

1   *Amitriptyline* This is the most well known and most widely prescribed tricyclic. It is extremely effective in restoring the mood system to normal. But sedation, and a very high risk of fatality if taken in overdose, makes it a dangerous drug to prescribe, particularly if suicidal thoughts are present.

2   *Imipramine* This is very similar to amitriptyline but has less of a sedative effect.

A second group of drugs used in the past were called the MAOIs. These drugs worked by blocking the natural breakdown of noradrenalin and dopamine at nerve endings. This build-up of neurotransmitters helped many with depression, but some of these drugs also interacted in the gut with common foodstuffs like cheese, sometimes producing a life-threatening increase in blood pressure. Due to their effect on the dopamine cable, they were particularly useful in improving symptoms of fatigue and loss of pleasure. Their use waned due to the seriousness of the potential serious side effects, however.

II   NEWER ANTIDEPRESSANTS

In 1988, depressive drug treatment was revolutionised with the arrival of SSRIs: selective serotonin re-uptake inhibitors. Their primary target is the serotonin mood cable; most SSRIs also target other mood cables to a lesser extent, with the exception of Citalopram and Escitalopram, which are exclusively selective to the serotonin cable. The first SSRI drug to be released was Prozac. This drug prohibits the re-uptake of serotonin. It demonstrated similar efficacy to tricyclics, but offered two major advantages. Firstly, it is safe in overdose, and secondly it has fewer side effects. The introduction of Prozac was followed by many similar serotonin mood cable antidepressants, which were modified to be more effective. Another major landmark in depressive drug treatment was the development of drugs that specifically prevented the re-uptake of noradrenalin.

It was hoped that these modern groups of drugs would turn out to be the 'miracle cure' for depression. Up to 30 percent of patients do not respond to them, however. They are also not without side effects. Nausea, tremor, anxiety, headaches and sexual dysfunction are commonly reported.

These drugs are not recommended for routine use, without specialist approval, for under-eighteens, as it is thought that, in some cases, they increase the risk of suicide in these individuals.

As a general guide, SSRIs are more useful than older antidepressants in treating mild to moderate depression, with the exception of Lexapro (Escitalopram), which has proven efficacy in the severly depressed. SSRIs are particularly useful if anxiety, sleep and appetite difficulties are present. Drugs that target the noradrenalin cable may be more useful in severe depression, where extreme fatigue and poor drive may be major problems. Despite their fairly numerous disadvantages, these drugs continue to transform the lives of people suffering from depression.

Here are some of the common modern antidepressants in use:

1   *Fluoxetine (Prozac)* This drug has proved a very effective and safe drug in the treatment of depression, anxiety and eating disorders over the past fifteen years. Some find that it has a very positive effect on their outlook on life. This has led to a growing debate (particularly in the USA) as to whether the drug is sometimes being used for the wrong reasons. This drug has been used in the under-eighteen age group usually under the care of a specialist.

2   *Escitalopram (Lexapro)* This drug is the most recent addition to the SSRI group and is different to the other SSRIs as it is a serontonin dual-acting agent, effective in all types of depression. It is now the drug of choice for the treatment of depression and anxiety. It has a favourable side-effect profile, with occasional nausea in the first week, but reduced sexual dysfunction compared to other SSRIs. It is generally fast-acting, well-tolerated, and effective in restoring normal mood and calming anxiety.

3   *Paroxetine (Seroxat)* This drug, which was a follow-up to Prozac, was initially greeted favourably. It then received a great of bad press because of its sexual and withdrawal-related side effects. Severe dizziness and disorientation can occur when the drug is stopped, so care is needed to do this very slowly. Concern has also arisen about its use in younger age groups (where some feel it may lead to an increase in suicidal thoughts), and in pregnant mothers, where it should be avoided.

4   *Venflaxine (Efexor)* Unlike the three previously mentioned drugs, this drug targets both the serotonin cable and (at high doses) the noradrenalin cable. It is effective in treating depression in those with poor drive or motivation. It has similar side effects to the SSRIs in low doses, but sweating, constipation and headaches can be additional problems, particularly in higher doses. Its effects on the noradrenalin system in higher doses also require careful monitoring in the elderly and in those with cardiac problems.

5   *Mirtazapine (Zispin)* This drug also targets the serotonin and noradrenalin cables. It is a very useful medication, but side effects like weight gain can be a problem. It is often used as a second-line drug where sleep difficulties and weight loss are a problem. One of the advantages of this drug is an absence of sexual side effects.

6   *Duloxetine (Cymbalta)* This is a very new drug, similar in type to Effexor. It is claimed that the side-effect profile of this drug, especially concerning sexual dysfunction, is more favourable. It will take some time, however, before this claim can be borne out in clinical practice.

This is only a sample of the many drugs of this type. A list of all these drugs ca be found at the end of the book.

The biggest advancement that these drugs have brought is the ability of the gener al practitioner to treat depression without the need for referral to a specialis Nowadays, only serious or resistant cases need to be referred. This has helped t demystify depression as an illness.

COMPLEMENTARY THERAPIES

Complementary therapies (which accept the relevance of traditional therapies like dru treatment and psychotherapy but hope to assist or complement them) are frequentl favoured over alternative therapies (some of which reject the role of traditional med cine completely and suggest alternative approaches) because they do not encourage the abandonment of conventional medicine completely – a dangerous approach to take when a patient has severe depression or is suicidal. There is much to learn from complementary medicine. Firstly, it takes a holistic view of the person, looking at their body, mind and spirit. Secondly, it provides more weapons in the growing arsenal of treatments for depression. Thirdly, it encourages the person to play an active role in their own treatment and recovery. Finally, it brings in other cultural influences, which can be helpful. Complementary therapy should only take place under the guidance of a trained professional. It should also, in my opinion, be exposed to the same rigorous controls as conventional medicine. Complementary therapies used to treat depression include the following:

I   MASSAGE

Massage is one of the most well-established forms of complementary treatment. The healing power of touch is thought to reduce stress and depression. Various forms of massage are available, including aromatherapy massage (where selected aromatherapy oils are blended together and used in the massage), sports massage and Indian head massage (a massage which concentrates solely on the head and scalp). Massage helps the mood system by calming the stress box, which in turn reduces levels of stress peptides and glucocortisol. Regular massage is often suggested to those suffering from depression as part of their treatment.

II   REFLEXOLOGY

Reflexology is an Eastern therapy based on the concept of energy flow. Certain points on the feet and hands are thought to be connected to various channels of energy that flow through the body. By pressing and massaging these points, energy blockages can be released, and symptoms can be relieved. Some find this treatment effective in releasing stress.

III   RELAXATION EXERCISES

Relaxation exercises include yoga, pilates and meditation. Yoga and pilates combine stretching with the development of correct posture and breathing. Meditation involves deep concentration to clear the mind and block out all distractions. These ancient 'workouts' have a beneficial effect on many areas of the body, and are particularly helpful for calming the stress box. They probably lead to a reduction of stress peptides and glucocortisol. All of these therapies share a similar goal: by surrounding the mind in peace and quiet, the mood system is given time and energy to heal. Some find meditation particularly helpful in managing anxiety, as it teaches the person to eliminate the worries that plague them.

IV   ACUPUNCTURE

This has been used in the East for thousands of years. It is based on the Chinese principle that the whole body is mapped out by invisible energy lines. According to this approach, illnesses such as stress and depression originate when energy lines become blocked. Acupuncture involves using needles on particular energy points around the body, called acupoints. Neuro-imaging studies show decreased activity in the limbic mood system, particularly in the memory and hormone control boxes. Other studies have revealed an increase in activity in the serotonin cable, as well as in the level of brain endorphins, all of which contribute to a lifting of mood.

V   HERBAL TREATMENTS

There is a bewildering array of herbal remedies available for the treatment of anxiety and depression. Naturopaths are trained medical specialists who prescribe herbal treatments as part of a treatment regime. Herbal remedies can be just as effective as prescription drugs but they can also have similar side effects, and should be used with equal caution. It is therefore reasonable to suggest that herbal remedies undergo the same rigorous testing procedures as prescription drugs before being released on to the market. If this was the case, doctors would feel more comfortable about prescribing them.

The most widely known herbal treatment (particularly in Europe) for depression is St John's wort, derived from the plant *Hypericum*. This has mild-to-moderate mood-enhancing properties and mimics the action of SSRI drugs. If taken with SSRIs, the person may experience the serotonin syndrome (a range of unpleasant side effects, such as confusion, agitation, nausea, muscle spasms, difficulties with balance, high blood pressure and, in severe cases, seizures and coma, resulting from too much serotonin in the body). On its own, it seems to be free of many of the side effects associated with the SSRIs. If you are on prescribed medication, you should check with your doctor before taking any herbal remedies.

VI   DAWN SIMULATORS

These are very effective in the treatment of seasonal affective disorder, or SAD, which is discussed further in Chapter 2 below. This device is plugged into a bedroom lamp, and gradually increases the amount of light available before the person wakes up. This tricks the body into believing that it is summertime, and helps the mood system to fight the effects of SAD. This is a good example of the way in which a complementary therapy can be used to treat a mood disorder.

All of the above treatments are available for those with depression. The other more serious forms of intervention, such as psychological and drug therapy, are usually initiated by the family doctor or a specialist.

Each person is individual. What works for one person may not work for another. It is important to remember that all treatments take time, and that patience is vital.

TREATMENT OF DEPRESSION: THE DOCTOR'S DILEMMA

There has been widespread concern regarding the increase in the prescription of anti-depressants in recent years. Such concerns range from depression being over-diagnosed, to the drugs merely working as placebos, to whether or not they have a lasting effect on depression.

Depression affects a large number of people. Experts estimate that, contrary to the concern some have about 'over-diagnosis', many cases in fact go undetected. The Irish College of General Practice often talks about the 'pyramid' of illness. For illnesses like heart disease or diabetes, they feel that only 5 percent of those suffering from such illnesses are seen and treated by a specialist, 40 percent or so are diagnosed and in some cases treated by their family doctor, and the rest remain undiagnosed or are self-medicating. (Of those who are receiving help for mental illnesses, around 85 percent are treated by the family doctor.) If this is so, it is likely that we are not over-diagnosing depression but, rather, missing many cases! If we accept Prof. McKeown's figures of only two out of every four cases coming forward for help, and one in four getting adequate treatment, we still have a lot to do!

Due to the shortage of trained psychologists and suitably qualified CBT therapists in Ireland, psychological treatments are not easily accessible or affordable to many people who are suffering from depression. In these cases, especially when the patient is in great distress, the doctor has no choice but to recommend drug treatment as the first option. Those with moderate to severe depression may have been struggling with crippling symptoms for quite some time before coming for help. They naturally want to get better quickly.

Since referral to a psychologist or therapist within the health-care system can involve a considerable delay (if this option is available at all!), the doctor must prescribe medication to prevent the condition worsening. Where the GP is trained in CBT techniques, this is of help, but time pressures often limit the level of assistance he or she can offer in this area.

Doctors can also provide the patient with a complete array of treatment options. Diet, exercise, supplements, relaxation techniques, and temporary abstinence from alcohol are all practical steps that the person can implement themselves. Counselling can help the person to cope with stress or relationship problems. In many cases of mild depression, this may be all that is required.

Sometimes, as in moderate to severe depression, the person is so low and exhausted that only an antidepressant can bring them up to a functional level, as they may be too tired to try anything else. Medication is not a 'quick fix' and will not magic away life's problems. It is, however, of great help in many cases in reducing the crippling physical and psychological symptoms associated with depression, allowing the person time and space to review all aspects of their lives, including their thinking patterns.

If CBT and other psychological treatments were freely available and the person could afford them, the need for longer periods of drug therapy might be substantially reduced. To ignore completely the benefits of drug therapy would in my opinion be naive and dangerous, however. The ideal situation would be a combination of both, as part of a holistic package. Above all, the person must be allowed to have an input into their own treatment. They must take their lives back into their own hands.

Many doctors would like to have CBT freely available to all suitable patients, not just to those who are able to afford it. Money spent by the Department of Health in this area (in both training therapists and providing easy access to them for all Irish GPs) might swiftly reduce the need in some cases for drug treatment, and actually save money in the long run. It is also worth listening to the CBT therapists themselves, who feel that many patients benefit from drug therapy to start with as it assists them in reaching a functioning level where they can become more actively involved. Otherwise, it can be difficult for the patient to find the energy and motivation necessary for successful CBT therapy.

We would also benefit from money being spent on educating people about the importance of mental health, and the need for proper nutrition and supplements, and exercise. Finally, it might be time for the health authorities to fund self-help groups to investigate the possibility of bringing CBT help to their members.

VI   SOME COMMONLY ASKED QUESTIONS ABOUT THE
        MANAGEMENT OF DEPRESSION

The long-standing ignorance and misconceptions that surround depression has made people reluctant to talk about it. In my experience, these are the most commonly asked questions about depression:

What will happen if I go to see my doctor complaining of symptoms of this illness?

Many who suffer from this illness are often unsure about how to approach their GP and struggle to put into words how they are feeling. They may not attribute their symptoms to depression, and may ask about some other illness instead.

The simplest thing is to tell your GP that you feel down and despondent. You should not be afraid to do this: there is no shame in it. Your doctor will then start to ask you a number of questions relating to fatigue, sleep, memory, mood, anxiety, and thoughts of harming yourself. He or she will probably ask about the medical history of your family.

He may ask questions unrelated to depression, or carry out a blood test, in order to eliminate the possibility of other illnesses. He may inquire about your weekly intake of alcohol. Once he is satisfied that you are suffering from depression, he will go on to discuss the possible causes, and the treatment options that are available to you.

Your diet, exercise, and use of supplements may be discussed. He will probably advise you to reduce or cease your alcohol intake. In the case of recent bereavement or relationship difficulties, counselling may be suggested as the next step. If, however, extreme fatigue, poor concentration, sleeping difficulties, and acts or thoughts of self-harm are evident, the doctor will probably consider drug treatment or psychological therapy.

You may be considered to be a patient who requires urgent referral to a specialist. This is likely if you are suicidal, or if the doctor is unsure about your diagnosis. The doctor or specialist might recommend that you go into hospital for a while so that you can avail of twenty-four-hour care until you feel better. This is particularly the case with patients who are suicidal, as there will be health professionals present to help them deal with suicidal thoughts, and keep an eye on them. However, most people can be successfully treated by their GP.

If your doctor decides on drug treatment, he will probably prescribe you one of the modern SSRIs. He will then review you after four to eight weeks to assess whether the medication has relieved your symptoms. If he deems it necessary, he will increase the dose until a satisfactory response has been obtained. You will probably have to take this medication for six to eight months, to ensure that your illness is properly treated.

When you feel well enough, the GP may, if he feels it appropriate, refer you to a counsellor or psychologist for a course of CBT. If you are reluctant to take antidepressants, or if they have proved ineffective in the past, your doctor may well recommend this method of treatment. Unfortunately, this can depend on the availability of such services. You should feel much better after six to eight weeks of drug treatment, and it is at this point that you need to make the necessary changes in your life to ensure that you remain this way. You may decide to move from a stressful job to a less stressful one, to cut down on your working week, to spend more time relaxing with your family, or to examine your financial situation and organise your spending to minimise stress. You may re-evaluate your weekly intake of alcohol and decide to incorporate regular exercise, a balanced diet, and supplements into your life.

When you reach the end of your course of medication (providing that you feel that you are back to normal), the doctor will slowly wean you off it. He will then advise you to make an appointment to see him immediately if any of the symptoms return.

COMMON QUESTIONS ABOUT PSYCHOLOGICAL TREATMENT

How long does a course of CBT take?

CBT usually involves eight to ten sessions (although sometimes much fewer), working with either a trained psychologist or therapist, or more rarely a psychiatrist who specialises in CBT. Each session lasts for about an hour.

What about the cost and availability of these treatments?

The difficulty with CBT and other psychological treatments is that there is a huge shortage of trained professionals in this area. As a result, there are long waiting lists in the public system. Normally, you will be referred to a psychologist by a psychiatrist. If you cannot afford to pay privately, you could be waiting for a considerable period to see a psychologist. To go through the private system is a costly affair (around €80 to €100 per session), and beyond the financial means of many.

What about psychotherapy?

Sometimes a person with depression, particularly if it is chronic, will not respond to drug treatment or CBT. There may be unresolved childhood difficulties like abuse, violence or addiction. There is a need to return to these painful memories and deal with them before the person can move on. This can be a lengthy and distressing process. We described it earlier as 'psychoanalytical psychotherapy'. Some believe that this is the only way to treat depression. There is no doubt that the physiologies of some people's brains are directly affected by adverse life experiences: in such cases, this form of psychotherapy can be of great help.

Much of the time, however, the depressive trigger does not lie in the person's past, but in an obvious stress trigger in the present. Psychotherapy in this form as a treatment for depression, although extremely useful in some cases, must therefore be put into perspective: some studies suggest that CBT in particular may be more useful as a general psychological tool for the treatment of this illness.

Although there is a great deal of truth in this approach, it ignores the abnormalities present in the brain, often at an early stage of adulthood, of some people with this illness. If depression was purely the result of problems occurring during childhood, or was due to some other unresolved issues or conflicts, one must ask why many people with very traumatic backgrounds do not develop depression, while others with quite peaceful backgrounds do. This view also ignores the effects of our present environment on the genes of the mood system.

Interpersonal psychotherapy (which explores the effects of past and present relationships in the creation and maintenance of depression, and the effects of the latter on present relationships) is a much more useful psychological therapy. For reasons that have already been discussed, relationships can be a problem, both in the present and the past. Improving such dynamics can be of great help. The same problem exists here as with regard to CBT counsellors: a lack of personnel. A recent positive development is a trial that involves providing counsellors to GPs to help with this form of therapy. If this could be extended to all GPs, it would be of great help.

How long before these treatments show results?

Depression is usually alleviated within four months of beginning psychological treatments like CBT/IPT. Drug treatment starts to work faster, usually within two to six weeks, but after the first four months both forms of treatment are equally effective. CBT is effective in reducing the rate of relapse in depression, so the results are in some cases more long-lasting. These treatments, by helping people to change their thinking and behaviour, teach them how to cope with life. Many experts feel that a sensible combination of drug treatment and CBT would be the ideal scenario.

COMMON QUESTIONS ABOUT DRUG TREATMENT

Why should I take drug treatment at all?

Depression is an illness, bouts of which normally last between six and twelve months. Without intervention, the body would eventually repair the damage that has been inflicted on the brain and revert back to normal mood. However, depression can be so distressing and disruptive that restoring normal mood through some form of intervention is the only logical course of action. Secondly, the lifetime risk of suicide can be up to 15 percent in this illness. Thirdly, depression opens the body up to other diseases, such as coronary heart disease and osteoporosis.

Many people are apprehensive about using drug treatment for depression. If drug treatment is used appropriately, however, it is invaluable in relieving the symptoms of depression and allowing the person to function normally. Although these drugs can have some side effects, their short-term benefits usually outweighs these negative aspects.

The primary advantage of drug treatments is that it is the fastest method of relieving the symptoms of depression. The ideal form of treatment involves a mixture of pharmacological and psychological treatments: this gives the person the best of both worlds and maximises their chances of success.

Are antidepressants addictive?

This fear dates back a time when tranquillizers like valium and librium were widely prescribed. These drugs were often used to treat anxiety and were extremely addictive. This stigma spread to all other psychiatric drugs. In reality, whatever about other side effects, antidepressants are generally not considered to be addictive. They simply restore normal mood, and are usually taken for a specific period of time.

Only in a small number of chronic cases will it be necessary for people to take antidepressants for long periods. This does not mean that the person is addicted to them; rather, they function better on them. Upon discontinuing these drugs, users will not experience the cravings associated with withdrawal from an addictive substance.

Most people will simply take the prescribed course of treatment, and withdraw from the medication slowly over a period of time (giving the neurons in the brain time to readjust to the absence of the drugs). Sudden removal of antidepressants will result in symptoms of dizziness and light-headedness. This is often mistaken for evidence of addiction, but clearly this is not the case.

There has been a lot of bad press, with Prozac in particular, concerning addiction. It became an over-prescribed 'wonder drug' in America, and was often used to boost low self-esteem and make people more assertive, rather than being used simply to treat depression. This clouded the issue. In reality, Prozac is not addictive (if the correct parameters of addiction are applied) and is an easy drug to come off, with almost no withdrawal problems.

Many mistake the reappearance of symptoms of depression as a sign that they are addicted to the drug. This causes great confusion amongst those who may need drug treatment but are put off seeking such treatment by a lack of clarity in the media about the use of these drugs.

The antidpressant Seroxat is another example of such media misinformation. It received controversial publicity because when people suddenly stopped taking this drug, they felt extremely dizzy. Many people took this as an indication that the drug is addictive. Once again, although this side effect is a great nuisance, it does not necessarily constitute a symptom of addiction.

Are antidepressants simply placebos?

A placebo is a tablet with no active ingredients, normally given to a person during scientific research into a drug, to test what happens if the person simply 'thinks' they are getting better. The tablet will look identical to the one that is being tested. By comparing this effect with those who have taken the actual drug, researchers can find out if the drug is making any difference. Some maintain that all antidepressants work as placebos by making the person believe they are getting better, and that the brain responds by elevating mood. Many psychoanalytical psychotherapists quote this fact and dismiss such drugs as 'expensive, drug-company-driven products'. I have had to treat some patients who were attending such therapists and whose depression was gradually deteriorating despite such intervention.

Many people hear this argument from a media that is sometimes in thrall to alternative-medicine approaches – 'anything other than drug therapy' – and this can lead to confusion and uncertainty. Let's examine the scientific data. The placebo effect does indeed complicate matters. A certain number of participants in any study, who have taken the placebo, usually report that they get better. We must therefore be cautious in interpreting the results of all drug trials. A percentage of those who 'responded' to the pill (and indeed to all therapies) include those who experienced the placebo effect and those experiencing a placebo and real effect simultaneously. So it is difficult to extrapolate from the results. Moreover, in general, the more severe the depression, the less the placebo effect is likely to be of relevance.

The situation is particularly complicated in the case of depression, as believing that you are going to get better is one of the steps towards recovery. For this reason, the placebo effect may be larger in antidepressants rather than in other drugs, due to positive thinking. However, the fact that drug therapy seems to take effect in many cases by the end of the second month, whereas CBT, which is an excellent psychological therapy, can take up to four months, would suggest that drug therapy is having more than a simple placebo effect. It would also suggest that the placebo effect for CBT works along different neurobiological pathways.

How long does it take for these drugs to work?

It takes two to four weeks for an antidepressant to start relieving the symptoms of depression. Some patients may note an improvement in symptoms such as anxiety after ten to twelve days, but most people will need six to eight weeks of treatment before they feel 'normal' again. When this happens, symptoms such as fatigue, anxiety, forgetfulness, reduced concentration, low self-esteem and low drive are alleviated. The person will have regained a positive outlook on the future.

How long will I have to take these drugs?

For the vast majority of people, courses of treatment will last from six to nine months. The general consensus is that it is advisable to take these drugs for a minimum of six months from the time you feel well. Since this is normally two to three months, the usual recommended period is about six to nine months. After this, the majority of people can be slowly weaned off the antidepressants. This will usually be sufficient, but for about twenty to twenty-five percent of patients, drug treatment may have to continue for longer periods, and may sometimes (usually following specialist advice) be permanent. CBT, along with lifestyle changes and a healthy approach towards alcohol greatly reduces the need for such long-term treatment in this group.

Why does it take six to nine months of treatment?

The body seems to need around six to nine months of treatment to restore its physiology. It is unknown why this is the case. The most likely reason is that it takes a long time for positive internal biological changes to occur in the cells of malfunctioning neurons in the behaviour and memory boxes, and indeed in the whole mood system. After this time, the body's mood system is functionally (if not structurally) healed, and when the person comes off these drugs they will remain well. How long the person remains healthy will depend on how they deal with the stress triggers that caused the depression, learn new ways of challenging negative thoughts, perhaps embrace ideas like mindfulness or yoga, learn to treat alcohol with respect, and improved their diet and exercise routine. A healthy, relaxed, physically fit body, together with a well-nourished brain, are the enemies of depression.

What will happen if I stop taking the antidepressants too quickly?

Patients often stop taking their medication as soon as they feel better. The danger time for this is between two and three months. At this stage, they feel much better, and – usually because they feel 'guilty' about taking the medication, a feeling which is often exacerbated by media hysteria about the use of antidepressants – decide to cease taking them. This is a major mistake, and the person usually does not remain well for long. Such a situation is very frustrating for doctor and patient alike. It is very important when a person starts a course of drug treatment to make a conscious decision to finish the course, regardless of how well they feel after the first two months.

What side effects can I expect?

With the older drugs, sedation, dry mouth and blurred vision are common complaints. With the newer SSRIs, initial nausea (due to initial activation of serotonin receptors in the gut), sweating, tremors of the hands, and heavier periods in the case of females (through their effects on blood platelets) are all commonly reported side effects. (Nausea can be counteracted by taking the over-the-counter medication Motilium.) They often disappear after a while as the body adapts to the medication. By keeping in regular contact with your family doctor, such side effects can be monitored, and adjustments can be made if necessary.

What about sexual side effects?

Many people taking medication for depression suffer from a loss of libido, impotence, and delayed or abnormal orgasm. For some, this may not be a great problem, as they had no sex drive due to their depression anyway. However, after several months of treatment, people will generally start to feel better and will regain their interest in sex. It is then that any sexual side effects caused by these drugs may become an issue. Many people find these side effects so frustrating that they stop their medication. For the following six months of treatment, the following difficulties may be experienced:

(a) *Men may have difficulty producing or sustaining an erection* This can be remedied for the remainder of the course of drugs by supplementing with Viagra or Cialis. Others may experience difficulties with ejaculation. This is more difficult to treat. Some experts suggest ceasing medication at weekends, but there are risks involved, so consult your family doctor first.

(b) *Some women may have difficulty achieving orgasm* This symptom seems to vary from person to person, and some will learn to overcome it with relaxation exercises.

These sexual side effects can occur because the drugs, as well as targeting the serotonin receptors that regulate mood, act on other serotonin receptors in the brain which regulate sexual activity. These problems will disappear within a week of stopping the medication. Upon finding this out, most people will agree to finish the course. The sexual side effects for some are a small price to pay for keeping depression at bay; others cannot tolerate them and stop taking their medication. In the latter cases, CBT should be considered as an alternative, along with the usual lifestyle changes. The hope is that future drug treatments will eliminate these side effects.

Do antidepressants increase an individual's risk of committing suicide?

This has become an increasing concern, particularly with the widespread use of SSRIs. Initially, the concern was to do with the use of these antidepressants in the under-eighteen group; recently, this has been broadened to their use in general. This concern relates to the tendency of these drugs in some cases initially to increase agitation in some people, with an increase in suicidal thoughts.

The current expert view on the use of antidepressants in the under-eighteen group is that in some cases there is an inceased risk of suicidal thoughts and actions, hostility and impulsiveness. Because of this, it is felt that the use of these drugs should be confined to specialists. Even under specialist care, there should be strict supervision.

But what can we say about the use of antidepressants by adults? All antidepressants may increase the chance of suicidal thoughts being actualised, as the person's energy and drive improve at a faster rate than their mood. This has always been identified as a potential risk.

The question being asked about SSRIs in particular is whether the drugs themselves are prompting the creation of suicidal thoughts. The general feeling is that only a very small number of those treated with these drugs will experience intense agitation or thoughts of self-harm as a direct result of taking these drugs. Careful monitoring in the first two months should reduce any such risks, along with early identification of those who seem to be generally more at risk of self-harm. Personally, I have come across this problem only occasionally in practice, and in general feel that the SSRIs reduce the risk of suicide. Some international trials suggest that SSRIs actually reduce the risks of suicide, because they encourage increased activity in the serotonin cable. It is also important to note that depression itself creates impulsive suicidal thoughts and actions. Eliminating all antidepressants would deny help to many who are at risk from the dangers of depression, and would seem unwise.

The widely accepted current view is that the risk of suicide associated with antidepressants is not sufficient for patients to stop using these drugs. Until some more expert scientific data appears to change this situation, these drugs will continue (quite sensibly, in my opinion) to be prescribed.

Can mild depression be treated without drugs?

Many people ask this question; the answer to it is an unequivocal yes! For many people, a change in lifestyle, in the form of exercise, proper diet and supplements, and a good look at major stress factors, may be enough to turn things around. This may be helped by counselling and interpersonal therapy in some cases. Another common error is to mistake chronic stress for depression. We have already dealt with the signs of the former. It is only if these measures do not work, or if the depression becomes more severe, that drug treatment may be recommended.

Is it true that SSRIs are more useful for the treatment of mild to moderate depression?

This is true. Research has shown that SSRIs seem to play an especially useful role in the treatment of mild to moderately severe depression, particularly if sleep or weight is a problem – with the exception of Lexapro, which has proven efficacy in the severely depressed. The SSRIs are also of particular help in those with anxiety and depression, in younger age groups (the under-forties) and in the elderly (due to the fact that they are associated with fewer side effects).

Drugs which stimulate the noradrenalin cable seem to have a more powerful effect on those with severe depression. (In general terms, the more severe the depression, the more important noradrenalin and dopamine depletion probably are.)

Some experts feel that SSRIs are prescribed too liberally. My own opinion is that, if used sensibly, they can play a useful role in many cases, as long as all the lifestyle changes that we have already dealt with are also being made. They are not, and never will be, the answer to life's many and varied problems, however! They are simply one of a useful group of therapeutic options available to help those who are suffering from a bout of the Red Flag.

What happens when the course of antidepressants comes to an end?

Abrupt discontinuation of the newer drugs (apart from Prozac) will, as we have already explained, produce symptoms such as giddiness, dizziness, nausea and lack of coordination. When it is time for your doctor to end the course of treatment, he will plan a gradual reduction of the drug, reducing the dosage from its current level to zero over a period of four to six weeks. If treatment is reduced gradually in this way, the patient should experience no withdrawal symptoms. By then, the patient will hopefully be feeling much better. Once their mood has improved, further changes can be made in their life to tackle the initial stress triggers and lifestyle choices that may have been the cause of the illness.

Are there any new drugs or other treatment options for depression on the horizon?

I am happy to say that there seem to be many exciting new drug options coming in the next five years and beyond. As a family doctor, I feel that there are many drawbacks to the drugs that are currently available. We are grateful for and continue to use them, as they help treat many of the distressing symptoms of depression, but most doctors look forward to the possibility of newer and better options.

Much of the work is being done into drugs which might dampen down the stress peptide/glucocortisol barrage which seems to lie at the heart of the biological malfunctioning in depression. We talked earlier about CRH (one of the stress peptides), and it and a number of other substances (including one called substance P) are being examined with a view to tackling depression from a different angle. Some of these drugs are now in the pipeline.

One other exciting area is research into the role of dopamine in depression. Many people with this illness describe how current drug treatments numb their pain and help to reduce many of the physical symptoms of depression, but do nothing to help restore their sense of joy and pleasure in life. Some go further, and say that some SSRIs in particular numb their feelings completely. This is an issue that many psychiatrists and family doctors do not in my opinion understand or engage with to a sufficient extent. It is clearly of great importance to the sufferer, however.

The reason that these modern drugs are unable to improve this distressing symptom is due, in the main, to their relative ineffectiveness in directly stimulating the dopamine cable into action. Any effects on this cable are usually secondary in nature. This is because their main effect is on the serotonin cable, and even here their action is not very targeted. Drugs which affect the noradrenalin cable also suffer from similar limitations in relation to the dopamine cable.

Paradoxically, some of the older type drugs, such as the tricyclics and in particular the MAOIs, were probably more effective in targeting all the cables, including the dopamine cable, than some of the newer drugs, particularly the SSRIs. As we discussed earlier, however, the side effects associated with these drugs, especially MAOIs, greatly limited their general use. This was a pity, as the MAOIs in particular were very effective in stimulating the dopamine cable into life, with a subsequent lift in the patient's feelings of joy and pleasure. The main concern was their capacity to interact with parts of the diet to produce potentially life-threatening increases in blood pressure.

Research into treatment for Parkinson's disease has thrown up an interesting drug called selegiline (Eldepryl), however. As we have already seen, half of those with this illness also suffer from depression. This is not surprising, as a lack of dopamine is common to both. It was discovered that, in smaller amounts (between 10 and 20 milligrammes), this drug (which is at present being used to help those with Parkinson's) was effective in helping those whose depression seemed to involve the dopamine and noradrenalin cables in particular. The classical example of this type of depression is atypical depression, which we will discuss in the next chapter.

It is likely that selegiline will be available in the form of a slow-release patch over the next few years, and it may help many of those who suffer from both extreme fatigue and the dark emptiness to which a life without joy or pleasure can give rise. This drug has the major additional benefit of not interfering with the sexual life of the person who is being treated. As always, only time and research will demonstrate the role that this particular drug may be able to play in the treatment of depression. For the time being, although this drug is available for the treatment of Parkinson's, it has not yet been licensed in Ireland for depression.

There is also research going on into drugs which affect melatonin. This is an important hormone released by the brain at night-time, as sunlight diminishes in the evening, causing us to feel tired and sleepy. Its levels are low in the daytime and high at night. If we have to remain awake when it is in our system, we can become irritable, fatigued and very moody (which explains why shift workers often struggle with these symptoms). It also explains why depression worsens in the winter months, when people have higher melatonin levels and lower serotonin levels. It has been shown that serotonin and melatonin are intimately linked, with the latter being manufactured from the former. Some studies have revealed higher levels of melatonin in major depression, so obviously it is also being affected by dysfunction in the mood circuit. A drug called Agomelatonine (which acts on both the serotonin and melatonin receptors) in particular looks very interesting (see Appendix 1). Future research may reveal whether this hormone has a role to play in treating this illness. Other future areas of research may involve examining the causes and consequences of glial-cell shortages on the survival of neurons within key structures like the behaviour box. In the long run, this may prove to be the best long-term treatment for depression.

One important finding involves the recognition of the importance of Area 25 of the behaviour box in depression. A great deal of this work in this area has been done by the pioneering research scientist Helen Mayberg. She demonstrated that Area 25 seems to be over-active in most cases of severe depression and that, irrespective of the type of therapy used, activity in this area reduces if the depression is successfully treated. Because of this constant finding, many wonder if studying this area will lead to a major breakthrough in the treatment of depression.

One consequence of the interest in Area 25 has been the exciting (although hugely expensive) treatment option in the case of very serious depression not responding to any form of drug or psychological treatment. This form of treatment, known as 'deep brain stimulation', is similar to the treatment of intractable Parkinson's disease. It involves the surgical implantation of a battery-powered electrode into Area 25 of the brain of individuals affected by intractable depression. The electrode were then connected to a small battery placed under the collarbone. The electrode then sent out a constant low-voltage charge to the surrounding area. The person would have the capacity to switch the device on or off. The results were profound, and in some cases immediate.

This form of therapy is at a very experimental stage, but initial results look very promising, and this treatment may in the future play a role in very extreme cases of depression. Of great interest to many was the finding, made by Mayberg, that stimulating this area produced the same neuro-imaging changes as CBT and drug therapy combined!

Another interesting area of research is examining the way in which genetic differences between people with depression relating to how they will respond to various forms of drug treatment. Hopefully, this in time may help medical professionals to 'target' the correct treatment option for each individual. We may also be helped by neuro-imaging studies to decide who would be best treated by drugs, versus psychological therapy.

There are many other areas where further research into this distressing illness may throw up new drug treatments or other options which will hopefully improve the quality of life for many without creating problems in the form of unwanted side effects. For the present, we must make the best use of what is available, in the knowledge that better therapies are on the way.

Is there any way of using neuro-imaging to decide which patients using particular drugs or CBT will or will not respond to therapy?

A great deal of excellent work by Helen Mayberg has started to reshape the way in which we view depression. She has been at the forefront of the circuit concept and work into the importance of Area 25 and has done research where patients with depression were scanned before and after treatment. She has identified some key findings:

§ That those who showed more activity than others in Area 24 (see Figure 14) prior to treatment with drug therapy and CBT were more likely to respond to both, and vice versa. Obviously, if Area 24 is very under-active, the mood-circuit dysfunction is more severe, and therefore harder to treat.

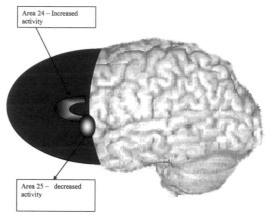

FIGURE 14: THE EFFECTS OF CBT ON AREAS 24 AND 25 IN DEPRESSION

§ That a drop in activity in Area 25 is common to all forms of successful therapy. Mayberg hopes that, by studying this gateway, we may come up with new information about both the causes and treatment of this illness.

§ That successful CBT showed an increase in activity in Area 24. This may be due to Area 24's role in the cognitive control of mood. (Area 25, in contrast, is more involved in the creation of low mood itself.)

§ That those who exhibited a good response to drug therapy did not show increased activity in Area 24 initially after the use of the drugs, but did so a year later.

§ That varying patterns of behaviour-box activity could assist in selecting the most suitable form of therapy.

§ That drug therapy and ECT worked on the brain stem and the limbic system, with the frontal mood department being affected by the positive changes in the mood circuit.

134

§   That CBT and psychotherapy worked on the behaviour box first, with the other changes in the limbic mood department, brain stem and mood-control boxes responding as the mood circuit settled down.

§   That it was possible to pick out patterns which made it more likely that changing therapies was less likely to be successful.

This is obviously a new and very exciting area of research, but we have a long way to go before we have worked out the whole picture. Nonetheless, in the future such mechanisms may prove to be of great help in 'targeting' specific therapies for resistant depression.

VII   OTHERS AFFECTED BY THE RED FLAG (THE CARERS)

The Red Flag causes a great of pain and suffering not only to those with depression but also to those who are close to them. The former may be angry because they hate themselves, and they may project this anger on to those around them. Often their silence, apparent laziness (due to extreme fatigue) and self-absorption, amongst other things, can be the cause of quarrels and disputes within the home.

This negative environment is fuelled by a lack of recognition of the symptoms of the Red Flag by both the person with depression and those close to them. The person with depression may blame those close to them for causing the problem. In fact, they are upset that their loved ones do not observe or appreciate the pain they are in. This hostility offends family members, who withdraw further, increasing the depressed person's sense of unworthiness, and lowering levels of mood and self-esteem further.

In reality, a person who is depressed is often not capable of communicating their problems to those who are close to them. This is partly because the ignorance which surrounds depression often takes away the family's ability to empathise with the sufferer, and to help them. It is important for those close to some who is suffering from depression to understand both the symptoms of and the various treatments for depression. A depressed person is greatly encouraged when they discover that they are suffering from an illness, and that it can be treated. This gives them the ability to say: 'This is how I feel, and I am not ashamed of it any more, because I know now that I have an illness. I am not weak, I am sick.' For the carer, knowledge of this illness educates them as to why things are the way they are: why their loved one is being hostile and pushing them away. It also plays a role in teaching them how they can help.

Depression occurs essentially because of a lack of communication in the brain, and is often accompanied by a similar lack of communication and understanding in society. If we can finally talk about this illness and what can be done to cure it, those suffering from it will finally realise that 'It doesn't have to be this way', and their loved ones will echo this epiphany.

2

SPECIAL SUB-GROUPS OF DEPRESSION

The previous chapter dealt with uncomplicated unipolar depression; patients in this group are generally treated by a GP, with occasional help from specialists in the field. The remainder, whose illness is more complicated in nature and difficult to treat, require intervention from a psychologist or a psychiatrist, or both.

I   DEPRESSION IN THE UNDER-EIGHTEENS

This is a unique group which has to be dealt with in a completely different way from their adult counterparts. The first crucial difference is that the body and brain of a child is in a gradual and constant state of transformation, which will eventually lead to the full formation of an adult body and brain.

A huge reorganisation of the brain takes place between the ages of twelve and eighteen. The production of sex hormones, and the immaturity of the frontal-lobe behaviour box, makes this a time a neurologically vulnerable one. The Red Flag of depression often initially emerges during this phase.

The young person has to endure many new stresses, which may include peer pressure, sexual discovery, physical changes to their body, increased independence, and the need to make decisions about their future. Combine this with alcohol and recreational drug use, and a breeding ground for depression is formed. Other illnesses, such as schizophrenia, may also begin to emerge at this time.

Not only are the mood departments underdeveloped in this group, but so too are the mood cables. This may explain why drug treatment is less effective – as well as being occasionally dangerous – and not routinely recommended in under-eighteens, although it can in some cases play a vital role.

This is an important group to focus on, because of the increased risk of suicide in males in particular. Nonetheless, it is important to note that more females than males in this group suffer from depression.

It is useful, in terms of symptoms, to divide this under-eighteen age group into two sub-groups, as follows:

1   DEPRESSION AMONG THE UNDER-TWELVES

Although depression is not common in this group, suicide by children younger than twelve is not unheard of. Members of this group will not complain of the symptoms of depression like an adult; the illness is more likely to manifest itself as an irritable, angry, apathetic and generally disruptive disposition. The individual also lacks interest in all activities. Features of anxiety, such as recurrent abdominal pain, headaches and limb pain, may also be present.

2   DEPRESSION IN THE TWELVE-TO-EIGHTEEN AGE GROUP

According to Prof. McKeown, community studies have shown that between 10 and 20 percent of adolescents will develop major depression, and there is evidence that the incidence is increasing. He also noted that having a parent with depression, particularly if it is recurrent, is the single most important risk factor for depression among adolescents. In the twelve-to-fifteen age group, the symptoms are closer to those documented above.

As teenagers approach the age of fifteen, symptoms of depression will start to resemble those found among adults. Common triggers include image obsession in girls and acne in boys. These individuals are inclined to look at themselves in a negative and critical manner.

A major risk factor during these years is separation or divorce in the family, and youngsters at this age are also acutely sensitive to peer pressure and bullying. They are also just starting to learn about their sexuality. Young girls feel under pressure to look like models from as early as the age of twelve; young boys feel that they must achieve and assert themselves, with the 'six-pack' physique almost mandatory. If they do not reach the goals that society has set out for them, they feel like failures, and their self-esteem may drop to a dangerously low level.

All these stresses and difficulties can combine to put a great deal of strain on the young person's stress system. Those who are genetically susceptible to depression become most vulnerable to the illness at this stage; alcohol and drug misuse exacerbate the problem. Some experts go further and wonder whether heavy alcohol or drug misuse may directly change the neurochemistry of the developing brain, thereby increasing the risks of depression and suicide.

It is advisable for parents to go through the Red Flag checklist for warning signs in their children; don't wait for them to come to you. Watch for withdrawal or isolation from groups, relationship problems, sexual-identity issues and alcohol misuse. Where there is a family history of depression, suicide or alcoholism, not picking up on these clues can prove to be a fatal oversight.

A major controversial issue is who should treat this group, and how they should do so. The physiology of this group, as well as the numerous influences on the maturing process from twelve to eighteen, means that the only person who is qualified to treat these teenagers is a psychiatrist. These individuals' mood departments and mood cables are too immature to risk routine drug treatment: it is not known what effect these drugs may have on the brain's development at this age. Many concerns have been raised about the possibility that the use of antidepressants of all types (although the modern SSRIs, especially Prozac, are the only ones that are generally used) in this age group may lead to an increase in suicidal thoughts and actions.

The present expert view is that, although these drugs can in some cases lead to increased agitation, suicidal thoughts and even suicide itself, their sensible use by experienced child and adolescent psychiatrists as part of an overall treatment package may, in severe cases of depression, reduce the danger of suicide. In mild to moderate depression, however, the consensus is that other therapies, such as CBT and family therapy, are more than adequate.

The modern approach to treatment involves a multi-disciplinary team consisting of a psychiatrist, a psychologist, a social worker and an educational expert to assess the child's problems in different areas and to isolate the the possible environmental and psychological causes of their depression. Once these causes have been discovered, they must be dealt with by the team. In more severe cases, this approach may include the child psychiatrist prescribing drug therapy.

This makes the child's environment favourable and free from stress, and this in turn helps the mood system to repair itself and continue to develop normally. The difficulty with this approach is that it requires time, money, resources and organisation: in many parts of the country at the moment, this service is just not possible. Another problem is the lack of child psychologists.

Of great concern to many family doctors, parents and those working with at-risk adolescents between the ages of sixteen and eighteen is the apparently nonsensical situation that only those under sixteen are eligible to be referred to such teams. Another concern is the lack of inpatient beds for high-risk young people.

The diagnosis and treatment of depression in this group is vital. Firstly, it is important to identify those who may be at risk from suicide. Secondly, this illness, if left untreated at this stage, when the mood system is forming, may in some cases continue for the duration of the person's life.

Many people spend decades suffering from depression, and remain undiagnosed and untreated until their thirties or forties. It has been shown that those who develop the Red Flag in their teens are more likely to suffer from recurrent bouts of depression later on.

If the multi-disciplinary approach can be so successful, why not apply it to the over-eighteen group? In adults, the mood system is fully formed. The mood cables and departments are operating normally. Many of the issues which affect this group become resolved as they approach twenty-five years of age.

To organise such a multi-disciplinary system for the adult population would be a massive undertaking and would take a long time to show results. Using antidepressants and psychological therapies in this group offers speedy and effective treatment. It is also easier for the adult to deal with any issues themselves, without a team of professionals doing it for them.

Recently, despite these observations, the Department of Health (in its 'Vision for Change' document) has decided to adopt this multi-disciplinary approach to the adult population. We will have to wait and see if this will become a reality!

Diet is crucial in the under-eighteen age group. The growing brain needs a diet rich in essential vitamins and nutrients and high in fish oils, which are easily available in the form of omega 3 from oily fish or other sources or in the form of supplements. Exercise is also important: apart from helping the young person's mood system, it reduces the incidence of obesity and diabetes.

II   DEPRESSION IN THE ELDERLY

There are also some key differences at the other end of the spectrum. The picture of depression in the elderly (defined as those over sixty-five) may be complicated by the presence of multiple other illnesses. For example, there is a high rate of depression among those recovering from heart attacks and cancer – two diseases that are common in this age bracket. Depression itself, as we saw earlier, can also increase the risk of both of these illnesses! So there is a huge overlap between our mood system and the other conditions that are common to the aging process.

There are two subgroups of the elderly suffering from this illness: those who have suffered from depression for the duration of their lives, and those who have become depressed for the first time over the age of sixty to sixty-five. The causes of depression are completely different for the two groups.

The first group may have suffered from bouts of depression since their early teens, and nothing has really changed by the time they reach the age of sixty to sixty-five. The stresses may take a different form: personal loss, loneliness, alcohol misuse and addiction, financial difficulties, and the loss of a job. The physiology of their depression remains unchanged, however, and by extension their possible treatment remains unchanged too: drug treatment, psychological help or counselling.

The second group (see Figure 15), however, may have suffered damage to their mood system because of a stroke, either small and silent, or large and paralysing. Out

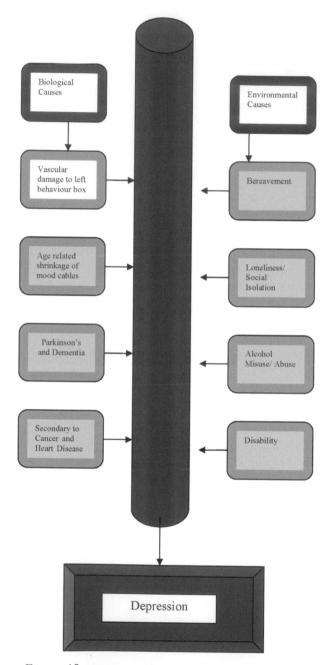

FIGURE 15: DEPRESSION RISK FACTORS IN THE ELDERLY

of the whole mood system, vascular damage to the connections leading to the frontal mood department (particularly the behaviour box) and the dopamine control box on the left side of the brain seem to be the most common. The end result of this damage can be depression. Aging in general also leads to a gradual reduction in both the number of neurons and in the blood supply to the brain, and this too may be a contributory factor. The mood cables themselves (the serotonin and dopamine cables in particular, and to a lesser extent the noradrenalin cable) begin to shrink as we get older, and this may also explain the high rate of depression in this group.

Two elderly groups that are particularly at risk of depression are those who suffer from dementia and those who have Parkinson's disease. Both of these illnesses occur as a result of abnormal degenerative and vascular changes in the ageing brain. In Parkinson's disease, for example, aa shortage of dopamine (which also causes difficulties with balance and movement) and serotonin in the mood cables they supply may lead to the appearance of this illness. Due to these unwanted biological changes, there is a high rate (up to 50 percent), in both of these illnesses, of the Red Flag of depression appearing.

The vascular damage to the mood sections mentioned above are of great relevance, as they help to explain the sudden emergence of depression in those who never before suffered from it. They are an obvious target for prevention, as treating illnesses like high blood pressure, eliminating high cholesterol and smoking, and using drugs like aspirin may reduce the risks of developing depression, as well as of suffering major strokes.

The real problem is the difficulties associated with the diagnosis of depression among the elderly. Too often, elderly people are dismissed as 'cranky' or 'senile', when a closer examination will reveal depression's classic calling cards. In general, the symptoms of depression are similar in both the young and the elderly: a lack of enjoyment in life, memory difficulties in particular (often confused with dementia), apathy, anxiety, and a preoccupation with minor ailments are often key findings in the elderly. Such people will often experience a substantial improvement in their quality of life when an antidepressant is prescribed.

The isolation of many elderly people is an important environmental factor for depression, as is the loss of a long-time partner. Another important factor is alcohol misuse and abuse. The lack of physical contact in many cases compounds the above factors. These social factors accelerate the arrival of depression in those who are biologically vulnerable to it.

Treatment of both types of depression in the elderly will usually involve drug therapy, and this therapy will typically be prescribed for longer periods than in younger people. SSRIs, because of their lack of cardiac side effects, are the drugs of choice. Elderly people should receive lower doses, and the maxim of 'start low and go slow' applies. Psychological therapies like CBT are also of help, but are frequently unavailable. Exercise is of great help, if it can be done. The role of alcohol, as always, needs to be carefully examined. Suicide (particularly in Asian countries such as China, where over-sixty-fives make up the bulk of suicides) remains a high risk in some cases.

Other ways of treating depression in this age group include:

1 Ensuring that the elderly person's diet is sufficient in the vitamins and nutrients which the mood system requires.

2 Exercise and supplements like B vitamins and omega 3 fish oils can be of great help. Massage and reflexology can also play a role.

3 Where there is social isolation, it can be extremely helpful for the elderly person to acquire a pet. The attention and affection which a pet bestows on its owner can have a beneficial affect on the person's mood system.

4 Encouraging elderly people to socialise in modern, well-run day-care centres. This makes them feel less isolated. In such centres, they can have conversations, eat together, and take part in activities such as painting, art work and pottery.

5 Encouraging, if possible, regular contact with children and young teenagers.

6 Family members should not be afraid to demonstrate affection by physically embracing the elderly person. Many older people are starved of this type of emotional contact. For those who have become isolated through depression, this can be a particularly nourishing experience.

All of these factors can contribute to the health of the elderly person's mood system. Another factor which exacerbates the problem of depression in the elderly is the way they are treated by society. They have become increasingly isolated and alienated from the modern world. Elderly people need love, warmth and physical touch, and deserve to be treated with dignity.

Finally, it is interesting to note that, in the elderly group, the physical changes that affect the brain and predispose them to the appearance of depression give rise to similar symptoms as those appearing in the fifteen-to-thirty-five age group. This is a powerful example of the importance of the brain in this illness at all stages of our lives.

III   POST-NATAL DEPRESSION

It is common for women to feel down and weepy from day three to day four following the delivery of a child. This low mood may last for days or weeks, but usually dissipates without any intervention. It happens due to a combination of 'coming down' from the high of having a baby, the body's sex hormones reorganising themselves after the delivery, and the stress of looking after the needs of the newborn baby. Most women, having gone through this phase, return to normal within a short period of time. Some women are slower to come out of this phase, however, and remain depressed.

It is likely that pregnancy, and the period of time after it, can in some people activate a latent genetic disposition towards depression. The symptoms of post-natal depression are identical to those of the Red Flag. Any lack of bonding with the new child occurring as a result of depression is extremely upsetting for the mother and is obviously not healthy for the child.

As with normal depression, the aim of treatment is to restore mood-system functioning within six to eight weeks. This can often be achieved quite effectively with the use of antidepressants and psychological therapy. Post-natal depression is normally dealt with by the family doctor. The time span of treatment is very similar to ordinary depression. Indeed, some experts maintain that post-natal depression is no different from ordinary depression and that the birth, together with the stress of the post-natal period, is simply a trigger for it.

One in every thousand cases of pregnancy-related depression will take the form of psychotic depression. In such cases, the woman suffers from serious delusions, often involving harming either the baby or themselves. This is a critical and dangerous situation and should be dealt with only by a specialist, in a hospital environment. It is extremely traumatic for the family involved. Most of these cases will respond to treatment, and the woman's life will return to normal. There is always the risk, however, of suicide, and, infrequently, infanticide.

Women with post-natal depression are also trying to cope with caring for a new baby. Some wait for three to six months before coming to their GP for help. If you experiencing any of the symptoms of depression, do not be afraid to come to your family doctor to discuss them. Your doctor will be able to assess the severity of the problem; antidepressants may not be necessary.

Mothers in other parts of the world have a much lower incidence of post-natal depression. One possible explanation is that mothers in the Western World are often lacking in the omega 3 oils (in particular DHA) which the baby desperately needs, particularly in the final stages of its development. When the baby has been born, the mother may suffer from a deficiency of omega 3 oils, and this may be a factor in the development of post-natal depression. Perhaps all mothers should be advised to supplement their diet with these oils for the last three months of their pregnancy and for the three to six months following the birth of the baby! Once again, only further research can throw more light on this area.

Another interesting, and almost completely overlooked, area is the effect of the arrival of a newborn baby on the emotional life of the father! It is felt by some experts that the high-stress phase experienced by the father in the first year of the infant's life may lead to many young males developing depression (which usually remains hidden). We could learn a great deal from a large research project looking at the mood status of such males. One wonders whether it is the stress rather than the hormonal changes that make both men and women vulnerable to developing the Red Flag during this phase.

IV   ATYPICAL DEPRESSION

Some patients will present with low mood but also with unusual symptoms which do not feature on the Red Flag checklist. These are:

§   Hypersomnia (sleeping too much)

§   Hyperphagia (eating too much)

§   Overwhelming fatigue, often termed 'leaden paralysis'

§   An ability to be cheered up for short durations by positive life events

§   Long-term sensitivity to rejection

§   Avoidant personality

This type of depression may be far more common than is currently believed. Some experts estimate that up to 25 percent of depressives may fall into this group. Others wonder whether we should really treat this form of depression as a special entity at all! It is thought to be associated with reduced activity of the noradrenalin and in particular the dopamine cable; this may explain the symptoms of fatigue and over-eating.

Atypical depression is often undetected, and these patients can be misdiagnosed as typical depressives. They are not likely to respond to SSRIs, however: drugs which affect the other two mood cables have a better chance of success.

A drug called Bupropion or Zyban, which is used in America for this form of depression, is also used here in Ireland to help smokers with their addiction. Earlier, we mentioned the drug selegiline (Eldepryl), which is being developed. This works on both the dopamine and the noradrenalin cables and will in my opinion offer much to those who suffer from atypical depression. CBT and psychotherapy can also be helpful in some cases, but many patients will need drug therapy as well as exercise-based behaviour therapy to ease the extreme fatigue in particular.

V   SEVERE DEPRESSION

Severe or profound depression occurs when there is a complete breakdown of the Red Flag mood structures and cables, often as a result of prolonged stress. A person with severe depression will present in a zombie-like state, with total depletion of their noradrenalin, dopamine and serotonin cables, causing visible difficulties in movement, thought and speech.

They suffer extreme fatigue because they rarely sleep. In some cases, delusions can occur. Any action becomes almost impossible. They do not hear what people are saying, because they are unable to focus on it. Thought processes are extremely delayed; the world appears to be moving in slow motion; tha passage of time is just pain, nothing else.

The total depletion of the serotonin cable puts suicide at the top of the agenda for these people. Sometimes, only their catatonic state prevents this suicidal urge from becoming a reality: it will take too much effort. Their dopamine system is also totally depleted, so their world is black, devoid of anything worthwhile.

Members of this group are clearly in serious difficulty: apart from being completely unable to function in the normal world, they are at great risk of suicide and other impulsive acts of self-harm. They are no danger to anyone but themselves, but the danger they pose to themselves is lethal.

Those belonging to this group are very sick, and should be immediately admitted to hospital. They may not respond to drug treatment at all. There has been such a depletion of the three main mood neurotransmitters – serotonin, noradrenalin and dopamine – and such extensive damage to the mood departments that these drugs cannot block the re-uptake of neurotransmitters, as they are not being released in sufficient amounts into the synapses.

Psychiatrists may decide that only ECT (electro-convulsive therapy) will be of any benefit. This is usually a last resort, and is carried out under general anaesthetic to protect the patient. ECT was the original treatment for severe depression, before the advent of antidepressants. An electric current is passed into one side of the brain to artificially activate the mood cables and departments. An appropriate analogy is that of a car with a flat battery. If it is attached to an active battery, the flat battery is reactivated by a charge from the active one, and the car begins to come back to life. ECT is normally given in a course of three treatments per week for a maximum of six to twelve sessions, depending on how quickly the person responds.

This process may seem scary and barbaric to many patients and their families, and remains a very controversial practice. In some cases, however, it remains the only form of treatment left, and seems to be effective. Often within a week, the person's mood system appears to kick back into life.

It is still uncertain exactly how ECT works. Many are of the opinion that it has a pronounced effect on the dopamine and noradrenalin cables. It has also been shown, through neuro-imaging, that ECT, like drug therapy, seems to act from the bottom of the mood system, activating the mood control boxes, and that Area 25 is also calmed. Some neuro-imaging studies have also shown no serious side effects. ECT is usually combined with drug treatment, which then takes over when ECT has brought the mood system back to life.

This form of treatment is only used in a tiny proportion of cases of the most severe depression. Maybe in an ideal world, deep-brain stimulation, as previously described, might be a good alternative. The psychotherapist may in particular object to the use of ECT, but what is the alternative when all other forms of therapy, including psychoanalysis, CBT/IPT and drug therapy, have failed?

A more advanced form of ECT treatment that is currently under investigation is trans-cranial magnetic stimulation. This involves a magnet stimulating the brain electrically, in the same way as ECT does; it is particularly aimed at the frontal mood department. Initial research into this treatment is promising: it does not require an anaesthetic and was initially thought to be as effective as ECT. Recent research, however, has dampened down initial enthusiasm, bringing into questioning whether it will prove to be of as much assistance as was formerly thought.

One danger in the area of severe depression is that, when the person starts to get better, they may become less sluggish and therefore more likely to act on suicidal urges. As a result, they are often safer in a controlled hospital environment until their condition has improved.

VI   Resistant Depression

This is another interesting group that the family doctor will refer to a psychiatrist. Up to 25 percent of cases of depression will not respond to treatment. It is not fully understood why some people are more resistant to treatment than others. There are, however, some common trends running through this group:

§   *The diagnosis may be wrong.* Certain illnesses, such as Bipolar Type 2 depression, and schizophrenia, can be difficult to diagnose. Many people suffering from these illnesses are misdiagnosed with normal depression. This may render their treatment ineffective, as bipolar mood disorder, in particular, may not respond to antidepressants. Another possibility is atypical depression, which will not respond to SSRIs.

§   *The person may not have dealt with underlying issues,* such as bereavement, loss or abuse. In this case, the stress system may be overwhelming the mood system to such an extent that treatment does not work successfully.

§   *The person may be confining themselves to a single form of treatment,* be it medication or therapy. For some, only a combination of drug and psychological treatment will treat their depression successfully. The real problem is the inaccessibility of the latter to the vast majority of patients!

§   *Non-compliance* Some people stop taking their medication, or take it only infrequently.

§ *The dose of antidepressant is too low.* This is a common occurrence, in my experience.

§ *The wrong antidepressant is being used.* Some types of antidepressants work on the noradrenalin cable, and others work on the serotonin cable. If one of these types of drugs does not work, then the other group should be prescribed.

§ *The patient is abusing alcohol* or other substances to combat their feelings of depression. This is quite a common occurrence. Alcohol is a depressant, and will limit the success of whatever treatment the individual is on; this can be dangerous if combined with drug treatment.

When depression is not proving responsive to any treatment, the GPr will usually refer the person to a psychiatrist, who may make the following changes to treatment:

§ *Review the diagnosis*

§ *Use psychological therapy* such as CBT or psychotherapy, depending on the nature and causes of the depression

§ *Review the type of medication or dosage*

§ *Prescribe a mood-stabilising drug* Lithium, which has been used for years in dealing with bipolar mood disorder, is sometimes used in cases of resistant simple depression. Another group of drugs which have been used with great success are anti-convulsants, which are traditionally used to treat epilepsy. Common examples include Tegretol, Epilim and Lamictal. They can be used with or without antidepressants.

If you have been suffering from depression, and treatment has not alleviated the symptoms of your illness, there are a number of areas you can address. These include:

§ *Diet* Are you eating a healthy, balanced diet?

§ *Exercise* Do you include exercise as part of your treatment plan?

§ *Alcohol* Are you using alcohol to block out the depression? Are you mixing drug treatment with alcohol?

§ *Relaxation* Are you taking time out every day to relax?

§ *Stress* What makes you stressed? How can you reduce this stress?

§ *Drug treatment* Are you taking your medication as instructed and finishing the course?

§ *Psychological treatment* Are you open to accepting help in this area? If you are, are you turning up for your sessions?

§ *Keeping an open mind with regard to your treatment* If you are currently using only psychological treatment, and it is not helping, are you open to the possibility of drug treatment also, or vice versa?

VII SEASONAL AFFECTIVE DISORDER (SAD)

Another variant of depression is a condition called seasonal affective disorder. It is well known that people become more depressed during the long nights of winter than during the long days of summer. It is known that around 25 percent of those with unipolar depression may deteriorate during the winter.

For some people, particularly in more northern climates, the darkness of wintertime creates a unique depression. People with SAD develop all the symptoms of depression, as well as a craving for food, with accompanying weight gain. Some experts feel that darkness encourages the brain to produce a neurotransmitter called melatonin. This has the general function of helping us to sleep at night. Light, on the other hand, encourages the production of serotonin. There is an important neural connection between the eyes and a part of the hormone control box which, as we discussed earlier, controls all our body rhythms/biological clocks. As daylight arrives every morning, it penetrates through our closed eyelids and activates this pathway (leading to increased serotonin-cable activity in this box), stimulating us to wake up. When darkness falls, this neural pattern is reversed, and the brain produces melatonin to encourage us to sleep.

In real life, artificial daylight (through our narrow-spectrum light bulbs) combats much of this natural pattern, in comparison to the world of our ancestors. Despite this, melatonin and serotonin are intimately interwoven into the normal circadian rhythms of our lives.

SAD seems to be caused by an excessive production of the former, and in particular a lack of the latter. Of great importance is the seasonal difference in production of serotonin, with higher levels in the summer and lower ones in the winter. It may be the case that this exposes a general shortage of serotonin in people with this condition. This may explain why they recover during the bright summer months and slip back into trouble in the winter. This seasonal difference may also apply to the 25 percent of people with normal depression whose condition deteriorates in the dark winter months.

It is also felt that a shortage of serotonin in the hormone control box in particular leads to a craving for carbohydrates, with resulting weight gain, during SAD episodes. This probably happens to us all during the dark months of winter but is a particular problem in those who suffer from depression.

Of note, melatonin is manufactured from serotonin! Numerous studies have been done trying to link melatonin and biological circadian rhythms, in order to explain this illness, but they have been inconclusive so far. At present, the role of serotonin seems to be more important than that of melatonin. SAD is almost certainly genetic. It is believed that the disorder is linked to problems with specific serotonin receptors (probably 5HT1A, 5HT2C and 5HT7).

Apart from difficulties within the serotonin system, it has also been shown that there are many similarities between SAD and atypical depression (so much so that some experts now feel that SAD should be considered as a sub-type of atypical depression) in that the noradrenalin and dopamine cables seem to be under-active during episodes, explaining the extreme lassitude, reduced motivation and libido, and hypersomnia so often seen in those with this illness.

Efforts have been made to treat this condition by exposing the person to bright lights for several hours, particularly in the morning. An effective way of treating this condition is to use a dawn simulator. The sufferer has a light installed in their room; this light starts to illuminate about half an hour before the person wakes up in the morning. The light simulates natural sunlight, and its intensity gradually increases, mimicking what would happen if the sun were rising at that time. This form of treatment is also sometimes effective in treating normal depression. I would highly recommend an American model, the 'Rise and Shine' bedside lamp, with its full-spectrum light bulb, for those who would like to try this form of therapy. It can be purchased online at *www.verilux.com*. (In Europe, it must be used with a 110-watt step-down voltage converter, which can be found in any good electrical store.) Research is continuing into dawn simulators, but they remain a more affordable and more practical treatment than moving to a country with a sunnier climate!

3

Bipolar Mood Disorder

Bipolar mood disorder, which forms a special sub-group of depression, is often confused with unipolar depression. People also refer to it as 'manic depression' and often view it as a form of madness; in fact, it is neither. Because it has been linked to high-profile creative people such as Spike Milligan, it has also been associated with genius. This illness is now better known as bipolar mood disorder, a term which describes it more accurately.

While the depression component of this illness is almost identical to that in unipolar depression, the mania component is its antithesis. In unipolar depression, the mood will swing from normal to low and back again, but will rarely become elevated. When looking at bipolar mood disorder, think of the North and South Poles, the two most extreme points on the Earth. Depression is down at the South Pole, and mania is up in the North. Normal mood resides in the middle, on the Equator. Sufferers experience not only depression but also its polar opposite.

Bipolar mood disorder differs in many ways from simple depression: in its causes, genetics, presentation and treatment. There are, however, a number of areas where the two illnesses overlap.

I   Symptoms of Bipolar Mood Disorder

Bipolar mood disorder can be divided into two main groups:

BIPOLAR DISORDER, TYPE ONE

Here, the person will have suffered at least one manic episode, usually associated with a period of low mood or depression. They suffer the usual symptoms of depression, which have already been dealt with, including:

§   Low mood
§   Sleep difficulties

§   Fatigue

§   Low self-esteem

§   Anxiety

§   Suicidal thoughts

Mania is the opposite of depression. It is defined as a distinct period of abnormally and persistently elevated mood lasting at least one week, and which sometimes requires hospitalisation. During this period of elevated mood, the person may display the following:

§   Extremely inflated self-esteem and mood

§   Decreased need for sleep

§   Talkativeness, and speech will often rhyme like poetry

§   Racing thoughts and ideas

§   High creativity

§   Inexhaustible optimism

§   Energy and enthusiasm

§   Anger upon being challenged

§   Indiscreet behaviour, with very poor judgement

§   Insensitivity to the feelings of others

§   Impairment of social function, particularly with regard to everyday activities

§   Involvement in pleasurable activities with no regard for the consequences, such as spending sprees, shoplifting, reckless driving, excessive sexual activity or impulsive behaviour

This change in mood usually causes difficulties in close personal relationships, and may result in the person becoming a risk to themselves or others. On occasion, the person may suffer from grandiose delusions ('I'm the Pope!') or hallucinations; this is why bipolar mood disorder is often misdiagnosed as schizophrenia.

A very unpleasant form of bipolar disorder, type one, is dysphoric mania. This is where the person gets a bout of depression during an episode of severe mania: instead of the person feeling 'on top of the world', they become extremely distressed, irritable and agitated, with racing and suicidal thoughts. This condition, which is also called mixed mania, probably constitutes up to 30 to 40 percent of cases of mania. It is more common in women, and is associated with a high risk of suicide and a higher rate of familial depression than uncomplicated mania. This condition will usually require hospitalisation (and occasionally, in very serious cases, ECT) and may be more difficult to treat successfully. It can be a very distressing condition for both the person and their family. It can also be present in a lesser form as dysphoric hypomania, where depression is present during an episode of hypomania (see below).

BIPOLAR DISORDER, TYPE TWO

Here, the person suffers mainly from bouts of depression, interspersed with periods of hypomania. Hypomania is a distinct period of euphoria lasting at least four days. During this period of elevated mood, the symptoms of mania emerge, although they are not particularly obvious, usually do not cause major difficulties in the person's ability to cope with normal activities (in fact, many feel that they cope better during such phases), and seldom require hospitalisation. The person will rarely suffer from delusions or hallucinations. A person with hypomania will have periods where they experience the following:

§   A sudden increase in energy levels

§   Racing thoughts

§   Increased talkativeness

§   Decreased need for sleep

§   Irritability and annoyance if confronted

§   Feeling on top of the world

Bipolar disorder, type two, may have a different biological source (possibly closer to that of unipolar depression) from bipolar disorder, type one, although this is an area where research is ongoing.

The main differences between the above symptoms and those of normal depression are the major fluctuations in mood, which are usually not seen in the Red Flag of unipolar depression. This suggests that something completely different is happening neurologically.

It is also important to note that low mood, normal mood and elevated mood are present at different times in the life of the bipolar depressive. There are huge variations in this illness from person to person. Bouts of low mood usually outweigh the highs by about three to one. A small number of people may get about four bouts or more of mania per year, which can cause chaos in the lives of themselves and those around them.

THE COURSE OF BIPOLAR ILLNESS

Bipolar illness usually appears in the teenage years; even when it is observed, it is often misdiagnosed as normal depression. It is only when the elevated mood periods are either admitted to by the individual or noticed by others that a new diagnosis emerges. Bouts of low mood, periods of normality, and occasional bouts of elevated mood merge to create the distinct pattern of this illness.

Unfortunately, there is often a substantial delay in diagnosis, due to the erratic nature of the illness. This can be further complicated by the concomitant presence of the Purple Flag of addiction. Some people with bipolar disorder may (through a combination of not presenting early enough and a delay in accurate diagnosis) have their illness remain undetected for up to ten years. In fact, only one in four bipolar depressives are diagnosed within three years of the onset of the illness. Most are labelled as normal depressives and treated accordingly – women in particular, as they are more likely than men to present with symptoms of depression.

This illness is not as common as unipolar depression, and it affects both men and women in equal numbers. The incidence of bipolar type one is around 1 percent of the population, and bipolar type two probably between 1 and 2 percent. Some experts feel that the true incidence of this illness may be substantially higher. It seems to be more common in urban than in rural areas.

The main difficulty with bipolar illness is the disruption it can cause to the social, working and relationship life of the sufferer. The condition is associated with a high rate of suicide. Between 20 and 50 percent of those who remain undetected or untreated will attempt suicide. At least 10 to 15 percent of people with this illness will succeed in taking their own lives.

There is also a strong link (in both the depressed and elated phases) to alcohol and substance abuse. The latter in particular is a major problem, with some placing the lifetime occurrence of alcohol and substance abuse in this group as high as 60 percent! Alcohol and substance abuse can sometimes be the triggering factors, particularly if drugs like marijuana or cocaine are used. Up to a third of those who suffer from this illness may struggle to function independently. Holding down jobs and establishing emotionally stable, permanent relationships becomes very difficult for many of them. Correct diagnosis and appropriate treatment can transform the lives of these people.

Over their lifetime, a bipolar sufferer will typically suffer eight to ten episodes of mood swings. Untreated episodes of mania may last from four to six months. In practice, the symptoms of mania are so severe that help is usually received quite quickly, so episodes may last only weeks. Episodes of hypomania are generally much more subtle and are of shorter duration, so they often go undetected.

Bouts of depression, if untreated, last up to nine months in people with biploar illness. One of the difficulties is that a patient who is treated with antidepressants may develop a subsequent bout of hypomania or mania as a result of the medication. A particular concern is where a person with dysphoric hypomania presents with appears at first glance to be simple depression, and is treated with antidepressants. The antidepressants can make them more agitated, and suicidal thoughts and actions may increase. The risk of suicide is greatest in the early stages of this illness (which is why early diagnosis is vital), and more often occurs in the depression or mixed-mania phases. Another problem is that patients sometimes do not respond to antidepressants at all in bipolar disorder.

There can be a delay of four to ten years between the first and second episode of bipolar disorder. Following this, the length of time between episodes will gradually begin to shorten. In some cases, the severity of the illness, especially if untreated, will worsen. In terms of the probability of recurrence, some estimate it at 50 percent for the first year, 70 percent by the fourth year, and 90 percent by the fifth year.

THE BIOLOGY OF BIPOLAR ILLNESS

Bipolar disorder is a very different illness from depression. Despite intensive and exciting research in this area, there is still no working model as to how this illness occurs. This is what is known to date:

(A)   THE MOOD DEPARTMENTS

Both the frontal and limbic system mood departments are involved in this illness. Recent research has focused on the role of the behaviour box and the stress box, and has reported the following:

§   A decrease in activity of the left frontal behaviour box in the depression phase of this illness

§   An increase in activity of the right frontal mood department in the manic phase of this illness

§   A reduction in size in some sections of the behaviour box: in one study, already discussed, a particular section (Area 24) shrunk by up to 40 percent

§   An increase in activity in the stress box

§   A reduction in volume in the following: the stress box, the pleasure box and, as noted above, various parts of the behaviour box, with a corresponding reduction in the number of neurons, neuronal connections and glial support cells

(B)   THE MOOD CABLES

These were the focus of attention for many years but research findings have proved insufficient in explaining the disorder. Findings to date include:

§ The noradrenalin mood cable is over-active in mania (explaining the reduced need for sleep and the unlimited energy seen in this group) and under active in the depression phase of this illness (explaining the usual depression symptoms of fatigue, difficulties with sleep, poor concentration and lack of drive)

§ The serotonin cable is under active during the depression phase. This explains why suicide thoughts and attempts are more common during this phase of the illness.

§ The dopamine cable is more active in the manic phase. This may explain the tendency to seek pleasurable activities. It is under active in the depression phase.

(C)   THE NEUROTRANSMITTERS AND RECEPTORS

A great deal of research has looked at the role of other neurotransmitters in bipolar disorders. The main findings are:

§ A reduction of GABA, the brain's calming neurotransmitter

§ An increase in intercellular G-proteins during mania, and a decrease during the depression phase

What are G-proteins? Some of the receptors activated by neurotransmitters, glutamate and serotonin in particular, release these proteins, which travel from the cell membrane to the genes in the centre of the cell. This in turn may lead to inter cellular changes, probably involving BDNF, which we dealt with earlier in the Red Flag. We still do not understand the role of the glial support cells in this process. The malfunction of this process may explain the volatility of cells of the mood system in bipolar depression.

(D)   THE STRESS SYSTEM

There is an increase in glucocortisol levels in both the low and high phases of this illness. The same risks that unipolar depression carries regarding heart disease, osteo porosis and a weakening of the immune system are also present with bipolar depression. The above finding lead to the following conclusions:

§ The depression phase of this illness is almost identical to that of normal depression.

§ The manic phase of this illness remains a mystery. The most likely explanation is that there are problems at cell-membrane level which make the cells of the mood system more vulnerable to becoming hyper-stimulated. The role of G-proteins, glutamate and glial support cells, in particular, may in the future be shown to play an important role in this process.

155

§   Some speculate that changes may happen in the womb, as the brain's mood system is developing, resulting in the emergence of this disorder when pruning of the brain begins in the twelve-to-twenty-five age group.

§   It is quite likely that stress may trigger mood changes, through the usual mechanisms.

SUMMARY

Bipolar mood disorder causes the following changes in the mood system:

1   Decreased activity in the left behaviour box during the depression phase of the illness, and an increase in activity of the right behaviour box during periods of elevated mood. The former explains the high rate of suicide among people with bipolar mood disorders.

2   Bipolar disorder affects the three main mood cables. The serotonin and noradrenalin cables are under-active during the depression phase of this illness. This gives rise to all the normal symptoms of depression. During the manic phase, the dopamine and noradrenalin cable are over-active. This explains the drive towards pleasurable activities during this phase, as well as the boundless energy and lack of need for sleep

CAUSES OF BIPOLAR DISORDER

It is widely accepted that bipolar disorder has an even stronger genetic foundation than normal depression. Between 8 and 9 percent of those with first-degree relations who have bipolar disorder will develop depression.

It has proved difficult to isolate the genes responsible for this illness. Initially, there was only one gene thought to be at fault, but recent research suggests that a number of different genes are involved. (For those who are interested, chromosomes 1, 4, 6, 14, 16 and 21 have been under scrutiny in this regard.) This would explain the wide variety of forms of presentation of this illness, and the fact that, although this illness is quite different from simple depression, there is a marked pattern of both illnesses developing in relatives of people who have this disorder.

It is more difficult to ascertain how stress triggers affect this illness. Stress and anxiety disorders are often linked to bipolar disorder. Presumably the stress system, including glucocortisol, is involved in kick-starting mood swings. The problem is that the understanding of the biological pathways is at present so limited that it is hard to quantify the role that stress triggers may play.

TREATMENT OF BIPOLAR DISORDER

Bipolar disorder is dealt with exclusively by a specialist, as it can be extremely difficult to stabilise the swings in mood. The mood, whether up or down, has to be brought back to a normal level and maintained there.

The first, and often most difficult, step in treatment is diagnosis. Bipolar disorder continually flies under the radar of even the most highly trained professionals. An episode of high mood, a bout of severe depression, or an attempted suicide often leads to the diagnosis. Severe episodes of either high or low mood may require a visit to hospital to help stabilise the person. Occasionally in severe depression ECT is required, and sometimes in severe mania high doses of tranquillizers may be needed to sedate the patient and bring their mood down to a normal level.

Most cases of bipolar disorder will be prescribed drugs by a psychiatrist, who may request the assistance of a psychologist. It is difficult to treat depression in people with bipolar disorder, as they often either do not respond to any form of treatment or respond too much, and drift into mania. As has already been stated, high mood is usually counteracted with tranquillizers. The tranquillizer Zyprexa (Olanzapine) is commonly used to stabilise elevated mood. Such drugs, while very useful in treating bipolar disorders, do have significant side effects, including weight gain.

Lithium has changed the lives of many people with bipolar disorder. This drug is very effective in treating the manic phase of the illness and, more importantly, is able to stabilise mood swings. Many will show a dramatic response to this drug in just one to two weeks. Lithium probably works at cell-membrane level (possibly on the G-protein messenger system), calming down cells which have become too agitated (and increasing their chances of survival), thereby helping sufferers to lead normal lives. Many now feel that this drug is the only one which is not only neuroprotective (i.e. encourages the production of internal cellular enzymes, which improve the neurons' survival) but which also increases the volume of key areas like Area 24.

The use of Lithium has to be carefully monitored through regular blood checks; it can cause some side effects, such as tremors and weight gain, but is usually well tolerated. Its use is nearly always initiated by the specialist, but is often monitored by the GP. Occasionally, the specialist may combine its use with antidepressants or may seek to stabilise low mood with antidepressants first, and then start the patient on a course of Lithium. Unfortunately, up to one third of patients do not respond to this drug.

The major problem with Lithium is that patients often miss the euphoria of the manic stage of this illness, or may feel that they simply do not need the drug. In both cases, patients may stop taking it, and the massive mood swings return. They may also cease taking it due to associated weight gain. Lithium also cannot be used during pregnancy, as it can cause foetal abnormalities.

Following the success of this drug came the discovery that some anti-convulsion drugs might mimic the action of Lithium. They achieve this by stabilising the cells of the mood system (probably by acting on cell membrane glutamate receptors). They may be used in the prevention of hypomania, mania or depression, either in conjunction with Lithium or on their own. The two main anticonvulsants used are Lamictal and Epilim:

§   *Lamictal* This is useful in preventing the depression episodes in bipolar type two disorders. It can be used on its own, together with antidepressants, and occasionally with Lithium. It can also be used safely during pregnancy.

§   *Epilim* This is useful in preventing the mania phases of bipolar disorder. Its main side effect is weight gain.

Stress triggers relating to bipolar disorders are handled in the same way as in normal depression. But the key to this illness lies in the use of mood stabilisers. There is also a great need for further research into possible drug treatments for this illness, with the aim of improving the quality of life of bipolar sufferers.

Bipolar disorder is a complex mood disorder: it is difficult to diagnose and understand and, in terms of treatment, is a challenge to both the specialist and the patient. Due to the high suicide rate associated with this disorder, however, and the degree of destruction it can wreak on people's lives, it is important that treatment takes place. This chapter will hopefully be of help to anyone who suffers from this disorder, or who has a family member or friend who suffers from it. Just as it is very important to be able to spot the warning signs of depression, such as low mood, it is also important to note that, on occasions, these warning signs can also be accompanied by elevated mood. If this pattern is observed, it is very important for the person to get help from their family doctor, and then from a psychiatrist. Bipolar disorder is highly influenced by genetics. As in the case of unipolar depression, all of us have a responsibility to try to understand the condition and help those who suffer from it in any way we can.

III

THE YELLOW FLAG

ANXIETY

1

ACUTE AND CHRONIC ANXIETY DISORDERS

Anxiety is a universal phenomenon, occurring in response to a situation which demands our absolute attention, usually when we feel threatened. These situations are usually temporary, and so is the anxiety that prepares the body to tackle them. Anxiety is best described as an uncomfortable state of hyper-alertness due to fear.

When it increase to a certain level, however, anxiety becomes an illness. For these people, anxiety is constant, out of proportion, disabling and exhausting. It controls what they can and cannot do in their lives and, more often than not, makes them too tired to do anything.

Anxiety disorders are very common: at least 5 percent of people will suffer from such a disorder at some stage in their lives. Unfortunately, just as in the Red Flag of depression, the Yellow Flag of anxiety often remains hidden. The two most common anxiety-related illnesses are panic disorder and phobias.

PANIC DISORDER

Episodes of this disorder are referred to as panic attacks and are common problems, presenting to both A&E departments and family doctors at all hours of the day and night. Such an episode is a short period of extreme anxiety which can occur at any time. The person may experience some or all of the following symptoms:

§ A feeling that they are going to die

§ Profuse sweating

§ Palpitations (fast heartbeat)

§ Dry mouth

§ Weakness

§ Headache

§ Chest pain

§   Hyperventilation (rapid, shallow breathing)

§   Trembling or shaking

§   Fear of losing control or 'going mad'

§   Dizziness

§   Sensation of choking

When these symptoms occur suddenly and simultaneously, they are terrifying for the sufferer. The attack, depending on how the person handles it, may last from a few minutes to several hours. The attacks is usually not prompted by any particular outside stress, and the person may be involved in their normal daily activities when it occurs.

Someone encountering an episode like this for the first time will appear to be extremely ill to friends and loved ones, and they often are admitted to a casualty department for an ECG or chest X-rays, as many lay people assume that they are having a heart attack or a stroke. It is often very difficult to convince the person that they are in fact physically quite healthy. They often attend their doctor the following day, seeking assurance that all is well.

Panic attacks are completely unpredictable, and consequently often affect the person at the most inappropriate times and places. This leads to a constant fear and dread amongst those with the condition that another episode will occur at an inopportune moment. For instance, a panic attack may take place in a crowded area; this may lead to the individual being afraid of entering such an area again, in case an attack recurs. Fear of such episodes – the so-called fear of fears – can thus become nearly as great a problem as the panic attacks themselves.

This disorder will often appear for the first time in a person's teenage years or early twenties. For genetic reasons, women are more prone to developing the illness. Panic attacks often appear out of nowhere; if they are allowed to proceed in a normal manner, the attack will usually plateau in about twenty minutes. If the person takes avoidant action, such as using tranquillizers or alcohol, or attending A&E, however, the attack may last for much longer. Attacks may occur weekly or monthly, and on occasions more often.

The initial episode may follow a period of intense stress or pressure, but after this the illness takes on a life of its own. Without treatment, this chronic and unpredictable pattern of attacks will continue indefinitely, interspersed with a continuous apprehension as to when such attacks will strike again. The tragedy is that a few sessions of treatment can in many cases quickly banish them for good, but sufferers who are unaware of this fact may never come forward for help.

Panic attacks are often experienced in association with other illnesses of the mood system. These illnesses include addiction (particularly in alcoholics), depression and chronic anxiety.

II   PHOBIAS

Few people are without fear. Many people will suffer from an irrational fear of a place, crowd, object, animal or insect. There are numerous documented exotic examples of such random fears. The most well known one is agoraphobia, which is a fear of either open spaces or large crowds. An agoraphobic may be afraid to leave not only their house but even their room. Phobias affect a large number of people – more often women than men – and are frequently never discussed by the sufferer. Other common phobias are fears of heights, mice and spiders. A person who encounters the object of their phobia may experience the following symptoms:

§   Sweating

§   Palpitations

§   Shortness of breath due to hyperventilation

§   Weakness

§   A strong desire to escape

§   Dry mouth

Removing oneself from the situation is a common reaction, and one which provides immediate relief. This approach does not solve the problem permanently, however. The person may later encounter their phobia in the middle of a supermarket, for intance, and want to just drop everything and run. As a result, the life of a phobic can be very restricted.

Because of their irrational nature, phobias are often very embarrassing to the sufferer. They feel helpless, as they have no control over their body and mind when the phobia is encountered, and may as a result try to hide the problem.

A particularly crippling phobia is social phobia, where a person dreads meeting other people. Such people are painfully shy. Suicide rates are higher in this group than among people with any of the other anxiety disorders. The probable reason for this is that they cannot ease their burden by sharing it with anyone: the company of others is the source of the problem. This phobia usually begins in the teenage years.

III   CHRONIC ANXIETY DISORDERS

There are two forms of chronic anxiety: general anxiety disorder (GAD)and obsessive compulsive disorder (OCD).

1   GENERAL ANXIETY DISORDER

While we may find it relaxing to watch ducks gliding serenely across a pond, we fail to see the frantic paddling that is taking place beneath the surface. When we observe a GAD sufferer, we can be fooled by their calm temperament and fail to notice the panic they are feeling underneath. GAD sufferers may experience feelings of intense anxiety, foreboding and excessive worry about their health, their family and their job, and often have a sense of impending disaster. This illness is associated with other symptoms, such as:

§   Mental and physical fatigue

§   Poor concentration

§   Mind going blank in common social and domestic situations

§   Difficulties with memory

§   Restlessness

§   Sleep difficulties, and nightmares

§   Indecisiveness

§   Regularly avoiding situations in everyday life due to fatigue and worrying about their ability to cope

The sufferer is also very vulnerable to bouts of acute anxiety, with the following physical symptoms:

§   Tension headaches

§   Constant sighing

§   Palpitations

§   Stomach cramps and disturbance

§   Loss of appetite, with associated weight loss

Severe stress, particularly in relation to loss or major health or financial concerns, will lead to bouts of extreme inner anxiety. In such cases, all of the normal symptoms of GAD are magnified, with the person becoming quickly exhausted.

Many people with general anxiety disorder (who are often perfectionists) learn to conceal their condition well, to the extent that even close friends and loved ones may not be aware of the problem, or the degree to which the person is struggling with their daily life. The sufferer may not even realise they are suffering from anxiety. They will, however, identify the fatigue and the difficulties in concentration, among other symptoms.

People who suffer from GAD will go through periods where they cope reasonably well. Any form of sustained stress will bring their mood system down again, however. During these periods, their apprehension and worrying will intensify, they will feel fatigued, and they will experience difficulties concentrating and sleeping. Often people reach the conclusion that they are simply not coping, or are stressed out.

Two-thirds of those who suffer from GAD will also suffer at least one bout of the Red Flag of depression at least once in their lives. Many use alcohol as an escape from the inner turmoil and intensity they experience – with the obvious associated problems. The condition can present at any stage of life but most often appears first in the mid teens and early adulthood. Women are twice as likely to suffer from this disorder as much as men. The illness often remains unrecognised and undiagnosed until the person is in their thirties or forties, particularly in women. As the stresses in life start to take their toll, the person, if untreated, may find the symptoms worsening with age. This deterioration will usually continue for life until help is sought.

2   OBSESSIVE COMPULSIVE DISORDER

This form of anxiety has become increasingly recognised in the past ten years and it is now regarded as a separate illness, unique from the other forms of anxiety. OCD results in constant unwanted irrational and obsessive thoughts, accompanied by compulsive actions to satisfy the urges these thoughts are producing. These incessant thoughts and compulsions (which the person often tries to suppress or avoid) will cause major interference with the person's family and working relationships, not to mention their own psychological state. The obsessive thoughts use up the person's mental energy by causing extreme feelings of anxiety. The resulting tension is only relieved by 'doing what the thoughts demand', but this is incredibly tiring, as the thoughts are never-ending. Such obsessive thoughts may relate to:

§ Fears about health, particularly personal health

§ Fears of contaminating themselves

§ Fears of harming themselves

§ Sexual and religious obsessions

§ Constant fears that something terrible is going to happen

Examples of compulsive actions are:

§ Cleaning

§ Checking

§ Counting

§ Repeating

§ Arranging

What separates a person with OCD from someone who is simply very neat, or a 'clean freak', is repetition. They will check the light switch, or the lock on the front door, three or four, or even up to ten or more, times in a row, knowing full well that the situation has not changed since they last checked, but feeling an overpowering urge to check again anyway. They experience a sense of relief and security when they re-check something, but this is only temporary, and the urge returns again. Paradoxically, the more they check something, the stronger the urge to check it again becomes. It is like an addiction, where carrying out the act reduces the cravings for a while, but in the long run intensifies them.

The condition usually starts in the young adult, but many experts believe that, due to lack of knowledge or awareness of the condition, its existence may go unrecognised for up to ten years before diagnosis. The pattern of this illness can be very difficult, both for the person themselves and also for those who live with them. The individual usually faces a lifelong battle with their obsessive thoughts and compulsive behaviour. Men with OCD will usually start to act compulsively earlier in their teens, and women may present with the condition much later. Men tend to worry more about checking things, and women more about cleanliness. There are powerful biological causes of this behaviour. Sufferers usually have an above-average IQ.

People who have lived with an OCD sufferer often find it impossible to get through to them emotionally, so relationships within this group are regularly troubled. The constant battle with obsessive thoughts and acts causes exhaustion on the part of the sufferer or those close to them, as it take up a great deal of their time and energy. They know that their behaviour is stupid and irrational but are powerless to stop it.

The fear is that the Yellow Flag may turn into the Red Flag of depression. Some estimate that up to a third of those with OCD will experience a major bout of depression in their lifetime.

III   BIOLOGY OF THE YELLOW FLAG

What is the difference between stress and anxiety? With stress, the threat is immediate, whether it is acute (such as sitting an important exam) or chronic (dealing with financial problems due to unemployment). In anxiety, however, the body's internal stress system is constantly activated, despite the lack of an external threat. Since stress is a response to an actual external event, and anxiety is a response to an internal, imagined one, the fear that fuels anxiety can be constant and potentially long-lasting. Anxiety is the result of the emotional brain or mind taking over control from the logical brain. It is the power of the former that makes the condition so hard to treat.

The stress box in the limbic mood department (the emotional brain) controls the stress response and acts as a storage area for the emotions associated with bad memories, thereby helping to produce negative thoughts. We have already seen how, under normal conditions, the flow of information from the stress box to the behaviour box is much greater than the reverse. So emotions such as fear will always tend to overrule our logical brain. When the stress box becomes hyper-stimulated, trouble will inevitably loom.

Over-activity of the stress box is present in most anxiety disorders. A combination of genetic and early environmental factors causes subtle changes in this box, making it hyper-sensitive from the early to mid teens onwards. It is not only the stress box that is involved in anxiety, however: the rest of the mood system also plays a part.

(A)   Mood Departments

1   THE FRONTAL MOOD DEPARTMENT

FIGURE 1: THE FRONTAL MOOD DEPARTMENT

The behaviour box plays a role in sometimes inadvertently triggering the stress box to over-act, and in other cases failing to shut off inappropriate responses from the latter.

2   THE LIMBIC MOOD DEPARTMENT

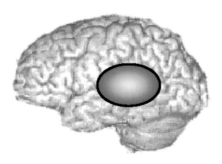

FIGURE 2: THE LIMBIC MOOD DEPARTMENT

In anxiety, the stress box incorrectly activates the whole stress system. It sends instructions to the adrenal gland, activating it. Over-activity in this box leads to the irrational fears and worries seen in some forms of anxiety.

3   THE ADRENAL GLAND

FIGURE 3: THE ADRENAL GLAND

In acute anxiety, the adrenal glands release adrenalin and noradrenalin in response to instructions from the stress box. When elevated, these produce the following symptoms:

§   Dry mouth

§   Profuse sweating

§   Headaches

§   Hyperventilation

§   Stomach upset

§   Palpitations

In chronic anxiety, the adrenal glands release glucocortisol.

4   GLUCOCORTISOL

FIGURE 4: GLUCOCORTISOL

This works with the stress box to produce the symptoms of chronic anxiety. When levels of glucocortisol are elevated, the person will experience some or all of the following symptoms:

§ Fatigue

§ Poor concentration

§ Difficulties with memory

§ Sleep problems

§ Anhedonia (inability to experience pleasure)

B MOOD CABLES

The two main cables activated by anxiety are the noradrenalin and serotonin cables. The noradrenalin cable is highly active in bouts of acute anxiety but may eventually become depleted in chronic anxiety, leading to fatigue and poor concentration. The serotonin cable is under-active in some cases of chronic anxiety.

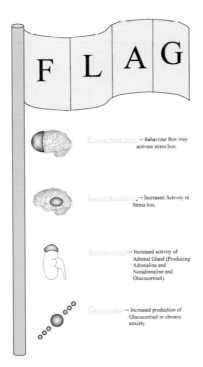

FIGURE 5

When all this knowledge is compiled, a model of anxiety can be formed (see Figure 6):

§ The behaviour box mistakenly activates the stress box.

§ The stress box, which is already predisposed to be hyperactive, completely over-reacts.

§ This causes the stress peptides to flood the brain and activates the noradrenalin cable.

§ It also causes the adrenal gland to pour out noradrenalin, adrenalin and gluco-cortisol.

§ In acute anxiety, this gland mainly releases noradrenalin and adrenalin.

§ In chronic anxiety, it mainly releases glucocortisol.

Most of the symptoms of anxiety are caused by the above mechanisms.

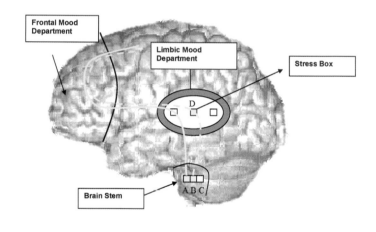

	A: Serotonin Cable → Reduced Activity
	B: Noradrenaline Cable → Increased Activity in acute anxiety but may become depleted in chronic anxiety.
☐	D: Stress Box – Increased activity.

FIGURE 6: THE MOOD CABLES IN ANXIETY

1   ACUTE ANXIETY DISORDERS

In phobias and panic attacks, the body's stress response is called upon by the stress box. The stress peptides and noradrenalin mood cable activate, and the adrenal glands release copious amounts of adrenalin and noradrenalin. The latter gives rise to symptoms that may include sweating, dry mouth, palpitations and weakness. This combination leads to the commonly expressed statement: 'I thought I was going to die!' When this activity recedes, the body disposes of the excess adrenalin and noradrenalin, and the system returns to normal.

If this is the case, what causes the 'fear of fears' that is evident in panic disorders? This is where a person remains constantly on high alert, fearing another panic attack. The memory box is the most likely culprit here, coordinating with the stress box to keep the fear of fear alive.

2   CHRONIC ANXIETY DISORDERS

In GAD, there is continuous stimulation of the stress box, adrenal glands and noradrenalin mood cable, and a constant flow of stress peptides and glucocortisol. All of these factors result in fatigue, poor concentration, difficulties with memory, sleep problems and other symptoms that have already been mentioned.

Constant worrying and a feeling of impending doom originate from the stress box, where negative memories are stored. In GAD, the stress box replays these memories over and over and projects them on to the future. Normally, this is prevented by the behaviour box, but in GAD the stress box runs amok.

OCD is a unique illness because it is biologically distinct from the other anxiety disorders. There are operational difficulties between parts of the frontal mood department and other sections of the brain. The secondary stress symptoms of OCD are mediated through the stress system, but the source of the illness is completely different.

SUMMARY

Anxiety can cause the following problems in the mood system:

1   Over-activity of the stress box in the limbic mood department (see Figure 2 on page 167). This leads to worrying, apprehension and a sense of impending doom.

2   Disruption of the noradrenalin mood cable (see Figure 5 on page 169). This results in poor concentration and fatigue.

3   Over-stimulation of the adrenal stress gland, leading to an excess of adrenalin, noradrenalin and glucocortisol in the body. This causes the palpitations, hyperventilation, sweating, dry mouth and stomach cramps often seen in acute anxiety, and the fatigue and poor concentration seen in chronic anxiety.

2

CAUSES OF ANXIETY DISORDERS

Scientific research over the past two decades has identified major anxiety as an illness rather than a personality trait. Genes, upbringing and environmental factors all contribute to the development of this illness. The biological model suggests that the stress box, through a combination of genetic predispositions and environmental factors, malfunctions when it is put under stress. It becomes hypersensitive to any stimulation, and this results in the symptoms of anxiety. This model is corroborated by psychological research, which suggests that many anxiety illnesses begin with difficulties or major stress periods in childhood. Genetic vulnerability to such stress periods during development may be a crucial factor. The final result is a stress box that is predisposed to hyperactivity in the presence of even apparently innocuous stress triggers. What follows is an assessment of the genetic and environmental influences on the development of these illnesses:

1   *Panic attacks and phobias* There is a moderate genetic component to these illnesses, particularly for panic attacks. Environmental factors also contribute.

2   *GAD* There is a moderate genetic vulnerability. (Almost 20 percent of first-degree relatives of people with GAD also have the condition, compared with 3 to 4 percent of those who do not.) It also seems that GAD and unipolar depression share similar neurological mechanisms. Why one person with such a vulnerability develops GAD and another develops depression is not known. Once again, environment plays a crucial role.

3   *OCD* There is a moderate genetic vulnerability. Environmental triggers also play a role.

ENVIRONMENTAL FACTORS

Recent neurological research into anxiety supports observations by psychologists that people at a certain time in their upbringing experience some major stress or loss which seems to act on susceptible genes to change the way in which their stress box and its pathways will respond in the person's adult life. By the time the person reaches their mid-teens or early twenties, their stress system is predisposed to malfunction, forging a lifelong battle with anxiety. What are these early stress triggers? They include:

§ Loss of a parent or sibling at a crucial stage of development as a child or adolescent

§ Emotional, physical or sexual abuse

§ Being reared in an authoritarian household

§ Coming from an addictive parental background

§ A major trauma in the life of the developing child

§ A very stressful or frightening episode at a vulnerable stage of development

3

TREATMENTS FOR ANXIETY DISORDERS

Many of the treatment options suitable for depression are also suitable for anxiety. Bouts of depression may last between six and twelve months, whereas anxiety disorders, if untreated, may be present for life. Treatment options for anxiety include:

1   *Exercise* This tackles many of the symptoms of anxiety. The chemicals it releases calm the stress box, aid memory and concentration, reduces the effects of external stress influences, and generally encourage the person to take a more positive approach to life.

2   *Diet* Many people with anxiety will go through periods of not eating properly. It is very important to have a healthy, balanced diet. Caffeine and other stimulant-rich drinks should be avoided, as they promote anxiety by activating the stress system. GAD sufferers can become dependent on caffeine to alleviate the symptoms of fatigue. This is counterproductive, as it will interfere further with sleep and increase anxiety, both of which will in turn increase fatigue.

3   *Supplements* Omega 3 fish oils in particular may help to alleviate some of the symptoms of chronic anxiety, particularly fatigue.

4   *Counselling* This is helpful in dealing with outside stress factors (rather than with anxiety itself), especially relationship problems, bereavement and addiction problems.

5   *Psychological therapies* The psychologist is the expert when it comes to dealing with anxiety disorders. Nowadays, many counsellors and psychiatric nurses are also trained in CBT techniques, as are an increasing number of family doctors.

The following therapies psychological therapies are commonly used:

(a)   *CBT* In the section on the Red Flag, we dealt with the various types of CBT, its neurobiological impact and its role in treating depression. CBT is also extremely useful in helping people to overcome panic attacks and deal with their phobias, and in reducing the symptoms of GAD. Here, the person's thinking and behaviour, both of which are negative and fearful, are challenged, and new coping skills are introduced.

CBT can be of enormous help in dealing with panic attacks in particular, often banishing them for good after a few sessions. At the end of this section, I include simple but very effective advice on how you can get rid of panic attacks for good using simple CBT techniques.

(b) *Relaxation exercises* Relaxation of both body and mind are of great help in dealing with anxiety. If people can consciously ignore their stress system by relaxing their body and mind, they break the cycle of stress and worry, take back control of their lives and are better able to deal with acute anxiety and GAD.

(c) *Psychotherapy* This seems to be the least effective psychological means of helping people to cope with anxiety. For some whose anxiety is rooted in a traumatic past, however, it may be of great help.

Before we leave this section, let's look at how CBT can help in preventing panic attacks. Before looking at such techniques, we must once again separate the role of the emotional brain or mind (the limbic system) from the logical brain or mind (the frontal cortex). The former often exerts a dominant effect over the latter. Let's look at some simple examples:

1   Imagine that you are walking down a dark alley which is poorly lit. You suddenly hear a loud noise. You instantly freeze, your heart starts to race, you feel goose pimples all over, your mouth goes dry, your stomach churns, and you rapidly turn to face the source of the noise. Then, out of the darkness springs a cat, and you start to relax, as you have logically located the cause of the noise.

The emotional brain was the first to respond to the sound. Without thinking, the stress system swung into action, and the logical brain took over later. This happens biologically because, if danger is sensed, the brain alerts the stress box first, so that we react instinctively, before identifying the source of the threat logically, through other pathways.

As we continue up the dark alley, even though we logically know that the cause of the sound was a cat, most of us will stay in a state of high alert, instinctively quickening our pace and look into shadowy areas despite ourselves. In short, we are unable to shake off our sense of unease until we reach the apparent safety of a well-lit area. All of this happens because our emotional mind overpowers our logical one. We know that there is no danger but cannot stop our emotions from taking over.

2   If I tell you: 'Close your eyes and don't think about bird droppings landing on your hair and face' despite your every effort to stop this image coming into your mind, your emotional brain will take over and you will be unable to do so. Once again, the emotional brain overrules the commands of the logical brain or mind.

3   Imagine your favourite football team being beaten by a last-minute goal. You will feel completely devastated. Although logically it makes no difference whether the goal was scored in the first or last minute of the game, the latter scenario makes us feel most upset. Once again, our emotional rather than our logical mind is in charge.

This is not to denigrate the importance of the emotional side of our lives. Life without emotion would be a colourless, drab place. Indeed, all of us constantly switch between the logical and the emotional during our daily lives: a healthy balance between both is vital. With these general concepts in mind, let's move on to examine in more detail what happens during a panic attack, and ways of dealing with them.

Let's imagine three different scenarios where a panic attack begins. In the first, we are sitting at home watching TV; in the second, we are in the middle of a busy office meeting; in the third, we are in the middle of a busy supermarket about to start the weekly shop. Although all three situations are different, the pattern of how the panic attack begins and progresses is quite similar.

§   *Stage One* We begin to feel the first symptoms of anxiety developing. We start to notice our heart pounding and our breathing becoming faster; we may start sweating and begin to feel weak. There is usually no obvious cause for this anxiety, but it acts as the initial trigger for the attack.

§   *Stage Two* Because there is no logical cause for the appearance of these symptoms, the person begins to assume that there must be a serious reason for how they feel. They may imagine that they are in the process of developing a major medical disaster, such as a heart attack or stroke, or that they are about to collapse and die. They may also become embarrassed that they are going crazy, or that those around them will see the state they are in.

§   *Stage Three* The feelings above further increase the anxiety symptoms, creating a desire to get rid of the cause of these feelings – namely anxiety, the initial trigger.

§   *Stage Four* This causes anxiety levels to rise further, by activating the body's internal stress system and finally kick-starting a full-blown panic attack. Here the heart races, we feel weak and faint, our stomach churns, we find it hard to breathe, and we experience an overwhelming sense of doom and disaster. The natural length of time it takes for the body to stop this panic episode is twenty minutes. If we did nothing at all, the attack would settle down and everything would return to normal.

§   *Stage Five* The real problem occurs when our natural sense of worry and desire to bring the attack to an end leads to so-called 'avoidant behaviour'. Common examples are using tranquillizers or alcohol; rushing off to the nearest A&E department, usually at the prompting of a well-meaning relative, friend or member of the public; trying hard to control our breathing during a panic attack; or running away

176

from the site where the attack occurred. If such avoidant behaviour is undertaken, the panic attack may last for several hours.

The key to all of the above is that the emotional brain or mind is ruling the roost. Our more logical brain has been silenced. In order to defeat panic attacks, we now have to put the latter back in charge.

Firstly, we have to eliminate all avoidant behaviour. The enemy must be faced head-on: running away merely prolongs the problem.

Secondly, we must never try to stop a panic attack when it is in progress, rather go with the flow (swim with the current rather than against it) and wait for it to settle naturally (as it always will) within about twenty minutes. The key to doing this is to accept that these symptoms, although unpleasant, will never do us any real harm. As I often say to patients: 'Emotions can sometimes be uncomfortable, but they are not dangerous'. Rather than trying to stop them, we should actually try to bring them on so that the problem can be addressed. Surprisingly, it is quite difficult to do this.

Thirdly, and most importantly, we have to return to Stage Two above. We have to start challenging the false perception that the physical feelings (such as palpitations and sweating) brought on by the initial symptoms of anxiety are indeed the precursor to something more serious happening. Although my heart is racing, have I ever had a heart attack during a panic episode? Of course the answer is no. Although I may feel as though I am going to collapse and die, has this ever happened? Once again, the answer is obviously no! Just because my breathing becomes shallow and fast, have I ever stopped breathing? The answer is once again no.

This is the key to eliminating panic attacks for good. If we learn to accept these feelings of anxiety as being a nuisance but not dangerous, then we stop becoming so anxious to get rid of them and start to dismiss them. This, in turn, reduces the build-up of anxiety that is necessary to trigger a full-blown panic episode. When our logical mind/brain regains control in this way, panic attacks become a thing of the past.

To summarise, in order to eliminate panic attacks, we must firstly stop all avoidant behaviour, never try to stop an episode if it does occur, and finally, and most importantly, logically challenge and remove once and for all the concept that the initial anxiety symptoms which can trigger an attack are in any way dangerous to our health physically or mentally. This all sounds too easy, but in practice it works amazingly well. Try it and see!

One final note of caution: sometimes panic attacks may be associated with other conditions, such as depression, alcohol/substance abuse, or general anxiety. Be honest with yourself. If you feel that any of these are present, go and have a chat with your family doctor. He will assess your symptoms and suggest further help. If you are unsure, reading the chapters on the various flags should clarify the situation. In general, the first step is always to deal with the panic attacks and then to move on to treating the accompanying illness.

If you continue to have difficulties with panic attacks, you should ask your family doctor for help. If he has the necessary skills, he may be able to help; if not, he can refer you to a cognitive therapist. For most people, if they apply the above simple principles their panic attacks will become a thing of the past.

VI   DRUG TREATMENT

Drug treatment has a place in treatment of the Yellow Flag, but most experts feel that it should only be used in conjunction with all the other treatment options. If combined with CBT and relaxation exercises, drug treatment can be of great help. In the past, however, the use of anxiolytic drugs (medications such as tranquillizers, used to calm down the symptoms of anxiety) did more harm than good.

TRANQUILLIZERS

These drugs combat anxiety by using the GABA receptors to relax the stress box: in effect, they force the brain to relax and stop worrying. They rapidly reduce all symptoms, and this makes them popular with anxiety sufferers.

The main group of these drugs are the Benzodiazepams. They were initially heralded as a revolution in the treatment and understanding of anxiety disorders in the late 1960s and early 1970s. They were potent annihilators of the acute anxiety symptoms seen in panic attacks, and allowed people with GAD to live without constant worry and fear.

They worked a little too well, however. The feelings of relaxation and pleasure induced by them created a generation of Valium, Librium, Xanax and Lexotane addicts. Tolerance to these drugs develops quickly and, as with any addictive substance, doctors had to keep increasing the dose to achieve the same effect. As doctors tried to wean patients off their addiction, the symptoms of anxiety were replaced by more serious physical and psychological problems. They also cause drowsiness and impair concentration. The drugs are very attractive to alcoholics and drug addicts.

As a result, the cure for anxiety ended up becoming a substance of widespread misuse and abuse. To this day, doctors still have certain patients whoare addicted to these drugs, and have been for decades. A further complication is that sudden withdrawal of these drugs in such people may lead to convulsions.

Nowadays, drugs such as Xanax and Lexotane are used by doctors on a very restricted basis. If used correctly for short periods, while other forms of treatment are being utilised, they can be very helpful. A simple example of their correct use might be in helping those with a fear of flying – although the CBT exercises mentioned for dealing with panic attacks could also be applied here. In short, these drugs are still useful, but the way in which they are prescribed must be carefully monitored, and their use stopped as soon as possible.

BUSPAR

This drug claims to have all of the positive and none of the negative effects of the aforementioned drugs in terms of dealing with GAD. It is not useful in acute anxiety, however. It stimulates one specific serotonin receptor in the stress box and takes about four weeks to start working; this sometimes makes it an unpopular choice among anxiety sufferers.

Its great advantages are the lack of any side effects or potential for abuse. Its main weakness is its inability to treat any associated depression, and the initial delay before it starts to take effect. This drug, when combined with CBT, relaxation exercises and exercise, can help some people who suffer from this illness. Since the arrival of the SSRIs, it is not used a great deal. It is still, however, a very useful drug in the treatment of GAD.

ANTIDEPRESSANTS

The genetic and biological pathways of depression and GAD are quite similar. It is therefore not surprising that antidepressants have been found to be of help in both acute and chronic anxiety.

The main drugs used nowadays are the SSRIs. These drugs have all been shown to decrease anxiety. When activity is increased in the serotonin mood cable by these drugs, the stress box and stress pathways are calmed. In practice, they are used regularly for short periods, together with CBT, to deal with panic disorders. They are also used in some cases of GAD and OCD for longer periods, sometimes for life.

In the case of long-term treatment, there is the issue of side effects, particularly sexual ones. As a result, psychological treatment should always be seriously considered in such cases, to try to reduce the need for such drugs. If drug treatment is considered to be essential, then Buspar might be a more attractive option.

VII   COMPLEMENTARY THERAPIES

Several complementary therapies can be very helpful in the treatment of anxiety disorders, as part of an overall treatment package. These include massage, meditation, yoga, pilates, reflexology and certain herbal treatments. Relaxation therapies such as yoga and meditation can be beneficial in calming the mind and body – something which is obviously particularly important in the area of anxiety.

Biologically, they seem to work by calming the stress box, and thus reducing level of glucocortisol. As certain anxiety disorders, such as GAD, can last a lifetime, it i especially important that the person look holistically at their own treatment an lifestyle. Those who suffer from such illnesses also need to learn to manage the stres in their lives more efficiently.

VIII COMMON QUESTIONS ABOUT THE YELLOW FLAG

Why treat it at all?

People who suffer from these illnesses dread getting up in the morning to face th world. Those with acute anxiety constantly fear another attack, and have difficulty deal ing with these attacks when they arrive. Those with GAD will suffer from constan apprehension and worry. They will also struggle with fatigue, poor memory and con centration, and sleep difficulties, all interspersed with bouts of acute anxiety. Many liv lives of quiet despair, always feeling a failure, unable to cope with any stress, and get ting over one worry only to be faced immediately with another.

If untreated, many people with GAD will struggle to hold down jobs or may us alcohol as an escape, with negative consequences. They will sometimes misuse tranquil lizers or alcohol in order to cope and will always remain at risk of developing a bout o depression at some stage in their lives, particularly after a period of severe stress Similarly with OCD, many who do not get help are strangled in their attempts to lea normal lives. Obsessive thoughts and actions become their lives, and everything else i secondary: the actions must be carried out first. Once again, their ability to form an maintain relationships, hold down jobs and cope with stress is severely compromised.

Another practical reason for treating anxiety when it is combined with stress is tha it affects the general health of the body. We have talked earlier about the effects o acute stress on blood pressure and the heart. We have also looked at the effects o chronic stress on heart disease and osteoporosis. GAD, as it follows the same pathway as chronic stress, may also lead to similar increased risks and, especially in the presenc of outside stress, may lead to the immune system itself becoming impaired. This make it more likely that, if the condition goes untreated, people with GAD may suffer from more viral and bacterial illnesses than other people.

How long will treatment last?

Assuming that the usual lifestyle changes, such as revising diet, taking exercise and sup- plements, and avoiding misuse of alcohol and caffeine have been looked at, the usua treatment package may involve drug or psychological therapy, or both. The length o treatment will depend on the type of anxiety disorder and its severity:

(a) *Acute anxiety* Panic disorders and phobias can be treated in most cases with six to twelve sessions of CBT. The former can sometimes be handled with as little as two to three sessions, particularly if the disorder in question is uncomplicated. Drug treatment in the form of tranquillizers should never continue for longer than the course of CBT, due to the risk of developing dependence.

(b) *Chronic anxiety* GAD is a lifelong illness. Relaxation exercises and CBT with a therapist can lead to a definite reduction in symptoms, however. The length of time for this treatment will vary depending on the severity of the condition.

If drugs are used, particularly the SSRIs, there is usually a trade-off between side effects, particularly sexual ones, and the efficacy of the drugs over a long period of time. Ideally, drug treatment should be combined with the above psychological therapies and withdrawn, if at all possible, when such therapies start to yield results.

In OCD, treatment in sufferers may continue for life. The use of drug treatment, particularly SSRIs, and cognitive therapy will vary from person to person, depending on the severity of the illness.

What are the side effects of treatment?

The side effects of the SSRIs have been dealt with in the Red Flag. The tranquillizers may cause drowsiness and impaired concentration and should only be used for short periods. If long-term drug treatment is necessary, it is better to switch to an SSRI or Buspar. Psychological treatment carries few risks when performed by a trained psychologist or therapist. If, however, a person is complaining of severe fatigue and memory loss, it may be better to use an SSRI first to try to restore normal mood, energy and behaviour before therapy can be really effective.

What will happen when I go to the doctor?

Many people worry that their family doctor will be dismissive and condescending when they admit to their irrational fears. This prevents many people from getting the help they need. Instead, just tell him how you feel. This will allow him to assess you, both physically and mentally. He will ask you a number of questions to clarify which type of anxiety disorder you may be suffering from. Sometimes, he may feel that the symptoms are more to do with stress than anxiety, and will discuss methods of dealing with this.

If he is satisfied with the diagnosis, he will firstly discuss with you the various lifestyle changes detailed above. He may also recommend a referral to a psychologist or trained CBT therapist, if one is available, or to a psychiatrist with CBT training. If appropriate, he may recommend drug treatment.

In general, acute anxiety is best dealt with by the psychologist or CBT therapist, and chronic anxiety through a combination of psychological therapy and drug therapy, to combat the symptoms of severe fatigue and poor concentration associated with severe panic attacks.

Above all, remember that the Yellow Flag of anxiety is an illness, not a weakness or a personality defect. You are neither mad nor insane. Quite the opposite, in fact: many people with these illnesses are often very sensitive and intuitive people. Your condition was created by an interaction between your genes and early environmental influences; you did not bring this upon yourself, and treatment is readily available.

IV

THE PURPLE FLAG

ADDICTION

1

THE CAUSES, SYMPTOMS AND BIOLOGY OF ADDICTION

The ability to feel pleasure motivates us to live a full and active life. Going for a drink, eating out in a restaurant, having sex, and placing a bet on the races are all examples of normal enjoyable activities. Despite the variety of pleasurable activities available to us, the stimulation of a single mood cable makes them all 'pleasurable'. When one constantly engages in any one of these activities to the detriment of everything else in one's life, however, the outcome ceases to be pleasurable. Eating to excess results in obesity, and drinking alcohol in excess gives rise to violence, vomiting and sometimes poisoning. In fact, the use of any drug in large quantities gives rise to a range of family, social and personal problems.

When a person feels compelled to engage constantly in a certain activity, to the neglect of everything else in their life, they can be said to be suffering from addiction. This is the term used to describe a physical or psychological dependence on either a substance or an activity; it is a worldwide problem.

Research carried out over the last five years has revealed a dramatic change in the understanding of what is happening in the body when a person is addicted. This research is badly needed, as the cost of addiction is borne not just by the medical services but by the families of addicts as well.

This chapter explains addiction, the biological factors associated with it, and the treatment methods that are available. The following chapter will focus on specific areas of addiction, which include alcohol, nicotine, gambling, drugs and food.

I   THE UBIQUITOUS ADDICTIONS

Smoking and alcohol are the most common addictions. Smoking in particular is highly addictive; the habit is usually begun in the mid teens. Alcohol, a depressant drug, is consumed to excess by many people, but about 10 percent of adult male and 5 percent of female drinkers will develop a serious dependence on it. Gambling is a hidden but prevalent addiction that is not as obvious as the first two.

The next most common addiction is drug addiction. This can take many forms. Some drugs, such as amphetamines, ecstasy and cocaine, are stimulatory; others, such as tranquillizers and cannabis, are depressants. Hallucinogens include LSD and magic mushrooms. Finally, there are the opiates, such as heroin. While drug use is fairly common among people in the fifteen-to-thirty-five age group, the actual number of addicts is not as high as the media would lead us to believe. Dublin city is a good example of this. There are approximately ten thousand heroin addicts living in Dublin. As this group is responsible for a great of crime, and is quite noticeable because many heroin addicts are homeless, it is understandable that it receives most of our attention. The problems associated with illegal drug use pale in comparison to the misery and social problems caused by alcohol in Ireland, however. Prescription drugs like Valium and sleeping tablets are also a major source of abuse, food addiction is widely under-recognised, and other forms of addiction, including shopping addiction, computer-games addiction and sex addiction, are also serious problems.

Two concepts that are commonly used when discussing addiction are tolerance and dependency. Tolerance refers to the diminishing pleasure derived from a substance through its constant use. (The corollary of this is the necessity to increase usage to maintain the pleasurable feelings.) Dependency relates to the unpleasant physical and psychological effects experienced when the drug or activity is withdrawn.

An interesting feature of addiction is that many addicts have more than one vice. This is known as cross addiction. Examples of this are an alcoholic who smokes, a gambler who drinks excessively, or an alcoholic who is addicted to prescription drugs. Addicts may succeed in stopping one addiction, only to switch to another (e.g. they stop drinking and start using tranquillizers instead). Many people who try to stop abusing alcohol will start to smoke even more. Even food addiction is often used as a substitute for alcohol or nicotine addiction. There is a biological explanation for this: all of these activities share the same brain pathways.

2   THE SYMPTOMS OF ADDICTION

Despite the diversity of addictions, the symptoms of addiction are fairly universal. Firstly, the substance being abused will be more important to an addict than anything else in their lives, be it family, friends or work. Secondly, they are usually fine as long as their addiction is being fed. If they are deprived of the substance or activity, they suffer physical (sweating, vomiting and tremors) and psychological (tension, anxiety, depression and suicidal tendencies) effects. The longer they engage in their addiction, the more they need to consume just to feel normal, let alone feel good. As a result, their addiction starts to take over their lives: unless they do it all the time, they feel terrible. Lastly, addiction damages the physical well-being of its victims, resulting in illnesses of he heart, lungs, liver and brain, and psychiatric illnesses such as anxiety, depression and chizophrenia.

3   THE BIOLOGY OF ADDICTION

All addicts behave in a similar manner, and this fact is known to any health profession-al working in the field. It is therefore little surprise that the latest research reveals that all addiction behaves in a similar biological manner.

One of the main boxes in the limbic-mood department is the pleasure box (see Figure 1). It has been known for years that the dopamine mood cable is involved in the process by which we experience pleasure. During normal activities such as eating, hav-ing sex, drinking and taking part in a sporting activity, the dopamine cable activates, as does the pleasure box itself (see Figure 2). Without this activation, our capacity to enjoy the good things in life would be seriously compromised. So from this point of view, the activation of the dopamine cable is vital.

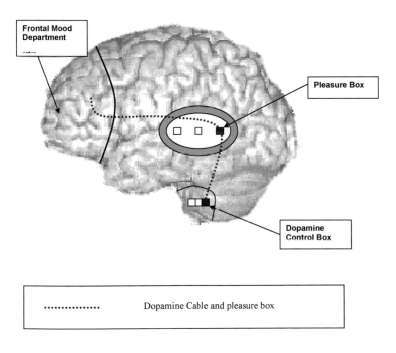

FIGURE 1: THE DOPAMINE CABLE AND PLEASURE BOX

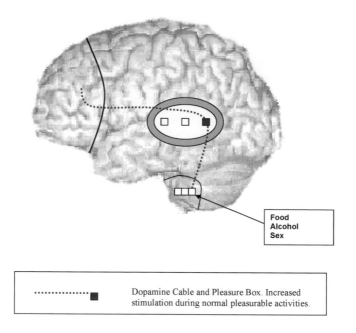

FIGURE 2: NORMAL STIMULATION OF THE DOPAMINE CABLE AND PLEASURE BOX

We as humans have for millennia found ways of artificially stimulating this cable to produce profound pleasure, however. To achieve this, some people misuse alcohol and other related substances; others may begin to gamble, shop, overeat or play computer games to an excessive degree. In those who are genetically or environmentally at risk of addiction, however, this persistent hyper-stimulation of the dopamine cable starts to cause subtle chemical and molecular changes in the neurons which make up the pleasure box.

When the person becomes seriously addicted, these changes become more permanent (see Figure 3 and 4). These aberrations cause the addict to crave the substance and become dependent on it. They also require the addict to use more and more of the substance in order to achieve satisfaction.

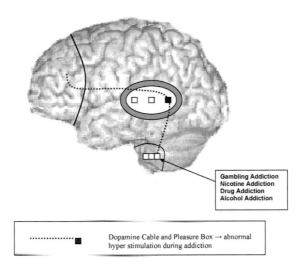

FIGURE 3: THE EFFECTS OF ADDICTION ON THE DOPAMINE CABLE AND PLEASURE BOX

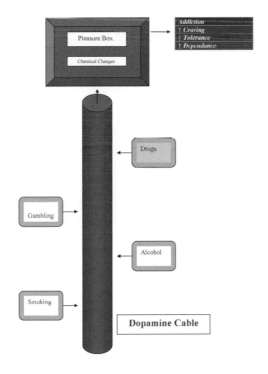

FIGURE 4: THE 'ADDICTION PATHWAY'

The biological composite of addiction is explained in the Purple Flag model below (see Figure 5). Purple is the colour of debauchery, which is why I have chosen it to depict addiction. Those who would like to know more about the chemical changes seen in addiction should go to Appendix 1 at the end of the book.

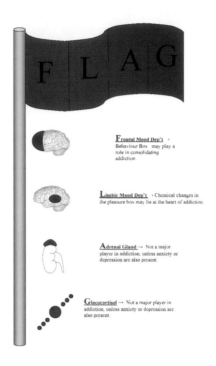

Frontal Mood Dep't ›
Behaviour Box may play a
role in consolidating
addiction.

Limbic Mood Dep't › Chemical changes in
the pleasure box may lie at the heart of addiction.

Adrenal Gland → Not a major
player in addiction, unless anxiety or
depression are also present.

Glucocortisol → Not a major player in
addiction, unless anxiety or depression are
also present.

FIGURE 5

Although the other mood cables (particularly the serotonin cable) and departments may be directly affected by alcohol and other drugs, it is the excessive stimulation of the dopamine cable and changes to the pleasure box which create the illness that is addiction. Experts are also looking at the so-called 'reward circuit' between the stress, behaviour and pleasure boxes (a part of the mood circuit we dealt with earlier) as being crucial in relation to the behaviour patterns related to this illness.

The chemical changes which cause the malfunctions in the pleasure box are the same for all addictions. This is a very exciting discovery, as it may lead in the future to the development of drugs that are capable of treating all forms of addiction. Once again, understanding the biology of our flag system may lead to a re-evaluation to how we treat addiction. Unfortunately, it may take many years to reach this point. For the present, turning the Purple Flag of addiction back to green is probably the most diffi-cult challenge of all.

4   COURSE OF THE PURPLE FLAG

Many addictions, like smoking, alcohol and illegal drugs, begin in the teenage years and early twenties. The process of becoming an addict usually takes a substantial period of time. Alcoholics generally take the longest to develop a problem – often after gradual increased drinking over a period of years. This fact should not go unnoticed as there is a time window present in such cases, which makes early intervention particularly impor-tant.

Drug addicts are more variable in the time it takes to develop a serious habit, and this can depend on the drug involved. Cocaine can be addictive from the first adminis-tration. Most addicts' lives involve periods where they feed their addiction, with paus-es in between. During these pauses, the addict will be restless, will have difficulty sleep-ing, and may even suffer periods of low mood. Again, depending on the substance involved, the length of these time periods last is highly variable.

Addiction is usually a lifelong illness. With assistance, some will be able to restrain their addictive urges and live a normal life. Although it may be controversial to say so, biologically speaking these people are still addicts – they have just learned how to man-age their illness.

The life of many addicts involves recurring bouts of addiction, which can destroy their health and their relationships. Some will die from the direct effects of the addic-tion on their physical health, and others from the White Flag of suicide. Most will live in unhappiness and loneliness until they reach a point where they seek help from the medical profession, addiction counsellors and their fellow addicts. The addict justifies their actions and delays facing the problem with the mantra: 'I will stop tomorrow'. Unfortunately, for many, tomorrow never comes.

5   CAUSES OF THE PURPLE FLAG

Addiction is now seen by most experts as being caused by a mixture of genetic and environmental factors. Many people can take drugs and alcohol, and in excessive amounts, without becoming addicted. Finding out why this is so is crucial to the under-standing and treatment of the illness.

I   GENETIC PREDISPOSITION

Although no specific gene has been associated with addiction, many studies suggest that it has a genetic component. Genetic vulnerability varies from person to person and in most cases is polygenetic in type. Even in the case of alcoholics, there are at least two subsets with a different genetic susceptibility in each.

There are two rival theories explaining the relationship between genes and addiction. The first states that genetic predisposition to addiction is a direct one based on malfunctioning genes within the dopamine system. The second theory (favoured by many therapists) is that genes play an indirect role, by creating certain vulnerable personality types. These types are more likely to experiment with pleasurable activities such as drinking and drug use than the norm, making them more vulnerable to addiction. It is quite likely that both of these mechanisms are involved and that only a full decoding of our genes will settle the debate.

II   ENVIRONMENTAL FACTORS

There is little doubt that environmental triggers play an important role in both the development and the maintenance of addiction. Very young people who start to smoke often move on quickly to abuse alcohol and are more likely to become addicts of some description. It has also been shown that those who start misusing alcohol under the age of fifteen have a much higher risk of developing alcohol dependence. Their brains are only developing at this stage of their lives, so such substances will have powerful effect on the genes which are in charge of the process.

Addicts also often emerge from addictive homes. There seems to be a potent combination of a genetic predisposition to addiction and unhappiness due to growing up in such an environment. In short, addiction breeds addiction.

Those reared in the following circumstances are more at risk of becoming addicts:

§   Homes and areas of poverty, neglect, unemployment and crime

§   Addictive homes, especially if the mother or father is the addict

§   Abusive homes

Those living in the following situations are also at risk:

§   Poverty, unemployment, lack of education and crime

§   Anxiety or depression which is self-medicated with alcohol or drugs

§   High-stress situations

Another important environmental factor is the cultural availability of the potentially addictive substance. In Ireland, for example, the easy availability of alcohol to all age groups, together with the widespread availability of opportunities for gambling makes these two into obvious sources of abuse. If a potential alcoholic lived in Saudi Arabia, for example, where alcohol is prohibited, it would obviously be more difficult for his addiction to actualise.

III   THE ADDICTIVE SUBSTANCES THEMSELVES

The neurons in the brain are not impervious to alteration by addictive substances. The brain is a plastic organ: it adapts to the situations it finds itself in. When alcohol and drugs are abused, the brain reacts by altering its own chemistry to compensate; this is where the problems start.

The substances therefore play an indirect role in the addictive process itself, by forcing the brain to make changes. The more the drugs are abused, the more likely it is that such changes will become permanent. Inevitably, the earlier the brain is exposed to drugs, the more likely it is that such changes will occur. Individual substances vary in their capacity to alter brain chemistry, and also in the speed that they do so. The primary site for such changes is obviously the pleasures-box/dopamine system.

A great deal of work is also going on to try to understand how these substances are, in some cases, able to cause permanent neurochemical changes to the behaviour, memory and pleasure boxes which make up the reward circuit noted above. This research may lead to new treatment options. When these three factors are combined, a model of addiction is formed (see Figure 6).

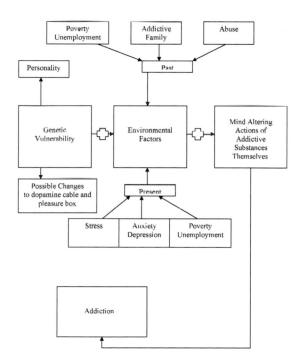

FIGURE 6: CAUSES OF THE PURPLE FLAG OF ADDICTION

It will take time for the whole jigsaw puzzle of addiction to be assembled. Within the next few decades, the complete genetic pathways relating to pleasure will be mapped out. The chemical process going on inside the pleasure box will also reveal the secrets of addiction. This, along with further research into how our neurons are altered by the drugs themselves, should create new ways of shutting down the whole addictive process.

6   THE 'ADDICTION CASTLE'

Addiction has a profoundly negative effect on the mental and physical well-being of its victims. As has already been seen, physical damage to the heart, lung, liver, pancreas and brain threatens the general health of the person. Psychological damage includes anxiety, panic attacks, depression and, sometimes, suicide.

The negative effects of addiction do not end there, however. Addicts will also have friends, families and partners, who must share in the misery of addiction. For every addict, there are five to seven people who will be indirectly affected by the addiction.

I would like to share with you a concept that I developed a long time ago to help people understand what it is like to be, or to live with, an addict. It is called the 'addiction castle'. This is a concept that has brought the addicts' loved ones to tears (sometimes joined by the addicts themselves) as, for the first time, they begin to understand what is happening to them or their loved one. This castle model works for all addictions (see Figures 7 and 8).

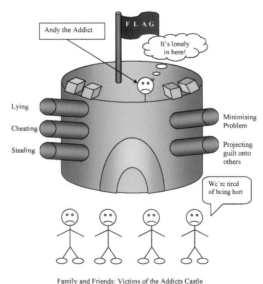

Family and Friends: Victims of the Addicts Castle

FIGURES 7: THE 'ADDICTION CASTLE'

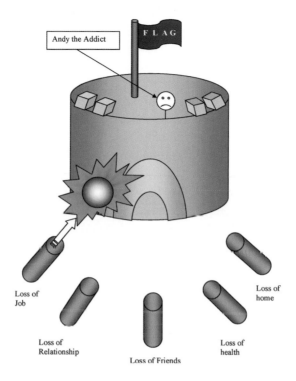

FIGURE 8: BREAKING DOWN THE ADDICTION CASTLE

Andy is an addict. As a result of the effects the addiction has had on his brain, Andy the addict has completely changed his behaviour and has decided to build a stone castle wall around him. He retreats into his lair and firmly closes the castle door behind him. In the middle of his castle, Andy lives in glorious isolation, cutting himself off from all of those around him, and then getting on with the serious work of feeding his addiction.

When Andy the addict enters his castle, the original, real Andy disappears from sight. It is also very lonely inside his castle looking at high stone walls and a closed gate, with only his addiction to keep him company. But Andy remains determined to defend his castle at all costs and has many weapons to make sure that his addiction is preserved.

Outside this castle are all those who care about Andy. They want to interact with Andy, but he is gone out of sight. All they can see are the stone walls, the closed gate and the castle full of weapons, all designed to keep them out.

His loved ones become desperate to reach him. Initially, they ring the bell at the gate, but they get no response. As the situation worsens, they then try charging the gate and the stone wall to try to break a hole in the castle and reach Andy. Then they bounce off the heavy wood and stone and get bruised and hurt in the process. Tragically, love has no boundaries, and this process is repeated over and over again until the loved ones spirits are broken from crashing into the stone of the addict's castle.

Eventually, somebody wise comes along and puts an arm around them, explaining that it is useless to continue like this and persuading them to withdraw or detach. They explain that only cannons will be able to blow holes through the stone walls. Only these and overwhelming loneliness, will encourage the addict to open the gate himself and look for help. Many, discouraged by this information and by the battle with the castle wall, will turn around and depart for good, abandoning Andy to his lonely vigil inside this stony retreat.

All addicts surround themselves with a defensive, wall-like castle and firmly shut the gate on those who are close to them. Signs of this wall are selfishness, self-obsession, and a complete denial that they have a responsibility to deal with their own addiction. The castle wall is built to protect the person's addiction at any cost. The weapons used by the addicts inside their castles are lying, cheating, stealing, minimising the significance of their condition, and most of all transferring their own guilt and blame onto those who are closest to them. Statements like 'I only drink because she nags me all the time' are examples of such behaviour.

Outside the wall are the innocent victims of addiction. They desperately want to reach their loved ones, who have closed themselves off in their castle. They get battered and bruised emotionally – and sometimes physically – from encountering the addict's defensive wall. Many feel guilty and responsible for their loved one's addiction: a sure sign that the addict has aimed well with his weapons. The families of those with addiction are often destroyed by this castle.

There are only two ways that Andy can be brought out of his castle. Firstly, Andy himself may get so lonely that he himself opens up the castle wall and comes out looking for help, and to find his loved ones. This rarely happens. The second way is for large cannons to be fired at Andy's castle; these weapons of destruction include the loss of a relationship with a partner or child, the loss of a home, the loss of a job, or severe illness as a result of his addiction.

These cannons, in some cases, can be enough to convince Andy that he must change his behaviour, and he may open up the gate and come out looking for help. Sadly, some addicts will choose to stay in their castle for life. They can die from either the side effects of their addiction, or sometimes they end their own lives as a means of stopping the loneliness and isolation of their life in the castle.

7   STAGES OF INSIGHT INTO THE PURPLE FLAG

Another useful approach in helping addicts and alcoholics in particular is to assess their level of insight into their own illness. I call this 'staging'. I classify the addicted into four main stages (see Figure 9). Stage 1: 'I have no problem!' Stage 2: 'I occasionally abuse alcohol or drugs, but so does everyone else, so it's not really a problem!' Stage 3: 'I am an addict. I accept that I have a problem but I can handle it myself!' Stage 4: 'Help!'

FIGURE 9: THE STAGES OF INSIGHT OF THE ADDICT

If the addict is at Stage 1 or 2, they are usually not ready to receive any help. I advise loved ones in these cases to detach themselves physically, emotionally and financially from the addict, if possible. This detachment has two important functions. Firstly, it safeguards the loved ones from future pain and hurt, as it means that they do not have to crash into the 'castle wall'. Secondly, it may force the addict out into the open. Life is no longer easy in his castle. The cannons are attacking his defences. I also refer the loved ones to self-help groups to get help from others who have been hurt by addiction.

If the addict reaches Stage 3, and in particular Stage 4, and the castle gate finally opens, help from doctors, counsellors and addiction self-help groups can start to restore Andy back to his original state. It often takes years, and even a lifetime, for addicts to go from Stage 1 to Stage 4. Many never get beyond Stage 2; others may stay stuck for long periods at Stage 3. In some cases, it can take many years before Andy can finally feel able to open the door and look for help.

8   TREATMENT OF THE PURPLE FLAG

Addiction is still very difficult to treat. There are two main reasons for this. Firstly, the biological changes that have occurred in the pleasure box, over a lifetime of addiction, become consolidated. The addict has been living for a long time with the cravings that these changes have produced. Secondly, the longer the addict has been living in his 'addiction castle', the greater the destruction he has caused both to his own life and to the lives of those around him, through neglect. This damage is difficult to repair, and it can take a lot of work to help the person to change the Purple Flag back to green.

If the addict begins to feel that there is nothing left for him to lose, he is unlikely ever to leave the comfort of his addiction, and will probably remain in his castle for life.

The journey to recovery can only begin when the addict opens up the gates of his castle and looks for help. When the addict begins the difficult road to recovery, he must accept the help of others, in particular other recovered addicts, in the battle towards health. He must also acknowledge the damage that he has done to those around him. The tragedy is that the lives of so many addicts and their loved ones are completely destroyed before they reach this point; death often becomes the final outcome.

Currently, it is very difficult to treat the addict before they reach Stage 3 or 4 of their illness. Therefore, it is not surprising that the success rate in the treatment of addiction, depending on its type, is as low as 25 to 40 percent. This is why research into the underlying causes of the Purple Flag is so important. The modern approach to addiction treatment involves two main steps:

1   Stopping the use of the addictive substance or behaviour

2   Changing the negative behaviour patterns that have developed in the 'addiction castle'

This second step is vital. Many addicts learn to stop their addiction but still have a tendency to remain 'in the castle' in terms of how they behave with friends and family. In order to recover fully, Andy the addict must, through counselling, learn to tear down the walls of his 'addiction castle'. Only then can he fully reintegrate back into a happy and fulfilling life with his loved ones. Only then can the Purple Flag be changed back to green.

The above treatment approach is now very community-based. Firstly, the addict must be dried out, i.e. removed completely from the addictive substance and behaviour.

This can generally be achieved by the family doctor, but in some cases admission to hospital may be necessary.

Secondly, the addict must work with specialist counsellors to help break down his castle walls. This will involve accepting the power of the emotional pleasure–driven emotional brain over the more logical one. They also have to learn new coping skills to deal with the problems and difficulties of life without the crutch of their addiction. They must also come to terms with the damage they have inflicted on their loved ones. This involves genuine self-acceptance as well as honesty about their previous behaviour in relation to them. CBT is now being increasingly considered as a treatment option for people suffering from addiction.

(One useful approach suggested by modern CBT therapists, and which I have found useful for patients, particularly those with alcohol addiction, is to encourage them to challenge their 'cravings' directly. This involves teaching them that cravings last for only five minutes! If they can learn techniques to beat these short bursts of longing, they can stay out of trouble. I often suggest texting a close friend, alcohol counsellor or AA colleague during such periods. By the time they have finished doing this, the craving has usually settled.)

Thirdly, he must learn to take part in addict self-help groups. Here he can lean on the collective wisdom of those who have spent their lives battling addiction. Most of these groups are founded on some form of spiritual basis, and rely on the ten-step approach as a road map to recovery.

Only a very lucky few have the opportunity to attend in-patient centres where this whole process can be accelerated. This is mainly due to the high cost of such centres. It has been proven that community-level treatment can, and does, work, however. Everything depends on the level of insight of the addict, and how serious they are about fighting their addiction. Drug addiction takes a longer course of counselling and treatment in comparison to other addictions: withdrawing from a drug like heroin may involve many years of help, for example.

It is also important to recognise the danger of cross-addiction. I have seen cases where one addiction is admitted to and treated, only to find a second, hidden one emerging later. Addicts are very good at fooling not only the doctor but also themselves.

9   ADDICTION: WEAKNESS OR ILLNESS?

The very word 'addiction' tends to evoke a strong reaction from the general public. Most feel that those who are addicted to alcohol, gambling or drugs have a weak personality. Many people think that addicts are entirely responsible for their own addiction. So is addiction merely a weakness which can be overcome?

A great deal of research has been carried out on the biological and genetic factors that underpin addiction. We now know that it is too facile to simply label addiction as a weakness. Addiction is an illness, caused by the exposure of a person with addictive traits to either substances or behaviour that can irrevocably alter that person's pleasure box in the brain. Such people are genetically or environmentally susceptible to the development of addictive behaviour.

We cannot choose our genes or upbringing; either of these can accelerate the addictive process. We *can* change our current environment, however. In diabetes, the predisposition is inherited genetically, but eating the wrong kinds of food and becoming obese will increase the likelihood of this illness appearing. On receiving the diagnosis, a diabetic could choose to ignore all medical advice, continue to eat the wrong foods, refrain from exercise, and refuse medications which would be of benefit, putting their health at risk in the process. This would of course be very foolish.

So, although the predisposition to develop an illness is usually genetically driven (in association with environmental factors), the person always plays an important role in how the illness is managed – to the benefit or the detriment of their health. Addiction is quite similar. A person does not directly cause their illness; they have inherited a strong predisposition (through genes or the environment, or both) towards it. By heavily misusing alcohol and drugs from an early age, however, the person increases the risk of this illness appearing.

There are also clear choices as to how they manage their own illness once they have been diagnosed. They can choose, as many do, to ignore all advice and help – to the detriment of their health, relationships and work prospects. Alternatively, they can choose to get help, and involve themselves in programmes which teach them how to deal with the cravings that this illness produces. This is the ground on which the battle against the illness must be fought.

Addiction is an illness, not a weakness. It is the way in which the sufferer deals with this illness that makes all the difference. If the addict chooses to hide in the addiction castle, they will spend most of their lives lonely and in poor health. Just as with diabetes and other illnesses, the addict also has the choice to get help from experts and fellow sufferers alike.

2

Individual Addictions

In this chapter, I will take a more detailed look at some individual addictions, such as alcohol, drugs, cigarettes and gambling.

1 Alcohol

This is the most prevalent cause of the Purple Flag. No other substance is so interwoven into the fabric of our society. In Ireland, we like to feel that we are world experts in this field. It is also a major problem in Britain and most of the northern European countries. Alcohol is a safe and enjoyable substance when used in moderation. But no other substance, with the exception of cigarettes, causes so much havoc when it is abused.

Why is alcohol enjoyable? Alcohol stimulates the serotonin and dopamine mood cables, and the pleasure box, so that the person feels quite euphoric. It also stimulates the GABA receptors; this has a relaxing effect. When used in moderation, alcohol helps us to relax and enjoy each other's company. If the 'mood machinery' is working normally, the effects are positive ones. Drinking does, however, affect our concentration and makes us more likely to become impulsive, so driving for example becomes hazardous with even small amounts of alcohol having been taken.

Excessive consumption of alcohol leads to loss of coordination, concentration and memory, and in some cases to complete memory blackouts. It releases self-control, and can lead to violent, impulsive behaviour. This is particularly dangerous for those who are already suffering from undiagnosed mood problems, and can facilitate self-harm and suicide.

The negative effects of alcohol can be seen on our streets, leading to an increase in assaults, rape, road-traffic accidents and suicide. On an average weekend night, A&E departments all over Ireland witness the fallout. Teenagers arrive to get their stomachs pumped. People are brought in bleeding and reeling from vicious assaults. Others, less fortunate, are dead on arrival from road-traffic accidents caused by people drinking and driving. A final group are admitted after overdosing on a deadly mixture of drink and drugs. Some of these may suffer from the Red Flag of depression.

Alcohol is attractive because of the feelings of well-being and relaxation it induces, making the person think that the more that they consume, the better they will feel. This is not the case, especially when the person is already suffering from the Red Flag of depression.

I   ALCOHOL MISUSE

Alcohol, when taken in moderate amounts, relaxes us by stimulating our GABA receptors, and makes us feel positive by stimulating our serotonin and dopamine cables and pleasure box. Once the amount of alcohol consumed becomes excessive, however, glutamate receptors in the brain are interfered with. As glutamate is important in almost every function of the brain, this results in chaos. We start to develop slurred speech and memory loss. We become completely uncoordinated in our movement and balance, our vision becomes blurred, and in some cases we become depressed and withdrawn.

A more serious side effect of alcohol is the removal of normal inhibitions. If we have a predisposition towards violent behaviour, alcohol reveals it. If we are depressed, alcohol may release suicidal thoughts and behaviour. Gross excess of alcohol can eventually lead to coma and death.

The results of alcohol misuse on a normal Irish weekend can be observed in almost every town and city in the country. Many people simply live and work to reach the weekend, so that they can meet up with their friends, go out on the town, and drink so much that they can forget about their problems for a couple of hours.

The side effects of alcohol inevitably emerge as the night goes on. A queue for a taxi or a takeaway becomes a flashpoint for a fight. Someone who was a normal young man at six in the evening has become an animal by 3 AM, kicking someone's head as they lie on the ground. This combination of alcohol and aggression has led to an alarming increase in serious assaults, rape and traffic accidents.

It is not only the younger generation who have an abusive relationship with alcohol; as a nation, we drink too much. Every Irish celebration ends up in the pub, from weddings to funerals, sports matches to birthdays. We have created and celebrated a culture which revolves around alcohol consumption. We turn a blind eye to the fallout.

One of the difficulties in confronting people of all ages about alcohol misuse is that those involved will quickly say: 'It's not a problem for me', 'I'm not addicted to alcohol; I can happily do without it if necessary', 'I don't crave it; I just go out with my friends at the weekend to enjoy myself.'

In the majority of cases, these statements are probably correct. Many can misuse alcohol but do not become dependant or addicted. If I injure or kill someone in a violent incident as a result of alcohol misuse, however, the damage to my life, and to the life of the victim and his family, may be just as great as the damage wreaked by addiction itself. If I spend my Monday mornings feeling down and hung over, alcohol misuse is intruding on my life.

Alcohol misuse has become one of the greatest problems facing medical personnel and police in the country. It is a factor in up to 40 percent of fatal road-traffic accidents, and around a quarter of male and a tenth of female admissions to psychiatric hospitals are due to alcohol-related problems. In our A&Es, drink-related admissions cause a huge increase in workload for the already harassed and overworked medical and nursing staff who have to man these 'war zones'. It breeds violence, mayhem and unhappiness, and is one intimate relationship that we could do without.

II   ALCOHOL ABUSE

This condition can be called by different names: alcoholism – an old term that is rapidly going out of use – alcohol abuse, or alcohol dependency syndrome, which is the most common definition. All of these terms refer to the same illness: the sufferer is addicted to alcohol.

Alcohol abuse differs from alcohol misuse in that the person, through a combination of genetic predisposition and environmental factors, has become completely dependent on alcohol. This means that withdrawal of this substance will produce physical (sweating, shaking, nausea, headaches, sleep difficulties) and psychological (craving, anxiety, panic attacks, depression) symptoms.

Most people who are at risk will move from simple misuse, to extensive misuse, to finally becoming completely addicted to the substance. Tolerance, craving and dependency or withdrawal symptoms are the main indications of alcohol abuse. The changes seen in the pleasure box after extended use of the substance are the notable biological feature of this condition.

Excellent research in Sweden in the 1980s and 1990s has shown that there are two different groups of people who abuse alcohol. Each group has a different genetic basis, presentation and behaviour pattern.

(A)   THE TYPE 1 ALCOHOLIC

This relates to a group of people who do not need to drink constantly in order to feed their addiction. They are often described as binge drinkers or, more accurately, as binge alcoholics. They are able to stay clear of alcohol for weeks, or even months. But eventually, they feel the craving building up, and they start with their first drink. Once the drinking begins, it may go on for days and nights, until sickness, or more commonly lack of money, brings the binge to an end. Such binges are often triggered by celebratory occasions such as weddings, holidays and birthdays. Funerals in Ireland are also high-risk events. The partners and families of addicts learn to dread these periods.

The genetic basis for this illness, although clearly of relevance, is much weaker than for Type 2 alcoholics. It is almost certainly polygenetic in nature (i.e. varying numbers of malfunctioning genes in the chromosomes are involved from person to person). It affects both men and women in equal amounts, and often starts over the age of twenty-five.

Family upbringing, particularly if alcohol addiction is present, has a much stronger influence in this group. If alcohol abuse is present in both parents, or if poverty is present, the risk of severe illness increases. Parents of Type 1 alcoholics are much more likely to produce offspring suffering from Type 1 rather than Type 2 alcoholism. The reasons for this seems to be a mixture of the genetic and environmental factors involved in the person's upbringing.

The type 1 personality is generally passive, introverted and perfectionist. They may express guilt about their binges when they are sober. Such concerns rapidly disappear during binges. They frequently suffer from symptoms of anxiety. In many cases, they may start to misuse alcohol in order to deal with feelings of being inadequate, or if they are having difficulties with coping. They develop craving and tolerance quickly. They are more likely to worry about their image; this is part of the reason why they try to hide their addiction. They are also less likely to get into trouble with authority figures. A favourite statement from this group is: 'I don't have a drink problem because I don't drink every day', which is clearly a form of denial. They spend their lives in an endless cycle of anxiety, craving and binges, followed by guilt. Stress is often a trigger for a binge.

This group will show dopamine-cable hyper-stimulation (which occurs during these binges), combined with the classical chemical changes in the pleasure box. It is these changes, both short- and long-term, which explain the craving, tolerance and lifelong nature of this illness.

The illness has a very damaging effect on the health, work and family life of the person. This group will have the usual 'addiction castle' symptoms of lying, stealing, cheating, and so on. But they are more likely to be secretive about their actions. This group are, however, more amenable to treatment and help than the Type 2 group. The addiction castle can be more easily breached by fear of losing family, housing, work, health or loved ones. AA is a particularly useful tool for this group if they eventually look for help and try to come to terms with their binges. One should not underestimate the power of their cravings, however, and many will struggle with this compulsion throughout their life.

These binges cause a great deal of damage to the person's health, in particular to the liver, pancreas and heart. Many will also suffer from the Red Flag of depression as a result of long periods of trying to cope with their illness. Sometimes, the Red Flag may follow the loss of family or work, as a result of their drinking. Suicide can eventually be the way out for many, especially if the Red Flag is already present.

This group contains a number of people who have been broken by life through abuse, loss or some other life problem. They may start to misuse alcohol as a way to cope, before moving on to binge drinking. Eventually, if they are susceptible (particularly if they come from a Type 1 abuse background), this turns into a full addiction.

Some similarly vulnerable people, initially suffering from depression, may also fall into this trap. In such cases, biological mechanisms take over, and a vicious circle of low mood, craving, binges and guilt take over. Many will become trapped in this cycle, eventually losing everything.

The female alcoholic in this group (many of whom may have a mother with the same illness) is particularly difficult to identify, and to treat. They are usually adept at hiding their problems and covering their tracks. Elderly females are exceptionally difficult, if not impossible, to help.

When people start using alcohol as a crutch, there is always a risk of developing this kind of addiction. If people are already susceptible, the crutch can become the main trigger. This is why the large number of people who misuse alcohol in Ireland is an extremely worrying phenomenon. As the numbers of people drinking heavily increases, so too does the risk of addiction. Misuse morphs into abuse.

(B)   THE TYPE 2 ALCOHOLIC

This alcoholic is driven to drink all the time. Symptoms of addiction can usually be seen before the age of twenty-five. This illness is strongly genetically inherited (up to 90 percent), and mostly involves males. It seems to be inherited as part of an overall personality disorder.

This group shows strong anti-social tendencies, often expressed in the form of violence, and has little remorse about the destruction that their behaviour causes in the lives of others. The combination of heavy alcohol use and violence often leads them into conflict with authority and the law. Some of the violence currently seen on our streets can be attributed to this group. Like all addicts, Type 2 alcoholics can be adept at minimising their own role in such situations, pushing the blame (and consequences) on to someone else. Sometimes, these violent impulses are self-directed, and suicide can be the final outcome. Drink-driving convictions are also common in this group.

In relationships, this group can cause major emotional and physical damage to their partners and children. The male children of this group run a greater genetic risk of developing the same violent destructive personality traits as the male parent, and of becoming young addicts themselves. The daughters of this group seem to inherit other personality characteristics, but not generally alcohol addiction.

It also seems as though environmental influences are far less important in this group than in Type 1 alcoholics. The fathers of this group will quite often have had similar personalities, and will often have a history of violence or conflict with the law.

This particular group of alcoholics can be classified as people who suffer from a strongly genetically inherited personality disorder, and who also happen to abuse alcohol (or any other substance they can get their hands on) because they find it pleasurable. They display the classical 'addiction castle' , and this, together with their violent anti-social personality, causes untold misery in the lives of those who are close to them.

The primary difference between this group, and those who misuse alcohol and the type 1 alcoholic, is their anti-social personality and continuous craving for alcohol. Lack of money is the only obstacle. They may lie, steal, cheat or use violence to get the money to feed their addiction. They will often also be abusing other drugs, like sleeping tablets, tranquillizers and street drugs.

Biologically speaking, the same addictive pathways involved in Type 1 alcoholism (with almost constant hyper-stimulation of the dopamine system and the pleasure box) are involved, but it is likely that the broader personality problems may have their origins in the serotonin cable (which may be under-active in some cases), and possibly in the early development of the brain.

Often, this group end up homeless or in prison (often for violent assault). Many reject any help or treatment. Their addiction-castle wall is almost impenetrable, and often remains so for life. A substantial number suffer from serious health problems. Many continue drinking even as they are dying from their condition. They remain impervious to the loss of everything, including their own lives.

The prognosis for this group is, at present, quite poor. This is because they suffer from both addiction and personality problems. Many will develop serious medical problems, with damage to the liver, heart and other organs, which may lead to their death. Others may commit suicide, usually in a particularly violent manner. Only a very few manage to break their addiction-castle walls, get treatment and end up living normal lives.

Not every alcoholic will fit neatly into either of the two groups above, but this general categorisation has proved to be of great help in improving our understanding of this illness.

It usually takes years for the full-blown emergence of alcohol addiction. Many are starting to look at this addiction as being part of a large spectrum of drinking problems, in all age groups. This starts with initial misuse, followed by increasingly hazardous, and then harmful, drinking, and finishes with eventual dependence or addiction. If one follows this approach, the major concern is the misuse of alcohol at younger and younger ages. Public discussion on the potentially harmful effects of alcohol on the developing brain and mood system must take place before the situation gets out of hand and a generation of alcoholics is forged. There is also increasing concern about the harmful effects of heavy drinking and addiction in the elderly, where the problem often remains hidden.

Some experts are uncomfortable with even describing alcohol dependency as an illness, and would prefer to call it a trait of particular personality types. Others feel that, if we could intervene at a much earlier stage in the cycle of development of this condition, many people would not reach a stage of full-blown dependency.

The example of being on a coach which stops regularly along its route across Ireland to allow passengers to disembark is often used by modern therapists. The coach is filled with heavy drinkers or alcoholics. It begins its journey in Galway and ends in Dublin outside the homeless shelter or the cemetery! The alcohol abuser, however, does not have to stay on the coach that is heading to ruin: they have the option of getting off anywhere along the way, and the earlier they do so, the less damage will be caused to themselves and their families. On the other hand, the closer they come to their final destination, the closer they are to ruin!

Encouraging as many heavy drinkers or alcoholics as possible to disembark early is now very much the target of many of those who work in this field. In my personal dealings with alcoholics and their families, I find that the 'coach' model seems to 'penetrate' the former, and the 'addict castle' the latter!

There is also a body of opinion that feels that early intervention might allow some heavy drinkers or alcoholics to continue to take alcohol in small amounts rather than having to face the prospect of abstinence for life. When alcohol dependency arrives, however (especially if serious physical or family difficulties are present), lifelong abstinence is usually the only solution.

Before leaving this discussion, let's examine what is happening in Ireland at present, bearing in mind everything we have learnt to date. Firstly, we have to accept that a huge cultural change has occurred in the past decade in relation to how we view and use alcohol.

Ireland has always had an alcohol problem, with its fair share of alcoholics of both types, but in the past, young people in particular had neither the money nor the possibility of drinking heavily before the age of twenty-one. Now, increasing prosperity, plus greater freedom of movement in the twelve-to-eighteen age group has exposed a much larger population of young people in this country to the perils of alcohol misuse and abuse than hitherto. Many Irish teenagers are holding down part-time jobs when they are still studying to help feed their weekend drinking – something which is evident on a Monday morning, as many teachers will testify to!

The official position that alcohol is only available to those who are over eighteen belies the truth of what is happening in practice. Underage drinking increases the potential risk of alcohol dependency. Common sense would dictate that the greater the number of people who are exposed to alcohol at an early age, the greater the number of people who become alcoholics at an early age – and this is what is happening.

From a biological point of view, this is inevitable. If the dopamine cable/ pleasure box is hyper-stimulated from an early age, the chances of dependency emerging increase. If, as we are seeing, regular binge drinking becomes the norm at an early age, we are much more likely to see Type 1 binge alcoholism appearing at earlier and earlier ages (sometimes before the age of twenty); once again, this is what is happening. There is also the potential for alcohol to alter the sensitive neurochemistry and neurobiology of the vulnerable developing brain in this age group.

This has many implications for us as a society. I often feel that the young person's peer group has taken control almost completely away from parents in this area. It now seems to be completely acceptable that Junior and Leaving Cert students be allowed to binge-drink as they see fit! Graduation celebrations have become orgies of alcohol.

What we are all forgetting is that the young people involved have immature brains and mood systems. The controlling influence of the mature behaviour box is not yet present, and pleasure rules. The risks outweigh the rewards. Because of these developments, the risk of future addiction, violence, accidents, depression and, most seriously, suicide dramatically increases. If we ignore the biology of the developing brain in this group, we will continue to pay a high price.

In older age groups, the combination of prosperity, high stress, an increasing acceptance of binge drinking, particularly among females, plus the easy availability of alcohol in off licences, pubs and nightclubs has led to an increasing risk of alcohol abuse (particularly of Type 1 binge alcoholism) in the adult population. Some experts think that we are at the start of an epidemic that will end up destroying many lives.

I am especially worried for the many young women who are drinking at levels they are neither physically (as women cannot process the same levels of alcohol as men) nor psychologically able to cope with. As this pattern often starts well before the age of eighteen, it is crucial that we try to reduce binge drinking at this stage. If we allow the dopamine system to develop a taste for alcohol at an early age, it is inevitable that the twenty-to-forty age groups will continue on the pattern. All of us have a responsibility in this area.

208

COMMON QUESTIONS RELATING TO ALCOHOL ABUSE

How big a problem is it?

At least 10 percent of our adult male drinking population, and 3 to 4 percent of the female drinking population, are dependent on alcohol – although even this may be a conservative estimate. At least another 10 to 20 percent is seriously misusing alcohol. There has been a gradual increase in the numbers of women developing serious drink problems in recent years.

It is estimated that around 25 percent of Irish adults drink above the recommended safe amounts of alcohol, and alcohol misuse is a factor in 25 percent of hospital intakes. Thirteen percent of patients attending A&E departments are intoxicated.

How is alcohol abuse treated?

Successful treatment for alcohol abuse depends on the level of insight that the person has into their own illness. Only those at Stages Three and Four are accepting of help and can really be reached by loved ones or professionals. The addiction-castle wall of the alcoholic is very resilient, and many will lose everything rather than open up the addiction gate and look for help.

The current community approach to this problem is firstly to detoxify the person. This means helping them to stop drinking by using a combination of tranquillizers and vitamins to help them survive the withdrawal effects. Usually, this is done by the family doctor, but occasionally, for safety reasons, it will have to be done in a hospital.

Following this, the person is encouraged to attend an alcohol counsellor, and to start involving themselves with a group like Alcoholics Anonymous. Most are apprehensive about the thought of opening up to such a group. Those who genuinely try to follow the twelve steps of AA will often do extremely well. Many will also need relationship counselling if there are relationship difficulties as a result of their addiction. Those with an underlying depression in particular will need further help.

In a small number of cases, in-patient care is greatly beneficial. This is costly, however, and is only available to a small number of people. Increasingly, however, employers are becoming involved in encouraging workers to get such help. A company may pay for such a course of treatment and allow the person to repay the cost to them over a period of time. In reality, very few alcoholics can afford such treatments themselves. Another problem is that many end up being admitted to treatment units when they are still not at a stage where they genuinely want help.

If drugs could be designed to reverse completely the pleasure-box changes, eliminating the craving and long-term dependence (while still allowing the person to enjoy normal pleasurable activities), the treatment of alcohol addiction could be

revolutionised. There are some drugs which are available at the moment (see below)
but none of them have yet achieved the goal of eliminating the cravings. Counselling
and self-help groups remain the cornerstones of treatment.

At present, the best strategy for dealing with alcoholism is early detection of potential alcoholics, and efforts to alter their habits in order to limit the risk of addiction. As
the brain is only fully mature by twenty-five years of age, however, it is difficult to reach
anyone under this age (particularly those under eighteen) with a logical argument.
Rather, one must appeal to their emotions, as this is the domain in which they are living. The drinks industry, for instance, is very aware of this vulnerability and is adept at
using this strategy in their marketing.

In the past, young people lacked the money, time and opportunity to drink at the
level that we are now seeing. Now, by contrast, they are quickly developing a taste for
alcohol at increasingly young ages. In the mid- to late teens, pleasure and experimenta-
tion are synonymous, especially if the money and opportunity to experience these
things are readily available. This is worrying, as the developing mood system is more
vulnerable to the effects of alcohol and other substances than the mature mood
system.

What, if any, drug treatments are available at present for alcohol addiction?

Although we are still some distance from a 'wonder drug' which would banish all addictive cravings completely, a number of options are available. A drug called Campral,
which acts on the GABA receptors, is sometimes prescribed for one year, in conjunction with counselling. Campral seems partially to alleviate the drive to binge-drink. It is
usually prescribed by a specialist.

An older drug called Antabuse is also occasionally still used. It is taken daily and
works by causing severe vomiting if the person consumes alcohol within three days of
taking the tablet. Although it is useful and of psychological help to spouses, who may
supervise its consumption, there are many drawbacks to its use. Firstly, many alcoholics
fake taking it, or 'forget' to take it; secondly, others will try and 'chance' drinking after
taking it, with some becoming violently ill and requiring hospitalisation; thirdly, it does
not deal with the cravings or the addiction-castle symptoms. If used sensibly in conjunction with counselling and AA, it has a role in some cases.

Finally, if the Red Flag of depression is also present (as is often the case), the use
of the SSRIs in particular has been shown both to treat the underlying depression and,
by stimulating the serotonin cable, to reduce impulsive cravings for alcohol. Patients
will often report a lessening of interest in the substance. Some will, however, keep
drinking even when on antidepressants. This of course makes the antidepressants less
effective, so the vicious circle of low mood, craving and drinking, followed by further

withdrawal anxiety and drops in mood, continues. Although the SSRIs are helpful, their use is usually linked to the concomitant treatment of depression, with the side effects of reducing craving as a bonus.

What about the addiction-castle victims?

People close to the alcoholic often require more help than the alcoholic themselves. The constant collision with the addiction wall leaves them bruised and battered, both emotionally and physically. They often present as tense, anxious and depressed, and despairing as to what to do. They feel responsible for the alcoholic's condition, and admit to feeling guilt about their role, as they see it, in causing such problems. Many are ashamed about admitting the problem to family members or friends.

In many cases, where the alcoholic himself is not prepared to listen, explaining the stages of insight to those close to him can be a great help. They then understand the situation. If the alcoholic is at Stage One or Two, it is best for families and friends to detach emotionally, physically and financially. This saves them from future emotional hurt and pain. It may also force the alcoholic out into the open, as life is no longer so easy for them. Talking to an alcohol counsellor and attending AA support groups such as Alanon or Alateen is also recommended. Such groups provide great support and strength from others who have experienced similar problems.

If the addict is at Stage Three or Four, they are ready to look for help. At this stage, the alcoholic counselling may be a vital link. It is also important to rule out or treat any associated depression.

In some cases, where the addict is clearly lost and unlikely ever to look for help, their relationships may irrevocably break down, leading to separation between them and their loved ones. Sometimes, this is the only possible solution for the partner of the addict, in order that they can rebuild and continue with their own lives.

How many alcoholics recover from their addiction?

'Recovering' here refers to stopping taking alcohol completely and making the changes necessary to live a fulfilled and happy life. The figures are not encouraging. Only about 25 percent of those with alcohol abuse will succeed in giving up alcohol for life. The rest will either never face their addiction or will spend their lives engaged in a tug-of-war between remaining sober and drinking heavily. In most of these cases, the drinking wins out in the end, and they lose their family and friends along the way. Some will die from complications due to their drinking. Others will end up homeless. Some will wave the White Flag and take their own lives. Many finish their lives lonely, embittered and stripped of all that they once held dear. The Purple Flag of alcohol addiction is a formidable one.

Is there a cost to the community?

The community pays a huge cost for this addiction. If one accepts that every alcoholic affects around five to seven people indirectly (i.e. family members, workmates, employers, friends, and so on), the ripple effect is enormous. Family breakdown, violence and road-traffic accidents and illness resulting from alcohol abuse take a huge toll on our social and health-care systems. When one adds in alcohol misuse, the financial cost of the use and misuse of this substance is enormous.

II   GAMBLING

This addiction, also known as 'gambling-dependency syndrome' or pathological gambling, is a concealed addiction that causes major loss and hardship to the families of the person involved. While alcohol and drugs grab all the news headlines, gambling-dependency syndrome is secretly destroying lives in our community.

Many people are surprised to hear the word 'addiction' associated with gambling because it is an activity rather than a substance. Gambling, like alcohol, may start as a form of misuse, but in vulnerable people the craving sets in and the gambler starts to behave like the alcoholic. Once the gambler starts, they are unable to stop until all their funds run out. Interestingly, a substantial number of gamblers will cross-addict with alcohol.

This illness follows the same neurological pathways that other addictions do, i.e. stimulating the dopamine cable and the pleasure box, with chemical alterations resulting in the pleasure box. It is the latter that produces the craving, which is only relieved when the person starts gambling again. The gambler gets a euphoric feeling from this activity and ignores all other parts of his or her life, to focus purely on their addiction. They also live in the addiction castle. There may again be a genetic predisposition for this illness, as some come from an addictive background. Once again, environment may play a role in such cases.

The main methods of gambling in Ireland are slot machines, horse racing and card games. In general, the addict will gamble on anything that is available. Young men, particularly those under twenty-five, seem to prefer slot machines, poker in particular. Members of this group are usually quite intelligent, and are convinced they can 'outsmart' the machine. Even if they win a substantial amount of money, they will usually keep playing until this money is gone. This is often followed by feeling down, and at this stage they often use alcohol to help them feel better.

A recent emerging problem is the arrival of internet gambling, where vast sums of money can be lost extremely quickly. This is believed to be a cause of increasing martial breakdown. The real risk here is the ability to run up huge credit-card debts.

As a group, gamblers are often tense, are superb liars, and are very good at stealing and cheating to feed their addiction. They will continue to conceal their illness until debt finally gives them away.

In the USA, it is estimated that between 1 and 2 percent of the population suffer from pathological gambling. Gambling is also a substantial problem in Ireland. Concrete figures are extremely difficult to obtain. Only figures from groups like Gamblers Anonymous on how many attend on a regular basis provide some clue as to the extent of this illness. A national figure of 20,000 was given to me on one occasion. For every one addict who is receiving help like this, there are almost certainly at least two or three who are not.

Gambling is particularly destructive to families and relationships. All finances are quickly (and often covertly) drained, leaving families in serious debt. This, combined with the constant denial of the gambler, living in his addiction castle, can lead to the breakdown of relationships. The gambler will risk losing everything – family, house and friends – to protect their addiction. They are usually good at holding on to their jobs, however: without this, they would have no money for gambling.

In terms of stages of insight, gambling is similar to alcohol. Those who reach Stage Four and are genuinely looking for help have a much higher success rate than alcoholics, however. This may be explained by the fact that, unlike alcohol and drugs, there is no direct chemical effect on the neurons of the pleasure box. The problem is that very few gamblers reach this stage. The treatment for the condition is similar to that for alcohol. If people can afford it, in-patient care in treatment centres such as the Rutland Clinic can be very successful.

Very few reach a stage where they look for this help – or indeed can afford it – however. For the rest, the main treatment will be attending Gamblers Anonymous. Many will do well by attending addiction counsellors as well. All addiction counsellors are now trained to help in the area of gambling as well as substance addictions.

One possible treatment option in the not too-distant future is the arrival of a sister drug to the one mentioned in the section on alcohol (Campral). This will probably work in a similar biological manner, to reduce the cravings associated with gambling. Once again, it will be combined with counselling. Although this approach looks promising, it remains to be seen how effective it will be in practice.

One further complication associated with gambling is cross-addiction with alcohol. Often the alcoholism kept hidden, while the gambling is treated successfully.

Many young men, fall into the trap of gambling abuse in the form of slot machines very early, in their mid-teens. Parents should always be vigilant for warning signs, such as behaviour changes, stealing, lying and denial. If large amounts of money are disappearing and the person does not appear to be using drugs or alcohol, it is possible that the person has a secret gambling addiction.

Those close to a gambler should study the addiction-castle model before they al: become seriously hurt by the behaviour of those they love. The addiction castle is ju as powerful with this addiction as with alcohol. The families of gamblers can also g help from addict groups and gambling counsellors.

III   NICOTINE ADDICTION

This is the most harmful and destructive drug ever sold to the public. It is responsib for more illnesses and misery than all the other substances combined.

Nicotine affects the same dopamine cable and pleasure box as all the other addi tions. The chemical changes in the pleasure box produce the smoker's intense craving The fact that a third of the population smoke, knowing full well what it is doing them, is testament to the power of this addiction.

Young people, girls in particular, think that smoking is attractive, and they like th fact that it helps control weight through metabolic enhancement and appetite suppre sion. In worldwide studies, this group seems to be impervious to all efforts to encou age them to quit.

This is due to the stage of brain development which they are at. They are quick addicted, often at a very young age, and the changes in their brain may become perm nent. A gene has been identified which predisposes some people to become addicte to cigarettes quickly. Thus, some will simply use nicotine and give it up after a whil Others will never break free from the 'death row' that is smoking.

To discuss the medical effects of nicotine addiction would require an entire boo A few key pieces of information, however, are useful to recognise. Firstly, nicotir increases blood clotting in the heart, brain and limbs. In those suffering from narrov ing of the arteries due to plaque, particularly in the coronary arteries, nicotine caus clotting or thrombosis, which can block such arteries and eventually lead to a hea attack. The graveyards are full of men and women of all ages who only smoked ten twenty cigarettes a day. Secondly, it destroys the bronchial tube linings of the lungs, fil ing them with thick, tarry material, and causing bronchitis, asthma and emphysem Thirdly, it attacks the lung-cell genes, increasing the chances of lung cancer. Lastly, destroys the blood vessels to the legs, increasing the chances of such long-term illnes es such as peripheral vascular disease, which causes pain and discomfort on walkin and gangrene.

Smokers destroy their bodies, and pay huge multinationals and their own goveri ments large amounts of money for the privilege of doing so. All the other illegal drug fade into insignificance in comparison with the number of people whose lives a destroyed by this substance.

The smoker also lives in their addiction castle and can only get help when they wa to open the door. Like all addicts, many will lose their lives before giving up their pleasure and craving. 'I might as well be dead', is what the family doctor often hears from someone when they are told that they have to give up smoking. Unfortunately, many get their wish.

Nicotine addiction is also a powerful indicator in young people of other possible cross-addictions, such as alcohol and marijuana. If young people do not smoke before the age of twenty-one, they have a lower risk of being hooked on nicotine or other substances. Smoking therefore does not just destroy the health of the individual, it also takes up a huge amount of resources within the health system, resulting in other illnesses not getting the funding and attention they deserve.

What is tragic about the illnesses resulting from smoking is that it is self-inflicted and avoidable. Sadly, smokers generally only start to take responsibility for their actions when serious illness or the threat of death starts to blast holes in the addiction wall.

In terms of helping people to stop smoking, numerous techniques have been employed. The commonest method adopted by health professionals involves the withdrawal of cigarettes and their replacement with substitutes such as nicotine patches (my preference), chewing gum, inhalers and tablets. My own approach is to explain that these replacements are worthless unless a genuine decision to cease smoking has been made. The logical brain must be actively involved in this decision, or the attempt to give up is doomed to failure. Nicotine patches are normally used for a period of eight to twelve weeks, with a gradual reduction in the strength of nicotine over time.

Smoking clinics are now in place in most hospitals. Holding them in hospitals helps to consolidate the link between nicotine and illness. Many patients with cardiac or respiratory problems are directed towards these clinics. They can, along with smoking help lines, be a great help to many.

Some nicotine addicts have tried hypnosis, with varying success. Some people are immune to hypnosis, and others seem to get only temporary benefit from it. My own feeling is that, until the logical brain has truly decided to stop, even hypnosis may be ineffective. It is amazing how the most seasoned smoker who has tried (apparently unsuccessfully) to cease smoking may do so instantly (and often permanently) after a bout of angina!

There can be little doubt that the smoking ban in public and work areas, now being adopted in many other European countries, has been a great success. The ban has been reasonably well accepted and enforced. Once again, the 'stick' approach to this addiction has been much more effective in changing people's behaviour than decades of trying to persuade them of the health benefits of ceasing smoking.

IV   SUBSTANCE ABUSE

This is an area which grabs all the headlines in the media when it comes to addiction. Experts in the field of addiction, however, know that alcohol and nicotine are the real problems. These two cause most of the carnage created by both misuse and addiction.

Many young people are being increasingly exposed to illegal substances, otherwise known as street drugs. Research has shown that, in Ireland, drug misuse is by far the most common problem among this group. In other words, many young people experiment with these drugs, but only a small number of them actually become addicted.

This distinction is vital, and is often not grasped by the public. Misuse of course carries its own risks, but compared to alcohol it is insignificant in terms of the damage done to the lives of young people. Parents worry about the dangers of drugs, but often ignore the more pressing and dangerous issue: alcohol. The real risk of drug misuse is that a small number of those who are predisposed, either genetically or through social circumstances, to it will move on into full addiction. In many cases, drug addiction is a downward spiral into illness and death.

Although it is cumbersome to detail the contents and effects of all illegal and prescribed drugs, it is important to have a general understanding of the more common misused drugs.

MARIJUANA

Also known as hash or cannabis. This drug is the most commonly misused illegal substance in Ireland. Its use is often concomitant with nicotine, as they are usually smoked together. Users will feel relaxed and sluggish, with some impairment of concentration and short-term memory. It is quite dangerous to use marijuana if one is driving a car. Large amounts can produce hallucinations. It seems as though there is a definite subgroup in those using this drug who are particularly vulnerable to developing psychotic reactions (losing contact with reality). This almost certainly has a genetic basis. The difficulty is that such people find this out only when they start to use it. Many psychiatrists are also becoming concerned about the increasing appearance of schizophrenia in young teenagers following the use of marijuana. Suicide can unfortunately be another result in such cases, as can violence towards others. Most other people will simply misuse this drug, but those at risk of addiction may eventually become hooked on it. This group can, in my experience, be extremely difficult to treat.

The main fear is that misuse of this drug can lead to psychotic reactions in those who are genetically vulnerable, and can lead to the potential abuse of other, more serious drugs. For parents, a good way to spot whether a young person is misusing this drug is the presence of scorch-like burns on their clothes. Most parents assume these

216

are due to smoking, but it is much more indicative of marijuana use. If this is accompanied by a change in behaviour or a disruption in school attendance or performance, one should start to ask questions. Often a timely chat can head off more serious problems.

COCAINE

There is increasing concern amongst medical personnel and the Gardaí that this drug is starting to become commonplace in Ireland. Cocaine can be extremely addictive from an early stage of use, particularly in those who are susceptible to addiction. This drug powerfully stimulates the dopamine cable and pleasure box, giving feelings of intense pleasure and confidence. It is usually sniffed up the nose (snorted) or smoked. A very addictive preparation smoked in poorer areas is called crack, and is almost instantly addictive.

Many young people and adults in the twenty-to-forty age group are experimenting with cocaine. Most will not become addicted, but unfortunately some susceptible people will. Chronic use of this drug will cause behaviour changes, impotence, paranoia and depression. Suicide is also a risk.

Those who misuse this drug will feel invincible, talkative and confident. They will also feel very sexually aroused. Overuse can lead to violent behaviour, paranoid thinking, and even schizophrenic-type symptoms. Withdrawal of the drug often results in depression and agitation.

There is great excitement among health professionals and others about the possibility of a new vaccination to help those who are addicted to marijuana. This will work by stimulating the body's immune system to attach a protein to the cocaine molecule, preventing the drug from being absorbed from the bloodstream into the brain itself. This of course prevents the drug from reaching the pleasure box, so the person gets no 'buzz' from using it. It is hoped that, in time, this may be used to help deal with other addictions, such as nicotine. Once again, understanding the biology of the mood system assists us in the treatment and prevention of this condition.

AMPHETAMINES

These drugs, also known as uppers, are, like cocaine, stimulant in type. Those who use them feel hyper-alert, and full of energy and confidence. Large doses can lead to major paranoid delusions, which may translate into violence. Amphetamines work by activating the dopamine and pleasure box, and also strongly activate the noradrenalin cable. The latter explains why users become so 'high'.

Withdrawal from this drug often leads to exhaustion and depression. Chronic abusers, at a later stage in life, are also at risk of developing Parkinson's disease. Of note, if amphetamine users are driving cars, particularly at high speed, their driving may be aggressive and dangerous. Though there are no figures available, it would be interesting to know how many road-traffic accidents are caused by the use of these drugs.

ECSTASY

This drug, commonly used by young people in nightclubs, is a mixture of a stimulant and a hallucinogen. Ecstasy 'hypes up' its users, making them extremely emotional, increasing their energy reserves, and allowing them to dance the night away, before they collapse into exhaustion as the effects of the drug wear off. This drug affects all three mood cables, literally driving the user wild.

Ecstasy is primarily a drug of misuse in Ireland, although a small number may become addicted. The real risk is death through dehydration, as several tragic young deaths have shown. Some young people prefer this drug, as it is cheaper, and will last the duration of the night better, than alcohol. This drug may also release very violent behaviour in some of its users, and in other cases unmasks schizophrenia.

HEROIN

This is the drug which lay people generally think of in relation to drug addiction. The classic picture of heroin addicts injecting themselves with dirty needles, prostituting themselves, stealing, being infected with HIV and hepatitis, and mugging others to get money to feed their habit is a strong stereotype. In practice, this picture is mainly confined to the bigger cities: there are an estimated 10,000 heroin addicts in Dublin today. The fallout from this addiction is all too clearly seen in the wasted bodies huddled on the city streets as night falls. A large percentage of these people are under twenty-five. This situation is the end result of a gradual progression from misuse to eventual abuse and addiction.

Not every person who uses heroin will become addicted, but misuse creates the potential in those who are susceptible to becoming dependent. Heroin addiction usually originates in areas where poverty, unemployment and lack of education are predominant: the drug is used to ease the pain and hopelessness of people's lives. Criminal gangs exploit this need, making massive profits from the misery of their victims. This group is in constant conflict with the law, are often homeless, and frequently end up in jail, where their habit is fed further. Many end up suffering from malnutrition, hepatitis, needle abscesses and HIV, and are likely to die from illness or suicide.

Heroin mainly affects the dopamine cable and pleasure box, so when chemical changes become permanent, the craving becomes absolute. Any act, criminal or otherwise, is acceptable to feed the addiction. Our present response is to try to substitute heroin with oral methadone, a replacement opiate. This has met with only limited success, however, as those who walk the streets of Dublin at night can attest to. Long-term

rban and rural treatment projects, with total detoxification for the individual, and a
ance to spend a number of years learning new skills and doing manual work, might
rove to be a more successful option.

TRANQUILLIZERS AND SLEEPING TABLETS

Tranquillizer misuse and abuse is, after alcohol and nicotine, probably the most
common drug problem in Ireland. It attracts little attention, because the drugs are not
legal.

As seen earlier in the Yellow Flag of anxiety, tranquillizers such as Valium, Xanax
and Lexotane, which ideally are designed for the short-term treatment of episodes of
acute anxiety, can end in lifelong addictions in susceptible people. This has been a par-
cular risk in the past. Sleeping tablets such as Normison and Rohypnol (the so-called
ate-rape drug) have also joined the list. Efforts have been made to make these drugs
more difficult to prescribe, because of the high risk of abuse of the drugs by addicts,
nd this has certainly helped to reduce the problem.

All addicts are at risk of cross-addiction with tranquillizers and sleeping tablets, par-
icularly alcoholics and serious drug addicts. A major problem is where they have been
prescribed by doctors for patients but have been diverted for sale on the streets.
Addicts claim that they can get whatever they want on the streets; it's just a question of
he price.

CROSS-ADDICTION

All addictions have a common biological basis. This is of course a result of the chem-
cal changes experienced in the pleasure box. It also explains the common scenario of
cross-addiction seen by family doctors in their surgeries. Addicts are very comfortable
slipping out of one mode of addiction and into another. Many will have two or three
addictions: alcohol and gambling, alcohol and sleeping tablets, smoking and marijuana,
cocaine and amphetamines, with tranquillizers to bring them down, and so on. I have
even seen food addiction creeping in to take over from other addictions. This makes
sense: the withdrawal effects of one can be eased by the administration of another,
regardless of which addictive substance it is. Above all, this shows that the Purple Flag
of addiction is truly an illness.

SUMMARY

Many of us are affected, either directly or indirectly, by the Purple Flag of addiction.
As a doctor, however, one can justifiably say that misuse of many of these substances
can cause as many problems as addiction.

Of great interest is the capacity of the various flags to interact with the Purple Flag.
For example, many people with the Red Flag of depression will use alcohol to numb

their pain. Conversely, many people with the Purple Flag of addiction will suffer sec ondary problems with the Red Flag of depression.

Many people with the Purple Flag of addiction end up giving up the fight and suc cumbing to the White Flag of suicide. Misuse of alcohol can also play a contributor role in suicide among those who are already thinking about it.

Some people with the Yellow Flag of anxiety will try to mask their symptoms wit either alcohol or prescribed drugs such as tranquillizers, and may become addicted as result. Up to 50 percent of sufferers from the Grey Flag of schizophrenia (this ment illness, involving loss of grey matter in the behaviour box, will be discussed later in th section on suicide) will become addicted to nicotine, alcohol, tranquillizers or othe drugs. This, unfortunately, increases their chances of committing suicide. The Purpl Flag of addiction is sadly often at half-mast, and rarely flies alone.

V

THE WHITE FLAG
SUICIDE

1

Niall's story

Loss, disappointment and difficulty are all part of the journey of life. Sometimes, these things can be overwhelming, and we just want to give up. Despite this, we usually make it through such periods, with the help of those who are close to us.

A small minority of people will find life too distressing, and see suicide as the only way of escaping the situation. Many of these people succeed in taking their own lives every year. They often leave devastated and confused families behind them, along with many unanswered questions. The answers are multifaceted, and modern research is gradually uncovering the mystery of why a person consciously kills themselves.

Suicide attempts are often a mixture of a wish to annihilate oneself and a cry for help. This duality of wanting to be destroyed and wanting to be saved reflects the state of chaos and confusion that the mood system is in at the time of the suicide attempt. Sometimes, the cry for help is answered; at another time, the suicide attempt might be successful. The only positive legacy of suicide is the opportunity of intensive research into these tragic victims, to try to understand why it happened in order to prevent it happening again. Although this is of little consolation to those who have had their lives shattered by suicide, the hope is that such research can prevent another family from enduring the same hurt in the future.

I'm going to start our journey into the causes of suicide by telling the story of Niall. I am grateful to his parents, John and Ann, for allowing me the privilege of telling his story. I hope that their bravery will help others.

On 15 November 2002, Niall left his home for a night out. There was little that was different about him that day, other than that he had had a bad cold, and his mother, as all caring mothers do, had tried to persuade him to stay at home for the night. Niall was anxious to go out, however, so his dad, John, gave him a lift into the town centre at around 9.30. Little did John, or indeed the rest of his family, know that they would never see Niall alive again. A terrible tragedy was about to unfold.

It is useful at this stage to describe Niall. He was a fine young man, nineteen year of age, with his life ahead of him. He was the second-youngest of a family of five chil dren, a warm, loving and caring family unit where everyone looked out for each othe Niall was a good sportsman and was well liked and respected by his peers and friend alike. He was a quiet lad unless he was out socialising, when he was known for his sens of humour.

He had finished his Leaving Certificate a year before and had been very disappoint ed about not getting an apprenticeship to be an electrician, something he passionatel wanted to do. He was advised to do an electronics course in the regional college t improve his knowledge, with a view to getting an apprenticeship later.

He was a normal young man in all other aspects. He had one close friend who ha moved out of the area the previous year, but had plenty of acquaintances. Like all lad of his age, he dated girls, but apart from a previous relationship a year before, had n major relationship going on at the time. He worked part-time, like most students, in th pub at the weekend, but did not take alcohol the nights he was working.

Niall had only started taking alcohol at the age of eighteen and was not a very heav drinker – unlike many of his peers. He did go out, however, usually once a week for night out, when he was not working. This usually involved meeting friends in the pu and then sometimes moving on to a late-night disco. But Niall never arrived hom drunk and was never in any difficulties in relation to misusing alcohol. He was a typi cal modern young lad, behaving in what would be seen by his peers to be a complete ly normal manner. In the days and months before his death, there was nothing to sug gest that Niall was unwell or was unhappy in any way.

The first warning of problems appeared in the early hours of 16 November. Nial had a good friend who worked with him. They regularly shared a taxi to work, or on night out. His friend rang Niall on his mobile to arrange to meet to catch a taxi home Niall answered, telling his friend that he was down by the river. His friend immediate ly sensed that Niall was in trouble, and rushed down to find him. On arriving at the river, his friend found Niall in a very distressed state, wanting to throw himself in. His friend managed to calm him down, and tried to find out what was wrong. When he was asked about several possible areas of difficulties or stress, Niall replied that none of these were the problem. His next words revealed everything: 'It's just me.'

Thinking that things were now more settled, and that Niall was calm, they began to walk back along the river in order to get a taxi home. Suddenly, Niall left his friend's side and jumped into the cold, dark waters.

The next six weeks were a living nightmare for Niall's mother and father, together with all his family, close friends and peer group, for the river refused to hand up its dead.

Days and weeks passed, and no body came to the surface, despite heroic efforts by the local search and rescue team, aqua divers, local people, fishermen and others.

His family waited in great sorrow, and with wonderful dignity, for Niall's remains to be discovered. A family of deep faith, they trusted in the power of prayer and the goodness of all those who helped them in any way. They also struggled desperately to come to terms with why Niall had taken his own life. How did this lovely, quiet young lad, so loved by them all, find himself late at night by cold, unforgiving waters wanting to end it all?

Finally, in answer to their prayers and all the hard work of all the rescue teams, Niall's body was discovered, tangled in moorings not far from where he had jumped in. The grieving family was able to lay their son's body to rest at last.

Niall's death had a huge impact on many in his town, and has acted as a catalyst for many new initiatives to try to ensure that his death would not be in vain. His father John, a wonderful and inspiring man, does not want other families to experience similar pain and loss, and also tries to help others who are attempting to come to terms with similar loss

If Niall's death is to have real meaning, why it happened has to be examined. The following chapter is a search for the answer to this question.

2

The Biology, Causes and Prevention of Suicide

Suicide Versus Parasuicide

The basic difference between suicide and parasuicide is that suicide is a wholehearted attempt to kill oneself, and parasuicide is not. 'Para' means 'faulty', indicating that the act was not intended to kill but to mimic suicide, either to get attention or partially to satisfy the suicidal urge which plagues the person. When one is addressing the issue of suicide in Ireland, these two distinct groups need to be examined.

Parasuicide

Each year in Ireland, a large number of people will engage in parasuicidal activity. It is very difficult to put accurate figures on this phenomenon (as many cases go unreported), but some estimates put levels in the tens of thousands (probably between 50,000 and 60,000). From a medical perspective, this constitutes an epidemic.

Around 11,000 of these cases of deliberate self-harm (usually the most serious) will reach the casualty department. Forty percent of these individuals are between the ages of fifteen and twenty-four. Although worldwide figures indicate a higher number of females committing parasuicide, there is a roughly equal number of men and women in this group in Ireland. Around two-thirds of cases will be from city areas.

Parasuicide usually involves an overdose of medication such as Paracetamol or tranquillizers. Alcohol is usually also found in the person's bloodstream. Another popular, but less common, method of parasuicide is self-mutilation, and this is done primarily by males. My own region, that of the former North-eastern Health Board, has the highest rate of hospital admission of parasuicides in the country.

Parasuicide has traditionally been viewed as a cry for help – an indication that one is feeling suicidal, but not an attempt actually to kill oneself. Common events such as relationship breakdowns can combine with alcohol and lead to parasuicide.

Although this is a rational approach, it is also a naive one. A person who is attempting suicide or parasuicide is not in a clear state of mind. To suggest that there is always a distinct difference between those who kill themselves and those who simply harm themselves ignores the nature of the illnesses which can spawn both behaviours. Some experts see parasuicide and completed suicide in many cases as being part of a spectrum of deliberate self-harm.

Twenty-five percent of suicides are preceded by an act of self-harm the previous year. The fact that the other 75 percent showed no previous warning signs is worrying, and makes the task of preventing suicide extremely difficult. (This statistic must be read with caution, however, as an act of preceding self-harm among the latter group may have simply gone undetected.) In either case, this highlights the importance of screening for suicidal tendencies. Three-quarters of the time, these tendencies will be practically invisible.

Self harm is also starting to emerge in younger and younger individuals. Children, particularly in the ten-to-fifteen age group, are committing parasuicide more frequently, which is a worrying trend.

At least 80 percent of those who attend A&E departments following parasuicide will be admitted for careful monitoring of their psychiatric state. Their assessment, and investigation into what makes them unique, is crucial in preventing further acts of suicide and parasuicide.

SUICIDE

Those who are successful in ending their own lives represent a major challenge for researchers. In most cases, it is difficult to know with any certainty why they did it, and how they came to find themselves in a situation where that was the only choice that was available to them.

Every year in Ireland, around 450 people will commit suicide (the figures are 444 in 2003, 457 in 2004, and 432 in 2005). This may be a conservative estimate, yet it is still greater than the number of people who die in road-traffic accidents every year. Despite the fact that, worldwide, more women than men commit parasuicide, men are five times more likely than women to complete the act successfully. In 2005, a disturbing statistic revealed that 40 percent of the deaths by suicide recorded were young males under thirty-five! In comparison, more women take their own lives between the ages of fifty and fifty-nine.

Ireland lies fifth in the expanded EU for suicide among males in the fifteen-to-twenty-five age group. Of all those who commit suicide, 25 percent will come from this age group. Another quarter will come from the twenty-five-to-thirty-five age groups (23 percent in 2003). The fact that these victims are so young makes their suicide even more harrowing. It is an important statistic to report: if a form of cancer was specifically targeting this many young people between the ages of fifteen and thirty-five every year, there would be widespread concern.

I often wonder whether these statistics are an accurate estimation of the scale of the problem. How can one tell whether the many fatal road-traffic accidents involving young males late at night are deliberate? Some experts suggest a figure of 6 percent. Others may choose to drown themselves, and as suicide is often so unexpected, it may be considered an accident, rather than a conscious decision on the part of the victim. Every one of these hundreds of suicides destroys a family.

Methods of suicide will range from hanging (around 50 percent of cases) to drowning (20 percent), to massive overdoses. Unlike parasuicide, these are serious attempts to end the pain for good. In many cases, there is no warning of the impending suicide attempt. Although the attempt may look like an impulsive decision, the person will probably have had a definite method in mind for some time. These impulsive yet thorough acts of violence towards the self are the subject of this chapter. We cannot defeat suicide if we do not understand it.

Professor Patrick McKeown, medical director and founder member of Aware, estimates (along with many world experts) that there is a prevalence of mental illness in up to 90 percent of suicides. In other words, suicide is rarely the act of a healthy mind. The majority (between 60 percent and 70 percent) of cases are due to depression. The remainder are a mixture of addiction (10 percent to 15 percent) and schizophrenia (approximately 10 percent). Sometimes there is a personality disorder involved. Professor McKeown also believes that suicides are often triggered by loss and fuelled by alcohol. This is a valuable breakdown of the statistics, which helps us to understand the causes of suicide better.

THE BIOLOGY OF SUICIDE

Suicide is the end product of an illness in which the mood system is, biologically, in serious trouble, with a resultant loss of the normal control mechanisms which are so important to our survival. The rational, controlling part of the brain is swept away in a torrent of impulsive, self-destructive behaviour, which occurs as a direct result of illness (usually interacting with environmental influences) attacking the mood system. This process is usually preceded and triggered by a massive surge in the activity of the individual's stress system. The final act is often aided and abetted by alcohol. This may be a revolutionary interpretation for some readers of this book, and I hope that it will bring a great deal of comfort and relief to families who have lost loved ones to suicide.

Post-mortem neurological research into victims of suicide has revealed some interesting results. Our understanding of this area has also been advanced by neuro-imaging research on those who have survived suicide attempts. Genetic research into families with a history of suicide has also been of help. This research is beginning to reveal what is happening in the mood system before suicide. What follows are the results of this research, and an attempt to explain the possible relevance of such research. Once again, the flag system is beneficial in understanding this process. In suicide victims, the Green Flag of normal mood is definitely not flying.

The neurological basis of suicide lies in the behaviour box in the frontal mood department, and in particular one key section, which for the purpose of this discussion we will call the 'impulse control centre', or ICC. (The technical name of this area is the ventral pre-frontal cortex.) The ICC controls our tendencies towards impulsive thoughts and actions. The normal functioning of this box and this control centre depends in part on information supplied by parts of the serotonin mood cable (see Figure 1).

FIGURE 1: THE ROLE OF THE SEROTONIN CABLE AND BEHAVIOUR BOX IN SUICIDE

Suicide victims, following post-mortem studies, revealed evidence of severe depletion of serotonin in the part of the cable supplying the ICC. This in turn leads to a reduction in the activity of this structure – a key finding.

This depletion of serotonin, together with under-activity in the ICC, leads to impulsive thoughts of self-harm that may make the urge to kill oneself overwhelming. This phenomenon seems to be common to all cases of suicide, whether the victim is suffering from depression, addiction or schizophrenia.

The behaviour box has three very important functions that are relevant to our discussion:

1   It produces positive/logical thinking, and is the rational, controlling 'boss' of the mood system

2   It prevents violent behaviour towards the self or others; this is the function of the impulse box

3   It overrules negative thoughts emanating from the stress box

In suicide, due to the reduction of serotonin in the cable which supplies the behaviour box, these three functions are impaired. This leads to negative thinking, so prevalent in this illness, and the inability to problem-solve or see a way forward, and also explains the increased likelihood of self-harm and suicide.

The stress box produces the negative emotional thinking, but the old saying that 'trouble happens when responsible people stand back and do nothing' is quite applicable here. The behaviour box normally prevents trouble from happening by overruling these negative thoughts, and controlling impulsive thoughts and actions. Without an adequate supply of serotonin, however, the effectiveness of this box is greatly reduced.

The entire stress system is also dysfunctional in suicide. Stress peptides are elevated, and the adrenal glands are over-active, producing too much glucocortisol. This stress barrage causes chaos throughout the whole mood system and seems, in many cases, to have been present for some time before the person died. The noradrenalin mood cable has been found to be depleted, and this is felt to be further proof of a period of severe stress prior to the event.

These facts help explain why suicide occurs. The severe attack on the stress system, combined with a malfunctioning serotonin cable to the ICC section of the behaviour box, go a long way towards explaining why some people suffering from depression, schizophrenia and addiction are more at risk of impulsive self-harm than others.

The mood department areas that are disrupted are as follows:

THE FRONTAL MOOD DEPARTMENT

FIGURE 2: THE FRONTAL MOOD DEPARTMENT

A starvation of information due to a depleted serotonin cable renders key portions of the behaviour box, in particular the ICC, ineffective and lets impulsive thoughts of self-harm run rampant. This situation is worsened by a stress barrage attacking the behaviour box – a barrage which is initiated by the peptide system. Of note, the frontal mood department behaviour box is still developing up to the early to mid-twenties, which may put those in the fifteen-to-twenty-five age group at a greater risk of suicide. It is also a major player in both depression and schizophrenia. This fact is reflected in the statistics.

THE LIMBIC MOOD DEPARTMENT

The limbic system is also very much involved in the neurobiology of suicide. This is inevitable, since depression is so often present. This system also plays an important role in schizophrenia and addiction.

FIGURE 3: THE LIMBIC MOOD DEPARTMENT

231

The stress box is over-active in suicide; this has been borne out in both post-mortem and neuro-imaging of high-risk groups. This box is normally restrained and regulated by the behaviour box. When this control by the behaviour box is undermined by illness (in the Red Flag, for example, we noted that Area 25, the 'gateway' between the mood departments, was over-active or 'open', allowing just such a negative flow of thoughts to run riot), feelings of helplessness and hopelessness dominate, and suicide becomes more likely.

This box is also commander-in-chief of the stress system, and as a result is the architect of the stress response which seems to predate the suicide attempt. It is the source of the flood of stress peptides and, through its links to the adrenal gland, the glucocortisol barrage, which in turn attacks the behaviour box and further depletes the serotonin cable which supplies it.

THE ADRENAL GLAND

FIGURE 4: THE ADRENAL GLAND

Studies have shown that these glands are often enlarged in suicide. Adrenal glands increase when the demand for the stress hormone glucocortisol is increased at the command of the stress system. For this gland to increase in size, it would have to come under pressure for some time. This suggests that the body was under constant attack from stress for a period of time preceding the person's decision to take his or her own life.

GLUCOCORTISOL

FIGURE 5: GLUCOCORTISOL

This stress hormone is present in higher quantities in the bodies of those who have committed suicide. This excess level of glucocortisol damages the two mood departments and mood cables.

When they are combined, these findings show the common biological predecessors of the White Flag of suicide (Figure 6). They also suggest that mood-system difficulties are present in the victims of suicide for a period of time before their death. Due to the severity of the underlying illnesses of depression, addiction and schizophrenia, it can be very difficult for the person to explain how they are feeling.

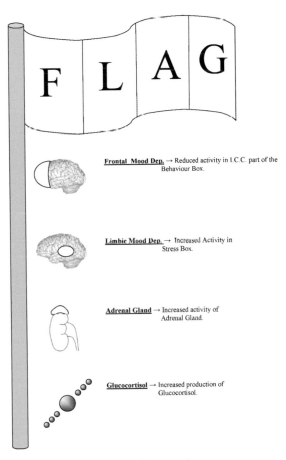

Frontal Mood Dep. → Reduced activity in I.C.C. part of the Behaviour Box.

Limbic Mood Dep. → Increased Activity in Stress Box.

Adrenal Gland → Increased activity of Adrenal Gland.

Glucocortisol → Increased production of Glucocortisol.

FIGURE 6

The link, for example, between the Red Flag of depression and the White Flag of suicide is obvious. Both display a reduction in serotonin-cable activity (due to serotonin depletion) and a constant stress response. In suicide, the depletion and stress barrage are particularly extreme. This suggests that in many cases suicide is simply the consequence of more severe (often hidden) forms of depression. This fact is borne out by clinical research.

But why is it that a greater number of people with depression do not experience severe suicidal thoughts, or that many more people who are experiencing depression, schizophrenia or alcohol or substance abuse do not take their own lives? The answer seems to lie in the ICC section of the behaviour box. Marked under-activity of this centre, and the serotonin cable supplying it, seems to a special risk factor.

This seems to be confined to a particular group who are at greater risk. So some people with this illness will not experience the same level of suicidal thoughts or behaviour. It may be that this impulsive self-harm trait lurks in the background and then, when depression arrives, with an accompanying general drop in both serotonin-cable activity and behaviour-box activity, it is unmasked. This trait also seems to be present in suicide involving the other illnesses mentioned above.

Research is already under way, particularly in the neuro-imaging area, into the behaviour-box changes which distinguish between the high-risk and low-risk groups, in the hope that we can pick out those who are at particular risk of suicide.

So there does seem to be a definite at-risk group in the community displaying a greater predisposition towards the above biological changes and corresponding symptoms. This group is probably created by a mixture of genes and environment, with the former probably being of greater importance.

There is some evidence, for example, that genetic deficiencies in a particular enzyme which helps to produce serotonin may exist in some families and individuals who are more likely to develop suicidal difficulties. Much more research needs to be done to pin down the genes that are responsible. It is important to note, however, that this underlying genetic potential is actualised by illness and major stress triggers in the person's life.

Whatever the underlying illness, these major biological disturbances help explain the stress, anxiety, severe emotional pain, and helplessness which precede suicide. Although suicide can seem sudden, impulsive, irrational and perplexing to an outsider, it is more likely to be the end result of a long period of severe emotional pain, low mood and stress.

In many cases, the final link in the biological chain of suicide is alcohol: the Great Pretender. For those who are battling low mood and suicidal thoughts, alcohol becomes a potent poison. Its short-term effects make it attractive to a person with depression: it reduces anxiety and lifts their spirits, but in the long term is equivalent to extinguishing a fire by throwing petrol on it.

Alcohol targets the section of the brain which prevents suicidal actions. It impairs the ability to make rational decisions, and to consider the true consequences of an action. By doing this, it removes the brain's last line of defence against suicide. Furthermore, as it is a depressant, it exaggerates the emotional pain the person is in. Thus it gives the depressive a greater motivation to attempt suicide, while removing any inhibitions they may have about completing the act. Under the influence of alcohol, the links binding those at risk to loved ones and the beauty of life are discarded, with the full impulsive suicidal drive from a failing mood system arriving – with deadly consequences.

Many who have survived major suicide attempts try to describe the pain and hopelessness they were feeling at the time. I have often been asked what biological changes bring these feelings about. I reply as follows: a constant stress barrage, excessive negative thoughts from an over-active stress box, a particular lack of activity in the ICC section of the behaviour box, and serotonin mood cable malfunctions. These cause low mood, anxiety, feelings of helplessness and hopelessness, impaired decision-making, and low self-esteem. For more on the neurobiology of suicide, see Appendix 1.

SUMMARY

Research into suicide has revealed the following:

1 The behaviour box, in particular one key section called the 'impulse control centre', in the frontal mood department (see Figures 1 and 2, on pages 229 and 231, respectively) is malfunctioning. This results in a lack of control by this part of the brain, which normally prevents suicidal thoughts and consequent impulsive actions.

2 The serotonin mood cable (see Figure 1 on page 229), which supplies this box is severely impaired. Many see this as the most important biological finding. This impairment contributes greatly to the breakdown of the behaviour box in suicide.

3 The limbic mood system (see Figure 3 on page 231), particularly the stress box, is over-active, giving rise to a huge surge through the stress system. The latter is also the source of many of the negative emotional thoughts of despair, hopelessness and helplessness that are so prevalent in those at risk of suicide.

4 The adrenal stress gland is often enlarged or over-active, releasing large amounts of the stress hormone glucocorticol and other stress peptides (see Figures 4, 5 and 6, on pages 232, 232 and 233, respectively). This may be the case for some time before the person's death. The stress box is the most likely culprit in initiating such anomalies.

Before leaving this section on the biology of suicide, let's match Professor McKeown's breakdown of the mental illnesses present in suicide with the above model.

DEPRESSION: THE RED FLAG

FIGURE 7

This is the most common illness (both on its own and combined with other illnesses, such as addiction and schizophrenia) present in suicide. In the Red Flag, all the mood cables and mood departments are affected. As this includes the serotonin cable and the behaviour box in particular, common sense dictates that suicide is a possible likely consequence of severe depression, especially if the person is in one of the high-risk groups discussed above.

It is quite likely that those who also have an underlying genetic predisposition to certain deficiencies in manufacturing serotonin, for example, may be more at risk of suicide than others. When depression arrives, with a secondary reduction in the activity of the serotonin cable, this underlying weakness may be exposed. This, as has already been explained, is why some people with the Red Flag seem more likely than others to self-harm.

One aggravating factor that may explain the number of suicides that stem from the male fifteen-to-thirty-five age group in particular is that these people are generally discouraged by society from openly expressing how they feel. Despite the fact that they may hate themselves, they put on a brave and unperturbed face that will not betray how they are feeling. They do not believe they can be helped anyway, so, as they see it, 'talking about it' will not solve anything. They may live in this sombre limbo state for a long time preceding suicide. When they cease to see a future for themselves and begin to review possible ways of ending their pain, suicide becomes a likely outcome. Clearly, in the Ireland of the new millennium, a great deal of work needs to be done to tackle this issue: 40 percent of suicides in 2005 were among males under the age of thirty-five.

The developmental immaturity of the frontal mood department will not help matters in the under-twenty-five group. Is this, combined with binge-drinking, the key to the increase in male suicides in this group? If illness combines with these factors, trouble looms. Binge-drinking interferes in particular with our glutamate system. Since activity in the behaviour box depends on glutamate, this can tip the already under-active section into serious trouble.

Men produce twice as much serotonin as women. This may partly explain why women are more likely to suffer bouts of depression. Is a major shortage of serotonin in males with depression more likely to lead to serious consequences, however? We can only speculate as to whether this biological difference is of any importance in explaining the disparity in suicide rates between the two groups.

Alcohol is a frequent and effective (albeit on a temporary basis) antidote for the symptoms of depression in those who are affected by it. It lifts mood and relieves anxiety, at least for a short period of time. Those suffering from depression will often seem quiet and self-absorbed, but will also expend a great deal of energy in order to appear 'normal' when they are with their peer group.

Many of our young men with the Red Flag are in pain, but hide it well through a combination of silence, seeming normality and alcohol. Some will spend a great deal of time on their own, sometimes in front of computers or video games or listening to music – anything to blot out how they feel. They are analogous to ducks on water, apparently floating effortlessly, but paddling furiously underneath.

The longer a person stays in this 'clandestine' state, the more prolonged the attack on the mood system by the body's stress system will be. The serotonin cable and frontal mood department begin to deteriorate under this pressure, and the behavior box malfunctions. The Red Flag turns white.

An important sub-group of the Red Flag, as noted earlier, are those who are suffering from bipolar mood disorder. These people, particularly those in a depressed or dysphoric state, seem to be particularly at risk in the earlier stages of the illness.

Because this illness is, in many cases, so difficult to diagnose, and because many may only present late, those who are at risk may never receive help. This, allied to their tendency to abuse alcohol and other substances, makes them a potentially high-risk group.

Obviously those in the fifteen-to-thirty age group are most at risk, because they will generally not recognise the symptoms, are slow to seek help, are in transitional stages of development, and are usually misusing or abusing alcohol. As a result, they are more likely to get into serious difficulties, often unnoticed by friends and family. Better training of both doctors and lay people in the recognition of the symptoms and signs of bipolar disorder, and indeed depression itself, might save many lives.

ADDICTION: THE PURPLE FLAG

FIGURE 8

Addiction leads in some cases to self-destruction, especially in the under-twenty-five age group. (In this group, the mood system, particularly the frontal cortex mood department, is especially vulnerable to addictive substances, as it is only slowly developing biologically.) Both alcohol and drugs (as dealt with in the Purple Flag) act primarily on the dopamine cable and the pleasure box, but they also interfere with many other parts of the mood system.

Addiction creates problems within the mood system, both in the form of direct biological effects on the cells of the mood departments and cables, and through the destruction of the fabric of the victim's personal life. There is also a robust link between addiction and depression – a fact that is only now being fully recognised.

Chronic alcohol and drug abuse destroys the life of the addict, adversely affecting their health, relationships, employment and financial security. Drug addicts will have to resort to crime to feed their addiction, ending up in conflict with those in authority, and subsequently being imprisoned, where their drug habit is likely to worsen. Homelessness is also a likely outcome.

Another often unrecognised risk factor for suicide is head injuries, which are common in this group due to falls and, in some cases, fights. Some experts feel that head injuries may damage crucial parts of the brain.

All of these factors obliterate self-esteem and lead to an overload on the body's stress system. In susceptible individuals, depression will result, along with a depletion of the serotonin mood cable, thus increasing these people's potential for self-harm. As the addiction worsens, so do the problems (both biological and social) facing the addict. Their general health, both physical and mental, declines. If they also harbour some of the at-risk traits that we have already dealt with, the risks reach a critical level. For some, there is only one way out: they raise the White Flag.

SCHIZOPHRENIA: THE GREY FLAG

FIGURE 9

Schizophrenia is a complex illness, and is usually treated by psychiatrists. This illness, which affects 1 percent of the population, is caused by malfunctions in the glutamate/dopamine neurotransmitter systems, combined with structural abnormalities in the frontal cortex and limbic mood departments.

Genetic contributions may combine with difficulties in the womb and delivery to cause these malfunctions. The condition usually presents in the early teens onwards. In this disease, a large amount of grey matter in the brain is lost during the ages of twelve to eighteen (which is why schizophrenia is referred to in this book as the Grey Flag).

Schizophrenia can cause damage to both the frontal cortex and limbic mood departments, resulting in a gradual withdrawal from reality. Delusions, auditory and visual hallucinations, paranoia, and thought disorders are among the symptoms.

Up to 50 percent of people with schizophrenia also abuse alcohol or drugs, and they are more likely to develop secondary depression alongside their existing illness. This group are at a high risk of suicide (especially early in their illness); despite their low prevalence in the population, they account for 10 percent of suicides. This mixture of alcohol and substance abuse, depression and schizophrenia produces a lethal cocktail which explains why the Grey, Red and White Flags often occur side by side.

PERSONALITY DISORDERS

There are two types of personality disorder which are susceptible to suicide.

BORDERLINE PERSONALITY DISORDER (BPD)

Among those with this disorder, women outnumber men by four to one in the USA (in Europe, the figures between the two sexes are more evenly spread). Ninety percent of such people come from a physically, emotionally or sexually abusive background. They have an unstable self-image and difficulties with personal relationships. They suffer from impulsivity, have difficulty in controlling outbursts of anger and in making key decisions, and regularly experience sudden shifts in mood. They live in a world of black and white, especially in their dealings with others. You may be their best friend one minute, and dismissed – or worse – the next!

Self-mutilation (cutting) is common, as are suicide attempts. The Red Flag of depression is commonly associated with this condition, as is anxiety. People with BPD regularly misuse or abuse alcohol and drugs, and can be highly manipulative.

They have been shown as a group to be very difficult to treat but, as noted in the Red Flag, DBT (dialectical behaviour therapy), as pioneered by the psychologist Marsha Linehan, has proved to be of great help, and is regarded by many as being the cornerstone of modern treatment for this condition.

Drug treatment with SSRIs has been shown to reduce the anger and thoughts of impulsive self-harm among people with BPD. If mood swings are a problem, mood stabilizers such as Lamictal or Lithium can be of great help. The risk of this form of treatment is the potential for a parasuicide attempt. Up to 8 percent of those with BPD, however, will be successful in committing suicide.

The serotonin cable has been shown to be depleted in those with BPD. Neuroimaging has also revealed excess stress-box activity and under-activity in parts of the behaviour box. This helps to explain the impulsivity, the links with depression, and the tendency towards self-harm among these people. Other biological features of BPD include an over-active noradrenalin mood cable.

ANTI-SOCIAL PERSONALITY DISORDER (ASPD)

This group is usually in conflict with the authorities from early childhood onwards, experiencing difficulties at school, at home and with the law. They tend to be violent, reckless and impulsive, abuse alcohol and drugs, and regularly assault others. They have a high incidence of both parasuicide and suicide. It is quite likely that the frontal behaviour box is once again involved in ASPD; a reduction in grey matter of up to 11 percent has been demonstrated in some cases.

Although the above personality types are more at risk of suicide than the population as a whole, it is important to understand that the majority of those who take their own lives will show no evidence of any major personality disorder.

THE CAUSES OF THE WHITE FLAG

To help understand the nature of the cause of the White Flag, it is useful to imagine a seed fed by fertilizers, sown in suitable soil, and germinated by the heat of the sun. The seed represents genes, and the fertilizer represents the stress triggers, which can be summed up in one word: loss. The fertile soil is the environment, and the sun represents alcohol.

THE SEED (GENETIC CAUSES)

Genes control all aspects of the mood system. In depression, addiction and schizophrenia, there are clear genetic predispositions. Genes are also important in the development of certain at-risk personality disorders.

In many cases of the White Flag (irrespective of any underlying illness), there may be a particular genetic predisposition for the serotonin cable to malfunction severely. Serotonin in the rest of the body (blood platelets) is at a very low level in suicide victims. Suicide tends to 'run in the family', and some interesting work has been done in such groups. We discussed earlier how one gene site involved in producing an enzyme crucial for the manufacture of serotonin has been examined to see if it could be the problem. This research revealed clear genetic differences between members of such families and those without such a history.

It is likely, however, that many more genes will be shown to play a part in the potential of an individual, irrespective of underlying illness, to self-harm. A full decoding of the body's genes will be necessary to reveal the full story.

THE FERTILIZER (LOSS)

The stress trigger activating many suicides is loss, of various types.

1   LOSS OF A RELATIONSHIP

There is an increasing trend towards marriage and relationship breakdown at all levels and ages in Ireland. Such separations are often associated with a great deal of bitterness and recrimination. Children are often used as pawns, forced to take sides between two people both of whom they love. This conflict and confusion may lead susceptible people to self-harm. Where there are children and young teenagers involved in the relationship, they too must struggle with the stress and loss of family security, and can be at risk.

For young men in particular (and young women to a lesser extent), the breakdown of a relationship is a serious stress trigger. In many cases, the response to the loss of a major relationship is to drink excessively. Alcohol will only worsen the situation, however, and make it more likely that the person, particularly if they are already vulnerable, will attempt some form of self-harm.

Although the break-up of the relationship will act as a trigger, the person may already have been suffering from poor self-esteem, low mood and an underlying genetic vulnerability for some time. The relationship may have been the only thing keeping depression and suicidal thoughts at bay, because it was a source of love and support. Therefore, once it ends, there is nothing to stop these depressive symptoms from taking over. Loneliness too is a common but often unwanted friend to those who suf fer from depression, and it often plays a role in the appearance of the White Flag.

2   LOSS OF LOVED ONES

Bereavement is a potent stress trigger which may lead at-risk people to suicide. Th death of a partner, child, sibling or close friend leaves a vacuum which is often fille only with pain and confusion.

Grief is a natural process that most people survive; this process usually consists c denial, realisation and, finally, acceptance. Sometimes, the grief is so profound that th body simply cannot cope with this process, and the person descends into depression The loss and depression combine to increase the risk of the White Flag of suicide. Th pain of bereavement can be so intense that death is seen as the only way to stop i Naturally, if the person is drinking, the coping threshold is greatly reduced. Wher brothers or sisters have committed suicide, or where a mother has lost her child, ther is an increased risk of suicide.

3   LOSS OF SELF-ESTEEM

Self-esteem relates to how we perceive and value ourselves. Losing one's sense of self worth removes another barrier towards suicide. It is a common result of bullying. Thi can occur anywhere where someone decides to assert their authority and make life misery for the person concerned, at home, in school or at work.

Children are very sensitive to bullying, and the trigger here must therefore be neu tralised as quickly as possible. If it is not, the annihilation of their self-esteem will lea to depression and possibly suicide, as a way of escaping the psychological torture the endure every day. It is important to ask young people about bullying, as they may b ashamed to talk about it. Bullying feeds on a feeling of helplessness. If children seen quiet, anxious or upset, the possibility of bullying must be addressed.

Bullying can occur in the schoolyard, on the way home from school, or in place where children play together. Children are often bullied by older siblings who are jeal ous of the younger child's popularity within the home. The bullying can be well hidde by those involved.

Bullying can also occur in the workplace, causing crippling stress and anxiety in th victim. This bullying can take the form of sexual harassment, or bullying by superior or work colleagues. In all of these cases, it can be difficult to know who to turn to fo help in dealing with the problem. The bullying may be too subtle to attempt legal actior over, but will nonetheless be extremely hurtful for the person involved. In this grouj also, suicide is in some cases seen as the only way out.

We mentioned in the Red Flag the particular problems experienced by youn; people in Northern Ireland who have been intimidated and bullied by paramilitar gangs. The profound effects of such thuggery have led many to take their own lives. This may be exacerbated by poverty and unemployment in some areas; all of these things reduce self-esteem.

Those incarcerated in prisons (particularly young men and women), those who live with addicts, and those who are victims of domestic abuse can also suffer a drop in self-esteem. The victims may feel that they are the problem and that the only way to fix the situation is to remove the problem through suicide.

Illiteracy is a little-noticed yet powerful cause of low self-esteem. People often leave school early for a variety of reasons, and as a result cannot read or write. I have counselled patients who have attempted suicide, only to find them deeply ashamed that they are illiterate. As this reduces their chances of gaining employment, they become frustrated and angry at themselves, and attempt self-harm. This issue must be brought into the open and addressed on a national level.

Low self-esteem is also a basic symptom of depression. Those with the Red Flag feel useless, worthless and deserving of their illness. They have no confidence in themselves. This may never be revealed to their family, and their inner world of self-hatred and low self-esteem ferments over time. As they feel that they are of no value, suicide does not seem like a big deal to them. Alcohol will help exacerbate their feelings of self-hate, and may remove any reservations they might have about completing the act.

4   LOSS OF IDENTITY

The role of men in society is not as clear-cut as it used to be. Women are enjoying new-found independence, financially and emotionally, as their roles in society have become more diverse. Men often feel that their role as provider and protector has been made redundant and are left wondering where they fit in.

Girls have always been more expressive emotionally, and more able to support each other when there is a problem, than boys. For men, to talk about one's emotions is seen not only as unbecoming of a man because it is somehow weak or effeminate but also as conveying a sense of incompetence when it comes to dealing with one's own problems.

This results in a feeling of dislocation from others, and a sense on the part of the man that he cannot cope with his problems. This reduces self-esteem substantially. Some men try to escape this dilemma by drinking excessively, but this often leads them to release their frustration in violent acts against themselves and others.

Females with depression are more likely to talk about their feelings and look for help. Men are more likely to try to deal with it themselves, increasing the risk of suicide as their mood system is gradually destroyed. Is this loss of identity, combined with a fear of talking about the problem, a major factor in the large number of suicides among young males?

5   LOSS OF EMPLOYMENT

For many people, their job is their identity, and the place from which they derive their sense of worth and satisfaction in life. To these people, the loss of their job delivers a devastating blow to their self-esteem. This can combine with the loss of financial security to make them depressed. This is particularly difficult for a person who is lacking in other skills, or who is of an age where they will find it hard to get work. The longer the period of unemployment lasts, the more under pressure the person feels. The body's stress system comes under attack as a result of constant anxiety about what the future holds, especially if there is a fear of having one's house repossessed.

Apart from these obvious financial concerns, the person begins to feel useless. The combination of financial insecurity, loss of self-esteem and loss of a defined role in life can lead the person to believe that they have failed their families and are of no use to anyone.

In some countries, such as Japan, this is exacerbated by an obsession with duty to family and a long tradition of seeing suicide as an honourable option. Although in Ireland the latter is not the case, there are still increased risks of depression and suicide in such cases.

6   LOSS OF FREEDOM

Prison is often the final stop on a difficult journey for many young men and women. A difficult upbringing and drug and alcohol addiction will clearly not help the self-esteem of these people either. Many feel they were born into a life devoid of hope or opportunity. The removal of their freedom through incarceration will only confirm this feeling of predestined suffering. Many will not be properly educated and may not be able to read or write. Some will already be suffering from the Red Flag of depression due to a combination of the above factors. Prison delivers the final blow to their self-esteem and suicide becomes an attractive solution. Our jails are also in many cases old and overcrowded.

These young people need professional help with their addictions, education deficit and mood problems – not a life behind bars. Prison does not solve any of their problems; it merely hides them and increases the risk of the White Flag.

Another group who are at high-risk of depression are the homeless, who have lost everything: their homes, loved ones, self-esteem and dignity. Many are dealing with chronic alcohol or drug problems and are suffering from the Red Flag of depression as a result. Others are suffering from the Grey Flag of schizophrenia, casualties of a poorly funded mental-health system.

Of the five thousand homeless people in Ireland today, 40 percent are thought to be suffering from mental illness. These people feel that no one will miss them, and that they are only a burden on society. They often take their own lives as a result

LOSS OF HEALTH

Many people with debilitating or chronic illnesses feel hopeless. Their sense of joy in life can be impaired, and they may feel that it is useless for them to go on living the way they do. Suicide may seem to be the only way out in some cases. Those who care for people with long-term illness are not immune from the stress of this situation either. They have sometimes made huge financial and personal sacrifices to care for loved ones. Loss of financial security, loss of freedom, and loss of self-esteem can also create a fertile environment for depression and suicidal thoughts to develop in the carer.

LOSS OF INNOCENCE

Those whose innocence in childhood is ravaged by sexual, physical or emotional abuse are at a lifelong risk of suicide. From an early stage of development in their mood system, this abuse creates a tendency towards living a life of anxiety, mixed with periods of low mood. This may facilitate suicide attempts later in life. The memory box in the limbic mood system has been shown in some cases to be reduced in size as a result of child abuse. Our past is indeed a part of our present.

THE SOIL (ENVIRONMENTAL INFLUENCES)

Just as a seed needs not only fertiliser but also suitable soil to flourish, so does suicide. A stress-free and supportive environment reduces the pressure on a person and their mood system. The opposite is also true.

MATERIALISM AND CONSUMERISM

The economy has undergone massive growth over the last ten years. This has been achieved at a high cost, however. Families and couples find themselves under increasing pressure to succeed financially in order to keep up with high mortgage payments and the rising cost of living. People are commuting longer distances and working longer hours. They find themselves under pressure to be financially successful, and often run into credit cards and other debt because they are living a life they cannot afford. This is another stress trigger.

Failure to reach these lofty financial goals makes young people feel like failures, unable to keep up with their peers. Sometimes, alcohol is used to blank out this feeling of worthlessness, leading in turn to a greater risk of self-harm. As long as self-worth is determined by the position you hold, the car you drive, or the house you live in, depression and suicide will be waiting for those at risk who don't make the cut.

2   SOCIAL ISOLATION

The French sociologist Emile Durkheim (1858–1917), renowned for his study and writings on suicide and religion, believed that the greatest deterrent to suicide in times of personal stress is a sense of identity and involvement with other people. Social isolation is a powerful environmental trigger in suicide. In many remote parts of the country, people are driven to the White Flag through a combination of loneliness, despair and depression.

Isolation need not only be physical. As technology advances, there is less and less need to communicate with other people, at least on a face-to-face level. This provides a dangerous breeding ground for depression and suicide. At home, televisions, DVDs and computer games have largely replaced conversation.

Technology eradicates the need for normal emotional expression, and can become a shield for many people with depression to hide behind. Watching television or playing computer games allows the person to avoid social contact, and their problems, and e-mail and texting reduce the need to talk in person.

For those who are feeling low enough to be considering suicide, it is vital that they can talk to someone about how they are feeling. They already feel lonely and isolated because of their illness. The silence that is promoted by technology ensures that no one will notice or understand the pain they are in. Without interpersonal communication there is no outlet for the person's emotions, and the White Flag can be seen as the only way out.

There are also worrying trends about overuse of the internet as a means of communication amongst our teenagers in particular. While the internet can be a positive development if it is used appropriately, many people worry about its potential for encouraging self-harm. One also must be concerned about the 'copycat' risks when suicide is glorified in communications between vulnerable twelve-to-twenty-year-olds. In general, there is concern that adolescents in particular are very vulnerable to the emotional 'hyping' or sensational reporting of suicide.

3   LOSS OF SPIRITUALITY

Ireland has gone from being a country that is heavily influenced and governed by the church to a more secular and affluent state. The church has been heavily hit by scandals of abuse and corruption. Religion has come to play a much smaller role than it did in the past. Are these changes, and the recent growth in suicide rates, just coincidence?

These changes in power and structure have had a number of important consequences. Firstly, the religious taboo which used to surround suicide has been broken. In the past, suicide was sometimes not mentioned by the family, due to the refusal

246

the church to bury the bodies of suicide victims in consecrated ground. As religion has come to play a smaller role (or no role at all) in people's lives, the concept of suicide as a mortal sin is no longer a deterrent to those who want to end the awful pain they are suffering. The documentation of suicide in the media has also contributed to the lifting of this taboo, with both positive and negative effects.

The second effect of this religious vacuum is more subtle, and difficult to quantify. An older generation still attempts to hold on to the value systems which they grew up with, but find it increasingly difficult to match these values with the world they are living in. The younger generation must devise their own value system, as they are not having one imposed on them. Materialism, money and hedonism, frowned upon by the old establishment, seem to many people to be the cornerstone of today's society.

Are they suitable and healthy replacements? Many experts agree that the dissipation of religious beliefs is removing a major inhibition towards suicide. If a person has no belief system, and consequently feels that life has no meaning, it is much easier for them to end their own lives in order to stop the pain.

THE SUN (ALCOHOL)

If the above ingredients are present in adequate amounts, all that is needed for the seed of suicide to germinate is the warmth of the sun. Alcohol is effective in helping people to forget life's problems and the pain one is feeling. As a result, it is a drug that is easily abused, especially in depressives. Alcohol frequently offers the final motivation needed to drive a person to suicide. It is a factor in more than 75 percent of young male suicides between the ages of fifteen and twenty-five. In one study carried out in my own North-east Region, alcohol was found to be present in more than 90 percent of male suicides in the under-thirty age group. It is particularly dangerous in the fifteen-to-twenty-five group, where its effects on the developing brain can be detrimental. It is perhaps little surprise that the more alcohol consumption per capita increases, the higer the suicide rate climbs, particularly in the younger age groups.

3

THE WHITE FLAG SUB-GROUPS

THE UNDER-TWENTY-FIVE AGE GROUP

In rare cases, children under the age of fifteen commit suicide. In 2003, 1 percent (suicides came from this group. Professor Carol Fitzpatrick of the Mater Chil Psychiatric Unit reported that, in the ten-year period from 1991 to 2001, forty childre under the age of fifteen committed suicide. She noted that a mixture of circumstance including relationship breakdown and a family history of depression and suicide, wa involved. The bulk of suicides in this group falls into the fifteen-to-twenty-five ag group, who make up 25 percent of the total number of suicides in Ireland.

Many will suffer from either diagnosed or undiagnosed depression, the latter by fa being the majority. Some are abusing alcohol to help cope with their problems. Thos who have been abusing alcohol or drugs from an early age seem to be a particularly a risk. Some may have had to deal with a family or personal relationship breakdown at critical stage of their development. Lack of self-esteem and lack of any belief systet are also key factors. Once a high stress trigger like the break-up of a relationship or th loss of a job is added, along with a binge of heavy drinking to numb the pain, suicid becomes a real risk.

In my opinion loss of self-esteem (often a warning sign of underlying depression loss of a major personal relationship and alcohol misuse, are the predominant risk fac tors in this group. In some cases the self esteem may be affected by prolonged alcoho or drug abuse. In others it may be severe bullying or abuse that starts the vicious circl In a small number of cases emerging schizophrenic illness will be the trigger.

This group is a naturally impulsive one. This is due to the delay in the maturing c their frontal cortex behaviour box. This is why impulsive suicidal behaviour is so com mon in this group.

Can we identify those at risk? This is the most important question asked in th book. The answer is yes, but with great difficulty. There are key warning signs:

§ Increased withdrawal in any form

§ Spending a lot of time alone in their room

§ Spending too much time communicating with the 'web'

§ Anxiety or agitation

§ Low self-esteem

§ Anger towards themselves or others

§ References to bullying of any form should be treated very seriously

§ A sudden increase in alcohol use (particularly binge drinking)

§ Fatigue, unexplained weight loss, or other common symptoms of the Red Flag

§ References to 'ending it all'

§ Listening to music which expresses suicidal thoughts

If we notice any of the above (or indeed any signs of the Red Flag) then we should inquire further.

There are also certain times in a young person's life which could be considered high-risk. At these times, parents, teachers, and friends, should be especially wary and vigilant. These include:

§ Recent break-up of an important personal relationship

§ Tragic death of a sibling through illness or suicide

§ Moving away from home for the first time to study or work (as this can be a time of loneliness and isolation from family and friends)

§ Failure in an important exam or job interview as this can damage self-esteem

§ If evidence of serious bullying is uncovered – this I feel is a key danger time, especially if the young person fears retaliation for opening the 'can of worms'

A sudden escalation of drinking is often a warning sign. As alcohol levels rise in this group, so do risks of impulsive suicidal behaviour. If a change in drinking habits occurs after a serious loss of any kind, then this risk is amplified.

If you are concerned, do not be afraid to openly bring up the area of depression with the young person. Ask if any thoughts of self harm are present in the young person's mind, better sooner than later. It's a fallacy to assume that such questions put the ideas into their heads.

Two useful questions to ask are: Do you see any future for yourself and if you were to harm yourself how you would do it? If the answers are that the person sees no future for themselves and if they share with you how they would harm themselves, then you know they are in serious trouble. The latter shows that they have thought a lot about the possibility. Often it will turn out to be a relief for the young person to share such feelings, and realise they are being listened to.

If worried do not hesitate to invade the young persons room or space to scan their diaries even if you feel very ill at ease about this. Talk to their friends, many of whom know much more about what is going on in the young person's life. Try and build up a picture of where the young person is at. Do not hesitate to openly discuss loss or to challenge the effects of alcohol and its negative effects. Above all, do not do nothing.

Often giving the young person a book about mood will help, as its may act as a vehicle to get them to talk about how they feel, and to help them realise they are unwell and there is something that can be done to help them. If they admit to a problem, encourage the young person to see the family doctor for further help and referral if necessary.

I know that there will be a special group of people who will be reading this section feeling a mixture of grief, loss and possibly guilt. These are the families of those who have successfully attempted suicide.

Many will carry a lifelong burden of guilt and a feeling of personal responsibility. To all of you I say; you must let go of this burden. In so many cases despite the best efforts of their families the young person will skilfully hide how they feel so they won't be a burden on you. They may even think their feelings are normal. Some will use turn to alcohol, making it difficult to separate the effects of the drug from the illness itself. Many have underlying (often unrecognised) genetic predispositions towards depression and suicide only triggered by loss, alcohol or both.

Young people in this group are usually moody and quiet anyway, and often misuse alcohol. As a result it is difficult to sift out those at risk. It's vital to accept that suicide is the result of an illness. You are not responsible for a young person losing their lives to this illness. The finger in many cases should be pointed squarely at alcohol. This substance is more responsible than any other factor for suicide in young people.

THE TWENTY-FIVE-TO-THIRTY-FIVE AGE GROUP

This is a subgroup of the White Flag of suicide that doesn't in my opinion get the attention it deserves. According to Irish suicide statistics of the past five years, almost as many people have died between twenty-five and thirty-five, as between fifteen and twenty-five, (in 2003, 23 percent). Once again, there is a predominance of males in these figures (four to one.)

The fifteen-to-twenty-five age group tend to grab the headlines. Loss of life is always upsetting, but is especially poignant when the person is so young. By the age of twenty-five, the mood system is fully mature. By this stage, most young people are relatively settled emotionally, and are looking forward to a life of promise in work and

lationships, looking forward to starting a family. They have left behind the impulsive
xuberance and emotional swings of adolescence and have developed a healthy balance
etween emotion and logic. So why do so many kill themselves?

MENTAL ILLNESS

ddiction, schizophrenia, and depression are the primary culprits. Severe abuse of
lcohol and substances over many years, may lead to depression and suicide attempts
1 this group. Schizophrenia, particularly if untreated, becomes more pronounced, and
nis, along with alcohol and substance abuse, make this group prone to suicide.

The majority are suffering purely from the Red Flag of depression. As a family doc-
or, I am often astonished at the number of young men who appear in their late twen-
es and early thirties; opening up for the first time in their lives about the emotional
urmoil they have been in since their mid teens. They have suffered for over a decade
efore finally being able to say 'this is how I feel'.

There are many more in the 25-35 age group who are in pain and are not seeking
elp. Why is this the case? Is it a reflection of the intolerance society shows to those
vho admit to suffering from this illness? Or is it due to the lack of awareness of the
Red Flag of depression?

Depression remains hidden, concealed under a mask of normality. The deep-seat-
d emotional pain experienced by many in this group, is analogous to a tumour grow-
ng inside them that is killing them slowly.

Those within this group, who have already been successfully treated for a bout of
he Red Flag in their early twenties, and find themselves suffering from a relapse, may
eel totally dejected. They wonder what point is there in seeking help again. They just
eel like they are complaining and annoying everyone again. This negative thinking can
ead them to view suicide as the only way out.

Negative thoughts are the chains that bind someone with low mood. People suffer-
ng from depression believe that it is normal to be in such pain, and that they don't
leserve to feel any better. If they open up they will only be ridiculed anyway, which will
nake them feel worse again.

Negative thinking is a warning sign that the mood system is damaged. If more peo-
ble were aware of this, it could become easier for young people (especially men) to
come forward for help. Otherwise the Red Flag will continue to be the main provider
of future victims to the White Flag.

2   ENVIRONMENTAL FACTORS

By the mid to late twenties, most young people have a general idea of where their careers and lives arc going. This is also the time when many will settle into long-term relationships. In our society, there is the assumption that people will have 'sorted themselves out' by this age. This has become an increasingly unrealistic goal for many. Those who haven't achieved these goals feel like failures. They may feel quite lost, unsure of where they are going, envious of others who have succeeded in finding their path in life.

When a person is already feeling down, the knowledge that everyone around them is buying houses, starting families, rising up the career ladder and seemingly happy, it is difficult to see where their own role lies. This uncertainty and frustration can develop into suicidal thinking and behaviour.

The nature of relationships too has changed dramatically over the last twenty years. They are now more numerous and fluid. Sometimes they involve children and sometimes not. Some young men, in particular, are unable to cope with this emotional turbulence. Many place too much of their emotional future in relationships, which later break down, and then struggle to cope with the consequences of such a split.

Loneliness too plays a part. This can apply as much to remote rural areas as towns and cities. As society grows more fragmented and technological, many find themselves isolated and without anyone to talk to.

Loss of personal relationships, isolation, an absence of financial success, and depression, are some of the contributing factors to suicide in this group. Young men must be encouraged to vent feelings of loneliness and isolation. If they could open up in this way, many suicides could be averted.

3   ALCOHOL

Alcohol fosters suicidal thoughts and behaviour in this group also. For many it is the temporary cure for low mood, insecurity, alienation, and loneliness. Eventually it drops their mood further, and increases the risk of serious, impulsive suicide attempts.

For those who are unable to express themselves, alcohol is a deceptive friend, numbing the pain for a while, before encouraging them to express themselves in an extremely violent manner.

THE OVER-THIRTY-FIVE AGE GROUP

Here things become a little clearer. The primary cause of suicide in this group is the Red Flag of depression, with alcohol and substance abuse coming in a close second. It is more likely individuals in this group will come forward for treatment.

Often depression is triggered by the loss of a relationship, bereavement, or financial insecurity, with a subsequent loss of self-esteem. Again alcohol acts as a suicidal catalyst. In other cases, particularly in males 45 and over, living in very isolated situations (urban or rural) will be the main cause of depression and suicide.

In this group there are also cases of recurring depression with previous suicide attempts. Patients with bipolar depression also may fall into this group.

In the elderly illnesses like depression, dementia with depression, chronic illnesses like Parkinson's disease all increase the risk. Cultural differences can be of great importance. For example in some Asian countries the majority of suicides occur in the over-seventy-five group, the exact opposite of Ireland. Obviously different factors are at play in such cases.

Risk factors in this age group include:

§ Emotional isolation

§ Geographical isolation

§ Family history of depression or suicide

§ Recent major loss

§ Alcohol abuse

§ Increasing age (particularly men over 75)

§ Previous attempts at self harm

§ The presence of elderly depression or dementia with depression.

Once again, a better public understanding of the Red Flag and how it presents would encourage more at risk people to come forward for help.

4

THE PREVENTION OF SUICIDE

Can suicide be prevented? We may never be able to eliminate suicide from society completely, but a number of steps can be taken which will reduce the incidence of suicide by encouraging people to come forward for help. These are the factors which, in my opinion, need to be analysed in order to help prevent suicide:

1   MENTAL ILLNESS

There are three main mental illnesses:

(A)   ADDICTION

Addiction creates a downward spiral into hopelessness and despair, and is often linked to underlying depression. This combination can lead to suicide. Encouraging addicts to develop an insight into their illness and to seek help is a difficult task. If they have lost everything, are homeless or are in prison, the risk of suicide is very high.

Warning signs of suicide in this group are symptoms of depression, a complete disregard for personal appearance, and an increase in impulsive and violent behaviour. Other indicators are recent major loss, either of a relationship or of financial security.

Those who are in contact with such individuals should be aware of these warning signs, and encourage the person to go for help if necessary. The addiction wall of those who are suffering from the Purple Flag will often resist such help, however. Until new and improved ways of dealing with addiction are forged, this group will continue to be at a high risk of suicide.

(B)   SCHIZOPHRENIA

This illness is often very subtle in its presentation, and its diagnosis is delayed if alcohol or substances are being abused, which occurs in up to 50 percent of cases. Earlier diagnosis and treatment, and improved help and support for both patients and families from the community and health services, focusing particularly on those who are misusing alcohol and substances, could greatly reduce the number of people who take their own lives.

We can pick out some useful information from what is known about the risks of suicide in this illness:

§ Many who die by suicide do so at a relatively young age and within ten years of diagnosis

§ Many will have misused alcohol or drugs

§ They are more likely to have had a chronic course of the illness, with more relapses and hospital visits

§ They are more likely to be male

§ They are more likely to have a family history of suicide

§ They may be more impulsive or aggressive in nature

§ They may have concomitant depression

Although the above can act as a guide when it comes to identifying at-risk people, it remains quite difficult to prevent many people with this illness from attempting to take their lives.

The overall risk of suicide among people with schizophrenia is estimated to be forty times greater than among the general population, and thirty to fifty percent of people with schizophrenia will attempt suicide at least once in their lives. There is clearly a great deal of work to be done in this area!

c)   DEPRESSION

Depression remains the largest single driving force behind suicide. This includes both unipolar and bipolar depression. The major complication with regard to suicide is the symptom of negative thinking. People who suffer from this illness believe that life is hopeless, that treatment will be ineffective, and that it is a waste of time for them to talk about how they feel.

There are two sub-groups here: those who are receiving help, and those who suffer in silence.

THOSE WHO HAVE BEEN DIAGNOSED WITH DEPRESSION

Suicide victims in this group may have only partially responded to treatment, be resistant to treatment, have experienced major stress triggers such as loss, or may have been treated successfully, only to relapse into another bout. Some may be using alcohol to self-medicate, making impulsive behaviour more likely.

Preventing suicide in this group depends on a high level of involvement from family, friends, health professionals and others. Any statements referring to hopelessness or suicidal thoughts, even of the most trivial nature, must be taken seriously. Those suffering from depression must be discouraged from drinking. In the fifteen-to-thirty five age groups, any sudden change in behaviour can be a warning sign. There is some evidence that CBT is particularly useful in challenging the negative thinking that is so pivotal in this condition. People with bipolar disorder in this group need specialist help as they are very vulnerable.

II   THOSE WHO SUFFER IN SILENCE

The real difficulties lie with this group. It is difficult to fight an enemy you cannot see These individuals will rarely open up to those who are close to them, let alone to a doc tor. The solution to this problem lies in developing a common understanding of the Red Flag. Depression needs to be discussed openly, in homes, schools, colleges and workplaces, and in the media.

Aware, for example, are running a programme called 'Beat the Blues' in many schools. This is a depression-awareness programme that was started in 1994 and i designed for senior classes in secondary school. It is run by Aware's education officers who visit the school to provide information on depression, mental health and suicide show a video of young people talking about their experiences with depression, and fin ish up with a question-and-answer session.

Initiatives such as this one should be supported and encouraged: the emotional stig ma surrounding this illness needs to be lifted. In particular, we need to look at new and innovative ways of reaching the fifteen-to-thirty-five-year-olds. I feel that tackling this problem, and alcohol misuse, is the secret to reducing the number of tragic deaths among our young men in particular.

2   UNDERLYING STRESS TRIGGERS:

These can be summarised in one word: loss. Loss of a vital relationship, a loved one, a job, financial security, freedom, or of self-esteem due to bullying can all act as triggers If we are aware of the potential of the above to damage the self-esteem of a person and how, in those at risk, this can lead to suicide, we can be on the lookout for the warning signs.

3   THE ROLE OF ALCOHOL

To understand the role alcohol plays in suicide, one only has to look at the statistics The higher the alcohol consumption per capita, the higher the suicide rate. In Ireland for example, in 1960 total alcohol consumption per person in the over-fifteen age group was five litres per person and the suicide rate was 2 per 100,000. By 2000, the total alcohol consumption in the same group had risen to 14.2, and the suicide rate had increased to 11 per 100,000. (These figures are from the interim report of the Strategic

Task Force on Alcohol, 2002.) If a person is suffering from low mood and negative thinking, alcohol should be avoided completely. The over-reliance on alcohol in Irish society when it comes to dealing with various personal difficulties needs to be dealt with in order to reduce the risk of suicide among at-risk individuals. We as a society need to tackle this evil, and all of us must play our part.

THE ROLE OF CRISIS INTERVENTION

A person who is feeling suicidal is at a crisis point in their lives. They are in great inner pain from a diseased mood system. In the same way that severe chest pain can be a warning sign of a heart attack, this deep-seated pain is a warning of suicide. Crisis intervention plays an important role in two groups: those who make contact with a friend, relative or health professional before they attempt suicide, and those who survive a serious suicide attempt.

(A)   CRISIS INTERVENTION IN THE PRE-SUICIDE GROUP

Here, the person may open up to a friend, family member or, quite often, a Samaritan's counsellor. The aim of these interventions is to calm the person, to try to help them deal with any immediate stress triggers, and to advise them to avoid alcohol. The next step is to encourage them to seek help from a trained professional: a doctor, nurse or counsellor. Similar attempts to head off suicidal episodes are carried out by river-watch patrols, Aware, self-help groups in colleges and other organisations.

If you, the reader, ever find yourself in such a situation, stay with the person until help can be provided by a professional. Encourage the person to tell you how they feel, and to avoid alcohol. If you are suspicious that somebody may be feeling suicidal, do not be afraid to ask them directly if they are thinking about suicide. Often, the answer will be a relieved 'yes'.

Sometimes just being able to open up to another person, not necessarily a professional, can be the catalyst for the person to seek real help. I often feel that the busyness of our modern lives prevents us from offering the 'sympathetic ear and the caring word', which can often transform the lives of many of those who are suffering in pain and in silence. Is it the loss of this wonderful Irish tradition that is helping to fuel depression and alcohol misuse in our young people, which in turn is leading to so much tragedy?

(B)   CRISIS INTERVENTION FOLLOWING A SUICIDE ATTEMPT (PARASUICIDE)

There has been an explosion in positive measures by the Irish health system to follow up on those 11,000 people each year in Ireland who will attend casualty departments following attempted suicide. There has been provision of specialised personnel at hospital level, and most health boards have appointed a suicide officer to coordinate work in this area.

Once the person's medical condition has been established, they must be assessed to understand the particular crisis that led to the event. Was alcohol involved? Were there obvious signs of depression or other mental illness? The better the screening and subsequent follow-up by psychiatrists, GPs and counsellors, the more likely it is that a successful intervention will take place before a further suicide attempt is made. At present, up to 25 percent of suicides will come from those who self-harm , so they are an obvious target for preventative screening.

5   WHAT CAN BE DONE TO HELP?

(A)   AS INDIVIDUALS

§ Learn the symptoms of the Red Flag. Be vigilant and open to the possibility of this illness being present in yourself and those close to you, whether at home or at work.

§ Offer help and support to those who are suffering from illnesses of the mood system. If a friend starts to talk about feelings of hopelessness, do not be afraid to ask them about suicidal thoughts. Often, this may ease the person's pain by allowing them to express how they feel. Always follow this up by encouraging them to go for professional help.

§ Never add to the burden of those with depression by trivialising their condition or regarding them as inferior.

§ Never try to stop a person from using medication for depression or any other illness of the mood system. To do so may put them at risk. Courses of medication should be started and stopped only by a professional.

§ Make an effort to stamp out bullying in any form, and don't be afraid to challenge those who bully vulnerable people.

§ Have open conversations about mental illnesses with family and friends.

§ Examine your personal drinking habits, diet and supplements, and the role of exercise in your life. Encourage others to do likewise.

§ Practise the art of unconditional self-acceptance and encourage it in others.

§ Remember, if you can help even one person who is at risk, you may save their life.

(B)   AT HOME

§   Look out for the warning signs (as already detailed) of depression and suicidal thinking.

§   Discuss regularly the whole area of stress and how to handle it.

§   Open up these areas as general topics for conversation.

§   Establish clear, healthy boundaries of behaviour, particularly in the area of alcohol.

§   Monitor carefully the use of computers by teenagers, particularly the use of internet chat-rooms.

§   Talk about the effects of alcohol on mood. Examine and discuss the role and importance of exercise, diet and supplements (particularly fish oils).

§   Do not be afraid to approach someone in the house who you feel is at risk.

§   If a family member with depression suddenly seems to become 'peaceful' after they had previously been very agitated, it may be that they have made a decision to attempt suicide. In such cases, do not be afraid of gently opening up this possibility with them.

§   Keep a lookout for any stockpiling of medication.

§   Try and improve the 'problem solving' abilities of our children and young adults.

Sometimes, it can be very difficult to see the warning signs of suicide in a person you live with: you are too close to them. Take a newspaper and hold it two feet in front of your eyes, and you can read it without difficulty; take the same paper and bring it right up to your eyes, and it becomes a blur. So too, the warning signs of depression, anxiety and potential suicidal behaviour can become blurred when you are very close to the person involved. This is why parents should try to keep in close contact with their young people's friends, as these people can be an invaluable source of information on their offspring's mood.

(C)   AT WORK

EMPLOYERS:

§   Become fully aware of the symptoms of these illnesses and the suffering they cause.

§   Offer help and support to those in trouble.

§ Acknowledge that, if the workplace is rigid, bullying or authoritarian, the self-esteem of employees will be damaged.

§ Be prepared to approach any employee who is at risk, in a caring and concerned manner, to talk about how they are feeling.

CO-WORKERS:

§ Treat co-workers with respect.

§ Never bully or ridicule those whose mood is clearly down. You may play a role in them ending their lives if you do!

§ Do not mock or denigrate those on drug treatments for depression.

§ Encourage open discussion of these subjects.

§ If a colleague seems to be in trouble, do not be afraid to approach them.

§ Do not put pressure on people to drink too much, especially in after-work drinking sessions; this can be a lethal trigger if the person is already feeling down.

(D)   IN SCHOOLS AND COLLEGES

§ As teachers, encourage regular discussions about these illnesses.

§ As individual teachers, try and build up some knowledge of depression.

§ Examine the role of relationships, alcohol and self-esteem in the development of mental health. Also promote the importance of diet, exercise and supplements.

§ Intervene quickly in any cases of alleged bullying. You may only get one chance to do so. Involve parents immediately.

§ Pay special attention to those who are having difficulties keeping up with school-work or attending school.

§ Be alert for those who may have slipped through the system and are struggling to read and write. Try to keep a close eye on children and young people from homes that you feel may be at high risk.

§ Encourage students to get together in small groups to discuss how they feel. This is an important tool in uncovering somebody who is at risk of suicide.

As part of the prevention package suggested by *Suicide in Ireland: A National Study*, published in 2001, the teaching of life skills was recommended as part of the school curriculum. These would involve coping skills in an emotional context, assertiveness, self-esteem and confidence-building.

Of note also is the active role that universities and colleges are taking in this area.

These institutions have many excellent self-help groups, some started by students themselves, which provide a safe and supportive environment in which those who are feeling down can express themselves.

(E)   AS A COMMUNITY:

§ Distribute information on these illnesses on a widespread basis, just as is the case with diabetes and heart disease.

§ Use the media to provide this information.

§ Encourage the media in particular to become fully informed about the Red Flag and to become more responsible in how they deal with it. For example, implying that the use of drug therapy is inferior to the use of psychotherapy (even though the availability of the latter is quite limited) may lead to confusion in the mind of a person with mental illness. As stated earlier, absolutism in relation to treatment must take second place to the diagnosis and acceptance of depression.

§ Encourage the media to avoid dramatising or sensationalising suicide. Much more emphasis should be placed on the extreme hurt and loss felt by those who are left behind. This may act as a deterrent to some people who are considering taking their own life. I feel, however, that recently the media has started to realise the importance of its role in this area, and to behave accordingly.

§ Treat bullying as something none of us will accept under any circumstances.

§ Encourage proper monitoring of the internet.

§ Support groups like Aware which do good work in helping those with mental illness.

§ Everyone needs to work within their own communities with young people to encourage people to take part in sport and other healthy options, and to keep an eye out for those who seem to be heading down the 'wrong roads'.

§ Try to foster a new approach towards good mental health.

§ Educate those who are most likely to come in contact with young people (males in particular), such as youth workers, those involved in sport, police and probation officers, on the symptoms of the Red Flag and at the signs of being at risk of suicide.

§ Target the common means of suicide. Control should be exerted over the sale of drugs like paracetamol, and the sale of ropes and pesticides to young males in particular, and guns should be tightly controlled. There should also be night patrolling of common 'suicide black spots', particularly rivers in major towns.

(F)   THE HEALTH SYSTEM

§   Constantly update skills to ensure that those at risk are picked up in time.

§   Provision and training of specialised nurses who will specifically deal with cases of self-harm in A&E departments.

§   Better training of family doctors in the recognition of symptoms of depression and the warning signs of suicide. This is seen by some as the linchpin of any approach to reducing the numbers of people who take their own lives.

§   Improve cohesion between crisis-management nurses in hospitals, GPs and psychiatrists, to ensure that nobody 'slips through the net'.

§   Provide a wider range of counselling services and psychological help (particularly CBT) to those who need it.

§   Target alcohol misuse as a priority area.

6   SPECIAL HIGH-RISK GROUPS

Certain groups are more vulnerable to suicide than others. These include:

§   Those with a strong family history of major depression or suicide

§   Those who have experienced the death of a sibling or a child

§   Families with histories of major upheaval through addiction, abuse and relationship breakdowns (particularly if acrimonious)

§   The homeless

§   Young people in prison aged between fifteen and thirty-five

§   Schizophrenics abusing alcohol or substances

§   Schizophrenics who are male, have a history of multiple relapses and hospital admissions, and are aggressive or impulsive

§   Those suffering from personality disorders

§   Those who are isolated, or have difficulties forming relationships

§   Those who express any thoughts of a suicidal nature

§   Parasuicides, i.e. those who have attempted suicide or self-harm before

§   Young people under thirty-five who are impulsive and violent, are abusing alcohol, and who may come from an addictive background

§   Young men under thirty-five, particularly if they are suffering from low mood, or who may be misusing alcohol following the breakdown of a serious relationship

§ Young men and women suffering from bipolar disorder, particularly if they are abusing alcohol

7   WARNING SIGNS OF SUICIDE

§ Increased levels of agitation or anxiety

§ Disruption in sleep patterns

§ Misuse of alcohol or substances

§ Recent loss of a serious relationship, especially if accompanied by an increase in binge drinking

§ In students, a drop in hygiene, and reduced performance or non-attendance at school

§ Withdrawal in any form from everyday social contact, particularly in men under thirty-five

Major signs of the Red Flag at any age include:

§ Impulsive, violent gestures

§ Any expression of self-harm or wanting to 'end it all'

§ A major change in someone who is known to suffer from unipolar or bipolar depression

§ A sudden peacefulness in somebody who has previously been very agitated or very down

If you notice any of the above warning signs in someone you know, encourage them to open up and talk about how they feel. If they are feeling down, or are having suicidal thoughts, they need to get help.

8   THE FUTURE ROLE OF BIOLOGY IN THE PREVENTION OF SUICIDE

Biology has helped us gain a more comprehensive understanding of these mental illnesses. The hope is that future research will help to identify those who are most at risk, amongst the many who present for help. Possible areas that may offer valuable findings in future are:

§ Conducting brain scans on those in high-risk groups to identify those with low serotonin levels or low behaviour-box/ICC activity.

§ Major research through both scanning and genetic testing on survivors of very serious attempts to self-harm. A large research project of this type, by Professor

263

Kevin Malone of UCD, is under way at present. It is hoped that the findings of this study will help reduce the number of suicides in future.

§ Looking at markers, such as the platelet receptors in our blood, as a means of identifying those who are suffering from low serotonin levels.

§ Genetic research into identifying high-risk genetic groups which could be targeted more effectively. Further research may also produce cleaner, more effective drug treatments for the treatment of depression, schizophrenia and addiction. This in turn may encourage sufferers to come forward.

I personally feel that we might learn a great deal about suicide through a major research project in Ireland (with the express permission of the families of those bereaved) to examine the post-mortem brains and bodies of those who died by suicide before the age of thirty-five.

Is there a unified theory of suicide?

Just as in depression and addiction, the possibility of putting together all the genetic, biological, psychological, social and other factors which cause suicide together into a unified theory has become the modern Holy Grail for those who aim to reduce the incidence of this illness. Once again, psychologists, psychiatrists, sociologists and biologists are all pooling their knowledge to make this happen.

So let's see what we know to date. As always, we start with genetics. Many studies have found that genes play a major role in a person's predisposition towards suicidal behaviour. Genes, along with environmental influences, play a key role in (i) predisposing us to the development of illnesses such as depression, addiction or schizophrenia (see the Red and Purple Flags), (ii) the development of at-risk personalities, (iii) determining how we will handle stress for the rest of our lives and (iv) the creation of specific biological weaknesses such as a lack of the enzymes needed to produce neurotransmitters such as serotonin.

Early environmental factors are the next part of the equation. Growing up with abuse, poverty, addiction or the loss of a parent or sibling (either from suicide or as a result of sudden death from other causes) at a crucial stage of emotional development creates the possibility, when combined with genetic influences, that the person may at some stage in their lives be more at risk of suicide.

As the person reaches adolescence and early adulthood, all of these factors combine to determine how well they will be able to cope with the stresses that this phase throws up: gradual separation from parents, dealing with the explosive nature of relationships and sexuality, bullying, loss of form, the pressure of exams and starting college or work, the emergence in some cases of latent illnesses such as depression and learning to handle the delights and dangers of alcohol – to name but a few. This mix of genes and early environmental influences will also determine how well these people 'problem-solve' when such stresses appear. It is now recognised that this is very important in suicide.

Suicide occurs at this stage mainly due to an emerging illness such as depression or schizophrenia. This often combines with an innate inability to handle stress or problem-solve (for all the reasons mentioned above) and a tendency to binge-drink as a means of dealing with all these issues.

This knowledge provides us with several different ways of trying to prevent suicide in this group. Improving our detection and treatment of depression, for example, would definitely reduce the risks, as would the teaching of better life-coping and problem-solving techniques. It goes without saying that reducing the easy availability of alcohol to young people in off licences and nightclubs would potentially save many lives every year. Other areas, such as diet and nutrition, may also prove to be more important than we imagine. A well-nourished, well-exercised brain may protect against many of the stresses to which the young person at risk is exposed.

As the person moves into their late twenties and early thirties, a similar combination of illnesses, life stresses and alcohol misuse or abuse come together to create the potential for suicide. Once again, an inability to handle stress, and poor problem-solving skills, are prevalent. In middle age, depression and addiction (sometimes both combined) often combine with social or personal isolation and alcohol to create a risk of suicide. The same lack of coping skills may also be present middle-aged people. In old age, apart from the presence of all of the above factors, physical damage to the brain, from vascular damage and major strokes to secondary illnesses such as Parkinson's disease or dementia, may also play a role in a person's potential risk of suicide.

In most cases, apart from illnesses caused by old age, certain biological and psychological traits are present. Many people, whether suffering from depression, schizophrenia or addiction, who take their own lives are impulsive, have difficulties coping with life's problems (sometimes even minor ones), do not handle stress well, have poor problem-solving skills, often end up 'in a corner' surrounded by helplessness and hopelessness, and tend to use alcohol as a crutch to deal with both of these things. This model fits with the biological model, where low serotonin (associated with impulsive behaviour) and a hyperactive stress system are the most important factors contributing to the risk of suicide.

In summary, suicide can occur due a cocktail of genetic, environmental and biological factors, all of which combine in different ways in individual people. Alcohol often plays a role in bringing this potential to fruition.

Can suicide be caused by alcohol alone?

This question is being increasingly asked by many experts, particularly psychiatrists who work with adolescents and young adults. Many Western countries have seen an alarming increase in suicide among the under-thirty-fives in particular in the past twenty years. Although illnesses such as depression are now being recognised much more than they were in the past, this does not in itself explain the increase. Although factors such as increasing consumerism, the dwindling of the influence of organised religion, the accelerating pace of life (with associated stress), the increasing rate of relationship breakdown are all important factors, it seems unlikely that these are enough on their own to explain the rise in suicides.

Attention has focused on one possible culprit, namely alcohol. It has long been recognised that the per-capita consumption of alcohol in a country is directly related to its suicide rate. As Ireland's alcohol consumption has spiralled, so too has its suicide rate. Nowhere has this been more evident than in the fifteen-to-thirty-five age groups, where binge-drinking has become a major problem. Inevitably, this has thrown up the possibility that alcohol alone may be the cause of many cases of suicide. It is very tempting to accept binge-drinking as the answer to the question as to why so many young people are dying so tragically?

The theory behind this scenario is that, in many cases, the person who is in the throes of a binge suffers from a sudden drop in mood. This in turn leads to an irrational urge toward self-harm. This is felt to be most likely to occur in the under-eighteen group, as their mood system is less mature, or in cases where the person is not used to heavy drinking. Some would extend this concept to include those in the twenty-to-thirty-five age group.

Biologically, this makes a great deal of sense. We now know that the developing brain is very susceptible to the effects of alcohol and drugs. When a young person begins to use alcohol, it takes only a small amount to make them drunk, because the liver and brain are not used to dealing with this substance. It usually does not take young people long to adjust, however, and after a while it require much higher alcohol consumption to produce the same result.

As the limbic mood system is ruling the roost in the under-eighteen group, it makes sense that the effects of alcohol would produce major shifts in mood, both up and down. As the frontal mood department is more immature at this stage, its control over mood would be less than when alcohol has not been taken. The ability of alcohol to inhibit the glutamate receptors is also widely recognised, and this effect is heightened by the inability of the young person to metabolise this substance. If we put all of these things together, the potential for binge-drinking both to depress mood and to reduce the brain's ability to overrule thoughts and actions of self-harm becomes clear.

It is also biologically normal for teenagers to experience short bouts of low mood as hormones associated with their physical and emotional maturing rush through their developing brain. Many psychiatrists feel that heavy binge-drinking during one such episode of low mood has the potential to develop into a sudden bout of dangerously low mood.

At first glance, this would seem to explain the vast majority of suicides among this age group. But although it may explain some cases, some important questions remain unanswered. For example, the number who binge-drink is far greater than those who take their own lives: why do we not see many more young people dying in this way? Is the psychiatric theory backed up by biological research?

We also do not have enough post-mortem evidence in this group to determine whether long-term evidence of an over-active stress system is present, or whether there is evidence of the low serotonin-cable activity noted earlier. If we postulate that such cases are caused by sudden drops in mood brought on by alcohol alone, we would expect such biological evidence to be absent. To answer this question biologically, we would need in-depth post-mortem evidence. We could also learn a great deal by scanning survivors of serious suicide attempts to see if there is evidence of serious depression or not.

If we look at the post-teenage group, it seems less likely that alcohol alone is the culprit, although the scenario (which would be unusual in modern Ireland) that a person who is completely unused to alcohol could experience such a sudden drop in mood is quite plausible. In practice, binge-drinking is almost the norm in this group, so most young people in this group are more likely to be more tolerant of such excesses. It seems more likely that, when the White Flag appears, illnesses such as depression have been lurking in the background. In such cases, alcohol is more likely to be exposing an underlying problem. Again, biological research would help to clarify the situation.

In older age groups, it is much more likely that illnesses such as depression and addiction are chiefly responsible for suicide. Once again, alcohol acts more as a catalyst than as a cause on its own.

If we put all that we know about suicide together, we can make the following tentative statements:

§ Binge-drinking in the under-eighteen group is thought by many to cause sudden drops in mood, with a greater risk of self-harm.

§ The biological model of the effects of alcohol on the developing mood system strongly supports this possibility.

§ The age of drinking heavily amongst our young people is dropping all the time, so tolerance to alcohol among this group must also be increasing. Other factors may therefore be involved.

§ Clinical evidence also points to the emergence of many illnesses, such as depression and schizophrenia, among fifteen-to-twenty-year-olds. Significantly, these conditions often remain undetected for some time.

§ We have insufficient post-mortem and other research in suicide victims in this age group to answer this question for certain.

§ In older age groups who regularly binge-drink, it is less likely that alcohol on its own is the cause of suicide, but this factor plays an important role in reducing the control of the brain that is so important in preventing self-harm.

§ The recent increase in binge-drinking in the under-thirty-five age group, allied to all the other factors already dealt with, is the most important reason for the increase in the number of deaths of so many young Irish people from suicide.

The question about the place of alcohol in the high rates of suicide seen in the under-thirty-five age group has to take centre stage in any discussion of suicide in Ireland. While young people in Mediterranean countries seem to be able to use alcohol wisely (that is, in small amounts and with food), in Ireland and Britain the opposite occurs. I feel that a major national debate on alcohol, as called for by President McAleese recently, is long overdue.

Personally, I would favour a ban on the sale of any alcoholic drinks other than wine in late-night discos; a ban on the sale of alcohol to anybody under twenty-one from off licences; the introduction of measures (as in Australia) making the sale of alcohol to those clearly inebriated the legal responsibility of the publican; a national TV campaign graphically explaining the place of alcohol in the death by suicide in young people; and, perhaps controversially, the raising of the age of legal alcohol use to twenty-one. I would favour this last measure on the biological grounds that, by that stage, the brain is maturing and is less vulnerable to the risks documented above. Such measures may seem draconian, but we have to ask how we are valuing the lives of our young people if we do nothing. Incidentally, these measures would also help to reduce the number of young death from road-traffic accidents.

Is suicide the result of illness, impulse or accident?

This is the question that is most often asked by grieving families and loved ones who have lost someone to the White Flag of suicide. Often, there are no obvious warnings that the person is in trouble; those left behind struggle to come to terms with the mystery of the death.

Illness and impulse are linked biologically. Imagine a lake, which on the surface appears calm and serene, masking treacherous currents underneath. Many who take their own lives may appear to be normal to those around them, but are in fact experiencing hidden currents of stress, low self-esteem, low mood and negative thoughts. Impulsive suicidal thoughts are not far away from breaking through to the surface.

1   ACCIDENT

In certain cases, suicide was probably not intended but became the outcome. Parasuicide can involve a mixture of alcohol and an overdose of prescribed medication. In this situation, it is inevitable that mistakes will happen: people who expect to survive are often not found in time, or miscalculate the amount of the substance they have taken. Ironically, if the cry for help is too loud, it may never be heard.

It is also possible that many fatal accidents that occur late at night and involve single vehicles are a result of impulsive, reckless behaviour (often alcohol- or drug-related), rather than being planned suicide attempts. Within this group, there may also be a number of young people who plan to take their lives (often fuelled by alcohol, relationship breakdowns and depression) in such a manner. Some experts feel that at least 6 percent of these cases may be genuine suicides. It is difficult to clarify this situations, as the person was alone, and there are rarely witnesses.

There are other situations where people throw themselves into rivers but immediately cry out for help. In these situations, it would appear that, where fatalities occur, they are more accidental than a suicide. Accidents are most likely to occur where large amounts of alcohol or drugs have been consumed. This may distort the person's normal, rational thinking, and affect their judgement.

2   IMPULSE

This is the most deceptive factor of all. At first glance, most suicides appear to be spur-of-the-moment events, where the person makes a sudden, unplanned decision to end the pain and take their own life. In other cases, there may be obvious evidence of pre-planning, often up to several days before the event, with written notes left behind.

To understand the role of impulse in suicide, one must understand the biology of suicide. In many suicide victims, a long period of stress, low mood and low self-esteem will have preceded the act. We have already explained how some people are more biologically at risk due to an under-active ICC. This group is already more likely to be more impulsive than other people. Eventually, in such cases, impulsive thoughts of self-harm may creep into the mind: these thoughts are initially rejected but finally embraced.

Impulsive behaviour, therefore, is often linked to fleeting, impulsive thoughts which may have been present in the person for a longer duration of time. These impulses merely need a catalyst – an emotional event such as the break-up of a relationship – for the irrational urge to become a reality.

Alcohol plays an important role in unlocking this impulsivity. Alcohol is very adept at turning off the frontal cortex behaviour box and allowing negative thoughts and actions to overpower the person's mood system – with fatal consequences. Many assume that it is the alcohol itself that produces the impulsive thoughts. This is not fully accurate: alcohol releases suicidal thoughts that were already there, hidden beneath the surface.

It is important to remember also that the frontal cortex mood department and behaviour box is not fully developed until the age of twenty-five. So, from fifteen to twenty-five, when the limbic mood department is raging with hormones, and feelings of low mood and self-esteem are common, the brain lacks the crucial set of 'brakes' to stop the person from inflicting impulsive behaviour on themselves or others.

One important exception is the use of powerful mind-altering drugs such as cocaine, LSD and magic mushrooms, where a major shift in neurochemistry may produce impulsive self-harm! This might happen in particular ithe person is using the substance for the first time, or in a young adolescent whose brain is still immature.

So, yes, impulse is a vital ingredient of suicide, but only when we consider the broader picture. Contrary to popular opinion, most deaths by suicide are not merely a whim or a spur-of-the-moment occurrence.

3 ILLNESS

This is usually the largest contributor to suicide. In most cases, suicide is not so much an accident or an impulse, but rather the consequence of an underlying illness attacking the mood system.

Most of those who die from the White Flag of suicide have the devastating turmoil of mental illness wreaking havoc beneath the surface of their seemingly calm exteriors. Many have very low mood and low self-esteem, and are in real pain. Others are suffering from the Grey or Purple Flags. In some cases, chronic stress, unemployment, bullying, or the breakdown of a relationship may, over time, combine with these illnesses to create a potential risk of suicide.

In such cases, impulsive, self-destructive thoughts start to intrude. The person's stress system is often over-acting; negative thoughts of hopelessness and helplessness take over. Solving problems becomes insurmountable. If we factor in the at-risk biological group's impulsive self-harm traits, these thoughts create the potential for suicidal action. It may then take only some relatively small event to trigger the conversion of such thoughts into action. When alcohol is added to the equation, tragedy can quickly ensue.

In general, suicide is an illness with impulsive traits at its heart; only on occasion can suicide be clearly recognised as being accidental. There is obviously ongoing research and debate into this subject. In my own career as a GP, I have learned a great deal from listening to people who have survived very serious suicide attempts, where death was truly the final goal. What these people have articulated to me supports the above concepts. In many cases, impulsive thoughts were usually restrained, but alcohol acted as a lethal catalyst.

To those who say that suicide is a 'coward's way out', I say this: suicide is often the final result of an underlying illness, with numerous stress triggers involved. Those who take their own lives simply want to end their pain permanently and may, in their confused mental state, give little thought to the impact that their death may have on those who are close to them. Those who have never experienced this pain will struggle to understand its intensity and the lengths to which people will go to end their inner torment. This pain, along with the release of impulsive thoughts and behaviour, lies at the heart of the White Flag.

THE LAST WORD

It is fitting that we leave this subject by once again recalling Niall's words shortly before his death: 'It's just me.' These words carry profound meaning for us all. They challenge us and point us towards the fact that we all have a responsibility to unlock the mystery of the White Flag.

We need to reach out with love and compassion to all those who feel down – particularly young men and women under thirty-five – and encourage them to come forward for help. We must talk about the symptoms of depression, its causes, and how it can be tackled. We also need to challenge the role of alcohol in our society. The task is huge, but the prize is beyond value: the lives of many of our finest people, both young and old. If all of us do our part, Niall's words may become a beacon of hope for many others in the future.

Appendix 1

For Those Who Want To Know More

Let me say from the outset that this section is not essential in any way to an understanding of the basic concepts of the flag system, which have already been discussed. I am including this section for two reasons: firstly, to validate scientifically the body of the text, and secondly to flesh out the underlying biological mechanisms relating to mood for those who are more scientifically orientated, who would like to know more about the subject, or who are involved in teaching and counselling people with mental-health problems or work in the medical or nursing professions. As a result, I make no excuses for using exact biological and neurophysiological names and concepts in this appendix. Some of these concepts are quite complex, and not everybody will feel able to tackle them; most will, however, be able to grasp the main points.

I will take each of the individual chapters on the various flags and explain in detail whatever underlying mechanisms I feel relevant. Most of this appendix is devoted to the Green Flag, which lies at the basis of all the others, and to the Red Flag.

Part I: The Green Flag

The Flag

As neurons are crucial to the functioning of the brain, and as a consequence of our mood apparatus, it is appropriate that we start our journey by looking in more detail at this unit. Neurons are basically cells which receive information, process it and pass on further information as a result. All cells in the body are tiny, fluid-filled units surrounded by a fine cell membrane which helps keep them separate from other cells. At the very heart of all our cells, including neurons, lies the nucleus which contains our chromosomes. As we have seen, these contain the genetic material which controls the functioning of particular cells.

The internal life and activities of the typical cell in the body is extraordinary. To begin with, each cell has about twenty separate sections, each with a different function. Messages are being constantly passed from the nucleus/genes back and forth to these sections, with instructions. All of the sections have their part to play. Some provide the energy for all the activities that are taking place within the cells, and others are involved in making the proteins and enzymes that are necessary for the day-to-day running of the cells; others parcel the proteins up into little bundles ready for transport, get rid of unwanted material, and so on. The nucleus is also in constant touch with the periphery of the cell, sensing and responding to its needs.

A simple example in the case of the neuron is the manufacture of a peptide like endorphin. The periphery of the cell sends a message to the central nucleus/genes. The genes send instructions to the ribosomes (the protein-making 'factory'), which in turn manufactures the neurotransmitter peptide, and passes it on to another section for 'parcelling' into little bundles surrounded by a substance that resembles clingfilm. Along comes the 'messenger boy', who in a sense throws it on his back and carries it step by step along one of the multitude of 'highways' which criss-cross the cell to reach the periphery of the cell. There it is dumped into a storage area, ready for use.

The structure of the basic neuron is shown in Figure 1. The main information collectors are the dendrites. The cell body contains the nucleus, which houses our genes and all the basic internal machinery of the cell. The axon is a long, tail-like structure that conveys information from the cell body to its terminal buttons. It is covered with myelin, which can be compared to the white protective structure surrounding electrical wires in our homes. Myelin's job is to speed up conduction of the nerve cells. The terminal buttons are the end points, where axons divide into many branches. Each branch ends in a small, knob-like structure. This in turn generally links up with dendrites to form the synapses we have dealt with in earlier chapters. The role of this terminal button is to release neurotransmitters such as serotonin, when the button is activated by an electrical charge surging along the axon itself.

So information is passed from the axon of one cell to the dendrite of another through chemical messengers released into synapses. This information is then passed to the cell body, which in turn sends its own message along its axon to its terminal buttons, and so on. This, at its most simple, is how the brain neurons talk to each other. A good analogy is to compare two people is a crowd where one person puts their lips close to the ears of the other person to pass on some important information. This information is assessed within the brain of the person, who then turns and puts their lips close to the ears of the next person and passes on the relevant information. Soon the whole crowd, one by one, has been told the message.

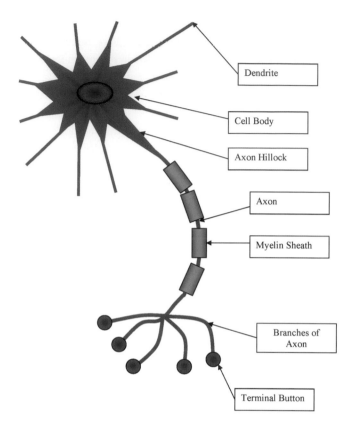

FIGURE 1: THE STRUCTURE OF THE NEURON

Although the cell body, through its genes, seems to be the boss of each neuron, what happens in the synapses at the level of the nerve-cell membranes plays a crucial role in how each cell behaves. It will be useful to look at this in more detail.

Each terminal button is full of little balls or vesicles, which in turn are full of chemical neurotransmitters. Many of the key neurotransmitters, indludling serotonin, dopamine and noradrenalin, are stored in these vesicles. When the axon is fired, these little bags release their supply of messenger into the synapse between the terminal buttons of one cell and the dendrite end of the next.

Within the cell membrane of the dendrite lie protein molecules, known as post-synaptic receptors. The chemical messengers link in with these receptors: i.e. serotonin molecules link up with serotonin receptors, noradrenalin molecules with noradrenalin receptors, and so on. Some of these receptors promote electrical firing of the cell.

Others have the opposite effect, and dampen down activity in the cell. Others, through more complicated reactions within the cell membrane, cause the so-called second messengers to travel to the internal genes of our cells. All of these kinds of receptors and responses are involved in the neurons of our mood system. There is little doubt that the answers to most of our questions concerning illnesses of our mood system lie in this complicated interchange between receptors and cell membranes, and the genes themselves.

What of the glial cells? There are three main types. Astrocytes are the most common support cell in the brain. Their main function is to provide structural support for the neurons, act as scavengers of debris and be critically involved in the metabolism of key neurotransmitters such as glutamate. In addition, they act as the barrier between the small blood vessels of the brain and the neurons themselves. *Oligodendrocytes* wrap themselves around the axons of neurons to form myelin, which increases the conduction of such cells. *Microglia* are also scavengers, and form part of the immune system which patrols the brain.

All of the above are essential for the normal functioning of the brain/mood system. Recent research involving astrocytes in particular is revealing the large number of roles that glial cells have. These cells may, for example, be involved in releasing their own neurotransmitters, have their own receptors, and influence both synapse development and the level of neurotransmitters within the latter. Many scientists believe that future research will demonstrate that astrocytes play a greater role in illness such as depression than has previously been thought.

OUR MOOD CABLES AND CONTROL BOXES

We have seen in the first chapter that one of the roles of the brain is to organise the efficient passage of information between departments by gathering neurons together into control boxes and cables. This is particularly so in the case of our mood system. In practice, the cell bodies are collected together in clusters, known as nuclei, with their axons, which are often quite long, wound together into long tracts, called cables. The axon cables then wind their way through the various departments in the middle and front of the brain. As seen in the first chapter, our mood system has three important control boxes (nuclei) and cables (serotonin, dopamine and noradrenalin). Let's look at these in more detail.

THE SEROTONIN MOOD CABLE AND CONTROL BOX

The cell bodies of our serotonin neurons are clustered together, particularly in the brain stem. The main control box is the *raphe nucleus*: a collection of nuclei in the brain stem. These pass information along the mood-cable axons to release serotonin and other transmitters at terminal buttons scattered along their paths. The serotonin that released in this way interacts with nine different types of serotonin receptors.

The serotonin mood cable tracks its way through the various structures of ou mood system, particularly the sections of the limbic system and the frontal corte mood departments. The key neurotransmitter involved in this process is serotonin. A we will see, serotonin's connections to the ventral pre-frontal cortex (PFC) are critic to our understanding of suicide. If anything interferes with the control box and moo cable, impulsivity, depression and suicidal thoughts may not be far behind.

II   THE NORADRENALIN MOOD CABLE AND CONTROL BOX

The patterns used are similar to that in serotonin. The cell bodies are once again co lected in nuclei or control boxes. The most important noradrenalin control box is calle the *locus coeruleus*. This supplies the thick band of axons which make up the noradren: lin cable. This band again passes through most of the departments of the limbic sy: tem and frontal cortex mood department, as well as many other parts of the brain. Th key neurotransmitter released by these axons is noradrenalin. The noradrenalin syste: is more pronounced on the right side of the brain than on the left. Starvation of sur ply of this neurotransmitter causes much of the fatigue and lack of drive we see in pec ple with depression. This cable is also involved in our response to stress and anxiet There are probably four main types of noradrenalin receptors.

III   THE DOPAMINE MOOD CABLE AND CONTROL BOX

Once again, in the dopamine mood cable the cell bodies are collected together to for: two main nuclei. The one which is most important in relation to the mood system called the Ventral Tegmental Area. Of note, the other main control box and nuclei he: is called the Substantia Niagra, and is involved in Parkinson's disease. Axons from th Ventral Tegmental Area (or dopamine control box) once again come together to for: a long cable, which extends through most of the limbic system and frontal cortex moo department. As before, dopamine is the main neurotransmitter, and is maintained an transmitted by this system. When this mood control box and cable is starved, we se the classical symptoms of lack of joy or pleasure in life that accompany depression. C note, the dopamine system is stronger on the left side of the brain than on the rigl side. If this cable is over-stimulated in susceptible people, the illness of addiction ma appear. This cable is also involved in the Grey Flag of schizophrenia.

IV   THE PEPTIDE INFORMATION SYSTEM

This differs from the above systems in that the peptides and wandering messenge: released by neurons at synapses roam off to stimulate more distant cells. In our moo system, these play a major role, particularly in the area of stress and how we deal wit

t. Key players here are corticotrophin release factor (CRF), which is released by some ey departments in our mood system as a response to stress; Substance P, which plays similar role to CRF; and endorphins, the feel-good messengers which are released par- icularly during exercise. Endorphins are an under-estimated tool in the treatment of lepression.

THE MOOD DEPARTMENTS

Ve have already dealt with these, but it may be useful to flesh out some of the details elating to them.

THE FRONTAL MOOD DEPARTMENT

The frontal lobe, which controls the behaviour end of the mood system, lies at the ront of the brain. It is primarily composed of the PFC, which is very developed in the uman being, compared to animals, for instance. This is the area which we have lescribed throughout as the behaviour box. It makes up 29 percent of the cerebral cor- ex and plays an extremely important role in all our thoughts, decision-making, plan- ing and impulsive behaviour, and in controlling our violent or suicidal thoughts and mpulses. Crucially, it is supplied by the three mood cables, particularly the serotonin nood cable. If this cable (and through it certain key sections of the PFC) is starved of erotonin, impulsive thoughts and actions may appear. As we will see later, this section of the brain is only fully mature by the age of twenty-five. In my opinion, this may be major factor in many of the mental-health problems we see in the fifteen-to-twenty- ive age group.

The PFC is divided into a number of different subsections: the medial PFC (which ncludes the sub-genual cortex), the orbital PFC and the ventro-lateral PFC. For the urposes of this book, I have included the anterior cingulate cortex (ACC) as being art of the medial PFC. This contains some of the key Brodman Areas, including Area 4 (rostral cingulate cortex) and Area 25 (the sub-genual cortex), and is one of the most mportant sections of the brain in relation to depression. A useful way of interpreting he functions of these two sections is to regard Area 25 as being important in the cre- tion of, and Area 24 as being involved in the cognitive control of, mood. Some regard he ACC as lying at the junction of the limbic system – and call it the para-limbic cor- ex. In practical terms, there is very little difference between them; for simplicity, I have ided with those who include the ACC with the PFC. More importantly, the ACC seems o lie at the heart of the neural circuit flow of information between the PFC and the imbic system, particularly the amygdala. It therefore has a crucial role to play in our :motional thoughts and behaviour. All of these sections of the PFC will be mentioned gain in our discussion of the Red Flag, but in general it can be said that they play a najor role in modulating emotional behaviour.

II   THE LIMBIC SYSTEM MOOD DEPARTMENT

The limbic system mood department, often called the emotional brain, is the main pla
er in the mood system, and lies at the heart of how we feel. It is composed of a nur
ber of different structures, all of which have different roles. It is situated in the midc
of the brain. Although we do not need to describe all the structures this part of tl
brain contains, some are very important:

(A)   THE AMYGDALA

This almond-shaped structure has been described earlier in the book as the stress bc
It plays a key role in activating stress pathways, and is involved in the creation, consc
idation and expression of emotionally arousing – and usually negative – memories.
has important connections to the various parts of the PFC, the hippocampus and tl
nucleus accumbens. The amygdala is a key player in the illnesses of anxiety and depressio
The fact that there are fewer neural connections between the PFC and the amygda
than vice versa is the reason why our emotions frequently overrule our rational brair

(B)   THE HIPPOCAMPUS

This seashell-shaped structure has been described earlier as the memory box. Its ma
function is to organise memories before they are stored in different areas of the brai
It is also important in helping the brain retrieve memories and put them in context, ar
for our spatial memory. When we are asleep, usually during REM sleep, the hippocar
pus switches on. This is believed to be part of the mechanism whereby memories a
consolidated.

The hippocampus is one of only two places where neurons are formed in the bra
– through a process called neurogenesis. This structure is highly sensitive to stress, ar
in particular to glucocortisol, both of which attack its sensitive mechanisms: dendri
connections between neurons and the manufacture of new neurons. This is why mer
ory and concentration are often seen to be adversely affected when a person is suffe
ing from extreme stress, chronic anxiety or depression.

(C)   THE NUCLEUS ACCUMBENS

This has been described throughout the book as our pleasure box. Strongly supplied l
our dopamine cable, it lights up whenever we are enjoying ourselves. If it is starved ‹
this messenger, as in depression or chronic stress and anxiety, lack of joy will follow.
has major connections with the amygdala, the hippocampus and the PFC – the s‹
called 'reward circuit' – and is also now seen as a key player in addiction.

All three of these structures are linked together in the brain in a neural circuit, with information flowing back and forth between the brain stem, the limbic system and the PFC. Dysfunctions in this circuit, together with its connections with the adrenal gland and glucocortisol, are responsible for most of the illnesses discussed in this book.

Another useful concept is to divide the various sections of the two main mood departments in the brain that are involved in normal emotional behaviour into the ventral and dorsal systems (see Figure 2). The ventral (meaning 'bottom') system links key parts of the limbic system, such as the amygdala, with the bottom sections of the PFC, such as Area 25 (the ventral subgenual anterior congulate), the ventrolateral PFC and the orbital cortex. This system has important links with the brain-stem mood-control boxes. Its functions involve identifying emotions and creating mood. The dorsal (meaning 'top') system involves Area 24 (the dorsal anterior cingulate), the dorsolateral and dorsomedial PFC, and the hippocampus. Its function is to cognitively regulate the moods produced by the ventral system.

FIGURE 2: THE VENTRAL AND DORSAL SYSTEMS

Of note, during periods of normal sadness, the ventral system is over-active and the dorsal system is inhibited. This is only temporary, and the balance is normalised when this period of upset is over. In depression, however, this balance is not restored

THE DEVELOPMENT OF THE MOOD SYSTEM

We dealt with this system in detail in the second chapter. There are a few interesting biological details worth mentioning here, however. Firstly, the limbic system is only slowly maturing from the age of twelve up to eighteen, mainly as a consequence of se hormones, underlying genetic predispositions and environmental factors. All of these come together in an explosive cocktail at this stage.

The hippocampus is very sensitive at this stage, and serious abuse of any kind may hinder its growth. This is likely to be secondary to a chronic glucocorticol barrage which is usually secondary to the stress induced by this abuse. Our amygdala too is ver sensitive during this phase of development, and may store up a lot of negative emotions associated with certain memories, which then may try to flood out later in our lives in the form of anxiety. A mixture of genes and environment are involved in this process. Our *nucleus accumbens* is also fairly immature during this stage of development Even at an early age, however, if serious misuse of substances is occurring, the warn ing signs of addiction may start to appear.

Our mood cables, like the rest of the mood system in the brain, are also maturing This, along with the graded development of our limbic system and the immaturity of the PFC, explains why many mood-altering drugs, such as the SSRIs, have been shown to be less effective in those under eighteen; some argue that, on occasion, they may do more harm than good. Lastly, our PFC is often quite immature in the mid-teens, and only slowly develops to full maturity by the early to mid-twenties.

Of interest to those who have children who suffer from attention deficit disorde (ADD), the reason that drugs can be used in this group is that they are normally aimed at the dopamine cable. It has been shown that many of the symptoms of this illness lie in underactivity of this cable due to a shortage of dopamine in its neuronal synapses To deal with this topic would require a book in itself!

A crucial question to be answered by researchers over the next few years is the nature of the development of the glial support system, particularly in relation to the astrocytes. (Fifty percent of the cells in the adult brain are astrocytes, so clearly they are of great significance.) We need to examine how stressful periods in the development of the child and adolescent affect these vital support cells, and how deficits in them in turn affect the health and survival of neurons and, in particular, the axon/dendrites connec tions. We need to understand better the genetic potential for an individual to develop difficulties within their glial system. We also need to learn how current stressors affec this system.

It is becoming increasingly obvious that depression in particular is intimately linked with such difficulties. As we have seen already in the Red Flag, these difficulties seem to be a cause of both structural and functioning problems within the mood system. I personally remain convinced that astrocytes will turn out to be the biological link which causes the mood circuits to go awry in this illness.

THE STRESS SYSTEM

It is particularly valuable to go into a more detailed analysis of the biology of our stress system, as it plays such an important role in our lives and in the health of our mood system.

Stress activates our limbic system, particularly the amygdala or stress box. This releases CRH, one of the roaming peptide messengers, and thereby helps activate two pathways in the brain.

The first, through activating two structures which form our hormone control box (the hypothalamus and the pituitary gland – often called the HPI axis) send information to the bloodstream through the adrenal gland, encouraging it to release glucocortisol, the main stress-related mood hormone. (Of note, the hyothalamus is of great importance in controlling the internal circadian rhythms of the body; both play a vital role in controlling the main hormone-producing areas of the body, including the thyroid, pancreas, ovaries and adrenal glands.)

The second pathway activates nerve pathways to our brain stem, through a separate nervous system known as the autonomic nervous system. This sends messengers to a different part of the stress mood adrenal gland, to release adrenalin and noradrenalin.

Our primary interest, in relation to mental illness, in how stress interacts with our mood system is in the area of chronic stress. This, through a glucocortisol barrage, hammers our three control boxes and cables. Because the three control boxes and the hippocampus are very rich in glucocortisol receptors, it is inevitable that an excess of this hormone has the capacity to cause chaos in the body's mood system. The serotonin system seems to be especially at risk. We saw the effects of this phenomenon in the first chapter.

It is interesting to note that our hippocampus (memory box) is particularly affected by stress. Neuron production can be affected, as can interaction between neurons, in illnesses such as chronic stress, anxiety and depression – with obvious consequences. Stress also attacks the PFC, particularly in people who are vulnerable to depression.

In relation to all of the illnesses affecting our mood system, the effects of CRH and glucocortisol on the neurons and astrocytes of these mood structures, control boxes and mood cables lies at the heart of the biological malfunctions. A great deal of work is being done on CRH in particular, as this substance seems to be a key player in kick-starting the whole process of mental illness. Whatever future research reveals, there is little doubt that the biological interaction between the stress system and the mood system will be found to be of great importance to our understanding of such illnesses.

THE GREEN FLAG

Our mood system is well when our biological flag is green. This means that our mood departments, control boxes and mood cables are functioning normally. In practice, this means that our *raphe nucleus,* plus its serotonin cable, our *locus coeruleus,* with its noradrenalin cable, and our ventral tegmental nucleus, with its dopamine cable, are all running smoothly.

Also, our stress system is not being over-stimulated, so pressure is not being placed on our mood structures. As a result, our mood stress adrenal gland and its hormone glucocortisol, in particular, are operating effectively. Peace reigns supreme.

We have dealt in great detail with the positive symptoms which biological harmony brings to our lives. The real struggle is, having found peace, how to keep it safely in our grasp.

Before leaving this section, it is worth briefly examining the importance of oily fish and the role of omega 3 oils. In the womb the foetus needs plenty of DHA. Its main use is in the formation of the retina of the eye and the in the grey matter of the developing brain (particularly the formation of synapses). The role of EPA has also been examined. We know that oily fish/omega 3 oils seem to reduce the risks of sudden heart deaths (by reducing arrhythmias), and probably through EPA seems to stabilize plaque in the coronary arteries most likely through its anti inflammatory properties. Apart from this, its importance to the cell membrane functioning of all neurons cannot be over emphasised. What's good for the brain is also good for the heart!

PART II: THE RED FLAG

SIMPLE (UNIPOLAR) DEPRESSION

In the last twenty years, a large volume of research has begun to shed light on the various malfunctions that occur within the mood system of a person who is depressed. Initially, almost all the attention was centred on mood cables: it was felt that the most likely cause of depression was a malfunctioning of these cables – probably due to a decrease in the amounts of serotonin/noradrenalin being produced by the neurons rving these cables. This possibility arose initially because drugs which increased the nount of neurotransmitters such as serotonin seemed to alleviate the symptoms of epression. One question remained, however: why did it take so long for these drugs work? It proved to be a difficult task to create a biological model in which neuro-ansmitter shortage alone explained all the problems seen in this illness.

Attention began to shift to the various other elements of the mood system. esearch involving EEGs (electroencephalograms, which measure electrical activity in irious parts of the brain), plus neuro-imaging (which examines the functional activity f various parts of the brain) of the person with depression, combined with post-ortem studies, began to reveal a great deal of interesting information.

First, electrical activity in the left PFC seemed to be markedly reduced in depres-on. Second, neuro-imaging showed a general increase in activity of a section 3rodman's Area 25) of the PFC behaviour box called the subgenual pre-frontal cor-x, particularly on the left-hand side. Neuro-imaging also showed evidence of an crease in activity in another section of the brain, called the orbito-frontal cortex, hich tries to counteract the typical negative thoughts probably originating in the mygdala. Third, major neuro-imaging research by Dr Helen Mayberg of the Department of Psychiatry/Neurology at the University of Toronto revealed that Area 5 was over-active in most cases of depression. This structure, situated deep in the FC, close to the limbic system, seems to act as a controlling gateway between the PFC nd the limbic system. Dr Mayberg demonstrated that successful treatment of this ill-ess, whether by drug therapy, CBT, psychotherapy, ECT or deep-brain stimulation, esulted in activity in this area normalising. Finally, research revealed decreased activity a the hippocampus (memory box) and other parts of the limbic system, and showed n increase in activity in the amygdala (stress box). All of the above fitted with the con-ept that biological difficulties within the two mood departments, particularly in rela-on to the behaviour, stress and memory boxes, seem to lie at the heart of depression.

Other research revealed that the stress system (the stress box, adrenal stress gland, nd glucocortisol stress hormone) appears to play a pivotal role in depression. It was ound that the stress peptides, particularly CRH, were often elevated in people with epression. In addition, blood glucocortisol levels were found to be elevated in 75 per-ent of people who were suffering from depression, depending on the severity of their ondition. Other glands involved in the stress response, such as the adrenal and thyroid lands, were also noted to be affected. We have already discussed the normal day/night luctuations of glucocortisol. In depression, this too was shown to be distorted, with a lay-and-night glucocortisol barrage appearing.

Another key biological fact noted was the disruption of the normal sleep mecha-ism. We all go through various stages of sleep every night. We are either in a state of dreaming (REM, or rapid-eye-movement, sleep), or not dreaming (non-REM sleep Sleep is important to us all: most importantly, it allows our brain time to heal the bic logical damage incurred during the day and provides an opportunity for us to reorgar ise our storage of memories.

In a healthy person, most of the dreaming or REM sleep occurs in the second pai of the night. In depression, this is altered, and it instead takes place in the first part c the night. The result is extremely disrupted sleep, as anyone with depression will attes to. This sleep-pattern disruption can also be seen in first-degree relatives of those wit depression, even when they are well. It seems to be a hidden marker of a basic undei lying potential problem within the mood system. Follow-on studies of such relative revealed the emergence of depression in some of them at a later stage.

Further neuro-imaging research has shown up other interesting data. In depressio (unipolar and bipolar), a reduction in grey matter and volume in parts of the orbital an medial PFC, and in the hippocampus, has been noted. One area that has already bee mentioned is the subgenual part of Brodmans Area 24 (at the junction of Areas 24 an 25), called sg24, where, in one study, by Dr Wayne Drevets (of the Department o Psychiatry and Radiology at the University of Pittsburgh) of familial unipolar/bipola mood disorders, 20 to 40 percent of the brain tissue was gone. In another study, com paring women following a bout of post-adolescence depression with another, mucl older, age group with a history of repeated depression, tissue loss of up to 19 percen in the same area was noted in both groups. What was of interest in this study was th very early presentation of the structural changes in the brain. These changes wer shown later to be unrelated to family background.

Post-mortem results supported these findings. Both demonstrated abnormal reduc tions in grey-matter volume, and in the number of glial support cells (particularly th astrocytes), together with dendrite/axon connections and, in some cases, the neuron themselves in various parts of the mood system: the sub-genual, orbital and latera PFC, the amygdala; the *nucleus accumbens*, and the hippocampus.

The loss of brain tissue in these areas seems in general to be due to a reduction ii the number of glial support cells which supply the neurons (although in many studie some neuron loss or dendrite reductions were also noted). The reason for the loss o glial cells remains a mystery: one body of opinion holds that some of the changes pre date the appearance of depression, or appear concomitantly, with the illness itself caus ing further damage.

Some researchers wonder whether impaired function or loss of glial cells may b the real cause of this illness. It is also possible that the body's own stress system coulc be involved in attacking its own glial cells. Perhaps to begin with there is a developmen tal (genetic or driven by early environmental stress) reduction of these cells in som eople and that, once stress appears, particularly in the fifteen-to-twenty-five age group, where maturing of the mood system is occurring, the mood system becomes dysfunctional. In other cases, an underlying vulnerability to stress may make these support cells open to damage when it arrives, setting off the biological cascade of the Red Flag, and leading to further activation of the stress/immune system, with further possible destruction or reduced functioning of these cells. This vulnerability may once again be the result of genes and environmental factors combining. The neuron loss in the hippocampus seen in those with depression is probably due to the effects of glucocortisol on neurogenesis. Importantly, these structural changes remain even after treatment.

The reduction in glial cells, particularly astrocytes, may be reducing the efficiency of the cells in the areas involved, by leading to a build-up of the neurotransmitter glutamate. (This happens because, when neurons release glutamate into a synapse, to stimulate the post-synaptic neuron, it is the astrocytes which subsequently clear it from the synapse, by absorbing it into itself and converting it into glutamine; it subsequently feeds this substance back into the cell of origin, where it is reconverted back into glutamate. If astrocytes are reduced, then too much glutamate builds up in the synapse.) This build-up of glutamate may cause the dendrites of these neurons to shrink (possibly by reducing the level of BDNF in the cell), reducing their capacity to communicate with each other. This is because BDNF is essential to the formation of new dendrites. If the growth of dendrites is impaired, neurons struggle to pass information efficiently from one to another.

Increasingly, experts feel that decreased levels of internal neuronal BDNF, probably fuelled by glial-cell shortages or malfunctioning (which may affect the activities of the neurons in several different ways) may lie at the heart of the neuronal-communication difficulties within the mood system.

Stress, in the form of stress peptides and glucocortisol, magnifies this situation, leading to further interference in the functions of the various sections of the PFC. The neural mood circuit becomes dysfunctional; the rest of the mood system is put under pressure and frantically tries to compensate. Repeated attacks of depression accelerate this process. This may be the reason that those who suffer from a number of bouts of the Red Flag seem to be more vulnerable to future episodes?

Our amygdala seems to be particularly active in depression: it is the most likely source of much of the negative thinking, poor self-esteem and anxiety that is seen in this illness. The normal modulatory effects of the PFC (particularly the orbital cortex) on the amygdala seem to be reduced in depression, increasing the risk of the negative symptoms noted above.

It may also be the case that Area 25 (itself involved in the creation of mood) is simply responding to all the difficulties that are occurring within the PFC, and that this part of the brain opens the floodgates (literally), giving the emotional limbic cortex free rein Area 25 plays a key role in connecting various parts of the PFC, the amygdala, the hip pocampus, the hypothalamus, and the brain-stem mood-control boxes.

As there are fewer neural connections between the PFC and the limbic system (par ticularly the amygdala) than vice versa, even in a person who has good mental health such effects will be compounded. Finally, the hippocampus is damaged by the stress barrage in depression, and there is also decreased neurogenesis. As the hippocampus also has an inhibitory effect on the activities of the amygdala, this may increase the neg ative effects noted above.

When one examines all this information, a clear pattern in relation to possible biologi cal pathways in depression begins to emerge. We probably develop, through a combi nation of genetic influences and early environment, a predisposition, when under stress, for various parts of our PFC (particularly on the left-hand side) to malfunction This vulnerability may vary widely, from those who will only suffer occasional episodes of depression, to those who will have constant bouts of the illness. Common sense would dictate that the latter may begin with, and subsequently develop, more chronic structural and functional changes in the brain.

Stress activates the amygdala (which itself has been shown to be low in astrocytes) to pour out stress peptides and glucocortisol, the latter via the adrenal stress gland. These substances attack the vulnerable left-hand side of the PFC, which begins to malfunction further. As a result of this reduction in its normal activity, the left side of the PFC lifts its normal inhibition of the emotional limbic system, particularly the amygdala, which in turn becomes more active. (Area 25 seems to be a crucial gateway in this process.) The mood circuit is now dysfunctional.

This in turn creates two main problems: the arrival of low mood, negative thoughts, poor self-esteem, worry and anxiety, and a further increase in the activation of the stress system. The latter results in a bombardment of the three main mood cables and boxes (the noradrenalin, dopamine and, in particular, serotonin cables). This leads to many of the symptoms that those who suffer with depression know so well, including fatigue, poor concentration, sleep difficulties, appetite problems, anhedonia, and poor drive and memory. As these cables begin to malfunction, the efficiency of the PFC and limbic mood departments deteriorate further, and the vicious circle continues.

Another result of the increased stress bombardment is the effects of glucocortisol on: (a) the receptors of the white blood cells, increasing the risk of infection and can cer, (b) the blood platelets, causing them to clump together, increasing the risk of heart attack, (c) the bones, leading to osteoporosis (thinning of the bones), (d) increasing damage to the hippocampus, further affecting memory, (e) increased risk, in those who are vulnerable to these conditions, of abdominal obesity and diabetes. Professor Ted Dinan of UCC has done some excellent work on the effects of this hormone on our general health. Lastly, and most seriously, the combination of a major drop in activity in the serotonin mood cable, together with reduced activity in the ventral portion of our left PFC may lead, in vulnerable people, to the arrival of suicidal thoughts and actions.

Can we match all of the twelve Red Flag symptoms of depression with the above biological data? Some may feel that this is an overly ambitious task, but we can at least speculate on the most likely causes of each symptom:

§ *Low mood* This is in many ways the most difficult symptom to place in relation to the biological data. The most likely culprits are reduced activity in the apical sections of the left PFC (involved in the cognitive control of mood), combined with increased activity of the lower sections of the PFC like Area 25, the ventrolateral PFC/orbital cortex, and the amygdala (involved in the production of mood).

§ *Fatigue* The reduced activity in the noradrenalin cable is probably the main cause of this symptom. Reduced activity of the dopamine system, the glucocortisol barrage, and reduced activity in the serotonin cable may also play a role.

§ *Sleep difficulties* There seems to be an underlying problem with the REM sleep pattern of those who are at risk of depression. During an actual attack of depression, it is probably the reduced general activity of both the serotonin and noradrenalin cables (which the body tries to counteract by increasing levels at night), together with high night-time glucocortisol levels, that gives rise to this symptom.

§ *Anxiety* This is caused primarily by the amygdala, which is over-active in depression. The inability of the PFC to switch off the amygdala is also a factor. It is helped by all the components of the stress system being over-active.

§ *Weight loss or gain* This is probably caused by the reduction of activity of the serotonin cable. The reduced activity in the dopamine cable and *nucleus accumbens* also causes problems by reducing the person's enjoyment of food and other pleasurable activities.

§ *Loss of self-esteem* This could well be the result of reduced activity in the PFC, together with increased activity in the amygdala. Both of these factors cause people to take a negative attitude towards ourselves. Reduced activity in the serotonin cable may also play a role here. The lack of control of the PFC over the amygdala probably contributes to this symptom.

§ *Lack of drive* Decreased activity of the noradrenalin cable is the most likely culprit here, allied to a reduction in serotonin-cable activity. The decreased activity in the dopamine cable and *nucleus accumbens* means that the normal enjoyment of everyday activities is further reduced, lessening the person's drive even more.

§ *Negative thinking* The amygdala is the most likely source of the problem here. Increased activity in this section leads to the generation of many of the negative emotional thoughts that are so prevalent in this illness. As these are normally held in check by the left side of the PFC, which itself generates positive thinking, it is likely that disruption of the normal activity of parts of the PFC plays an important role. It is also likely that the over-activity of Area 25 is crucial to the development of negative thinking.

§ *Poor memory* There are a number of potential reasons for this. First, reduced activity in the PFC may adversely affect short-term memory. Second, the hippocampus, the main organiser of memories prior to them being stored in other parts of the brain, is hammered by glucocortisol in particular. This part of the limbic mood department is important in that it constantly produces new nerve cells. In depression, this process, along with the formation of inter-neuronal connections is hugely disrupted, making difficulties with memory virtually inevitable.

§ *Poor concentration* Poor concentration is primarily due to a reduction of activity in the noradrenalin mood cable. This, combined with difficulties with PFC short-term memory problems, makes concentration on tasks very difficult. The PFC is particularly activated when it comes to taking on new tasks, so depressed activity in this area makes coping with new situations particularly difficult for people with depression.

§ *Lack of joy or pleasure* The dopamine cable and control box (the ventral tegmental area) is also attacked by the stress barrage of depression. This leads to reduced stimulation of the *nucleus accumbens* (pleasure box). Suddenly, life seems very grey and meaningless.

§ *Suicidal thoughts* These are created by reduced activity in the left ventral PFC, together with a marked depletion of the serotonin mood cable which supplies it. This combination is the most likely cause of impulsive thoughts of self-harm.

If we put all of these factors together with the effects of glucocortisol on our heart, bones and immune system, we have a possible biological picture of why we develop all the symptoms and signs of depression. Further research may confirm the validity – or otherwise – of this model.

We can also see how accurate the Red Flag model of depression is as a way of investigating mental-health issues. It is clear that this illness is caused by disruption to the two mood departments, combined with reduced activity of the three mood cables and mood circuit, and over-activity of the stress system, particularly the adrenal gland and the production of glucocortisol.

A final point here relates to older people. Elderly individuals who have no previous history of depression, vascular damage (related to arterial supply) to neural-circuit connections to the left side of the PFC and the left basal ganglia (the structure containing the ventral segmental area and the substantial nigra, the two dopamine-producing parts of the brain) in particular, combined with degenerative changes to various parts of the mood system (notably a shrinkage of the three major mood cable and systems), produces another version of the Red Flag, even though the underlying biological mechanism in this case is different. This, is in my opinion, is one of the most powerful illustrations of the central role played by the brain in depression, whether in the young or the elderly.

Before leaving this discussion on the biology of unipolar depression, it is worth distinguishing in more detail the difference between structural and functional findings relating to research into brain activity. Wayne Drevets and many others have done a great deal of valuable work in this area; I will try and summarise the main findings of their research. Once again, it is important to stress that a great deal of this research is ongoing, and is being constantly re-evaluated as more information comes on stream.

The sub-genual cortex (particularly sg24, at the junction of Area's 24 and 25), as we have seen above, has revealed volume reductions on the left side in particular. This structural change is felt to precede the appearance of depression in familial cases (relating to families with a very strong history of depression presenting under the age of twenty-five) and may (based on studies of twins) occur immediately after the first episode of depression in other cases. The cause of this volume loss is, as has already been noted, a shortage of both glial cells and dendrite/axon connections.

Functionally, Area 25 (the ventral sub-genual cortex) is overactive in depression and reverts to normal with successful therapy. It is felt that the increased functional activity of Area 25 due to its extensive connections with the amygdala, orbital PFC and mood control boxes may contribute to the vegetative/anhedonia symptoms of depression.

The rostral cingulate (Area 24) structurally is abnormal. Functionally, this area seems to be under-active in those with depression. It plays a role in resolving cognitive conflicts in relation to emotional stimulation (a process known as emotional monitoring). The degree of under-activity has been shown to be an excellent predictor of whether a person may turn out to be resistant to the drug-based treatment of depression. Those who show greater activity in this section prior to treatment have a better chance of responding to it, and vice versa.

Of great interest to many researchers was the difference between CBT/IPT and drug therapy on this area. The former caused the area to become more active, while the latter did not. This once again demonstrated how these psychological therapies work from the top (i.e. the cognitive part) of the brain down.

In structural terms, the orbital and left ventro-lateral PFC has revealed reductions in volume, again due to shortages of glial cells and dendrite connections, among other things. In some cases, these areas may be functionally over-active in people with depression. The orbital area links very closely to the amygdala and is extremely interactive with it. In depression, it seems as though the ability of the orbital area to modulate negative information from the amygdala is diminished, possibly due to the structural changes mentioned above. The over-activity of this part of the brain is related to its attempts to quieten the amygdala. Drug therapy, when it is successful, reduces activity in this part of the PFC, as its monitoring role over the amygdala can relax. (If the latter is less over-active, then the orbital area is no longer forced to calm it down.) In CBT/IPT, this area becomes more active, as it tries to overrule the amygdala's over-activity, which gives rise to so many of the symptoms of depression.

The dorsal anterolateral PFC has been found to lack both glial support cells and neurons. Functionally, it and the dorso-medial PFC have been shown to be under-active in depression, something which generally normalises following treatment. Again, these areas seem to play a role in controlling the negative emotions associated with this illness.

The amygdala has also been shown to lack glial support cells. Functionally, the more severe the depression, the greater the level of activity in this structure.

Structurally, all forms of drug therapy for depression, apart from, possibly, Lithium, cannot restore the volume (particularly glial-cell deficits) of the PFC but can help to improve dendrite connections. Functionally, however, such drugs can restore many areas of the brain to normal functioning, despite the persistence of structural deficits.

When one takes all of these findings into account, the case for combined drug and CBT therapy in particular is compelling. The former, by acting from the brain-stem mood-control boxes, the amygdala and Area 25, seems to kick-start the mood circuit into action, increasing the energy and concentration needed to become involved in the latter. which can activate more efficiently the cognitive areas necessary for it to succeed.

A fascinating review by Dr Mary Philips (of the Institute of Psychiatry in London) and Dr Wayne Drevets looked at the two neural systems involved in human emotional behavior and how they are involved in depression. The first, called the 'ventral system' (see Figure 2), incorporates the amygdala, the orbital and ventrolateral PFC, and the ventral sub-genual cingulate cortex (Area 25). In depression, the structural deficits, with a resulting increase in functional activity in the above, lead to a restricted range of emotions, with the emphasis on the amygdala perceiving negative rather than positive emotions. The second, called the 'dorsal system', incorporates the dorsolateral and dorsomedial PFC, the dorsal cingulate cortex (Area 24) and the hippocampus. In depression, structural changes lead to a functional reduction in activity of this system and to an executive functional inability to regulate the negative emotional thoughts and behaviour emanating from the ventral system.

The final result is persistent low mood and the disappearance of joy from the per-on's life. This approach seems to offer a particularly useful way forward, as it brings all the structural and functional changes seen in this illness into an easy-to-comprehend model. It also shows the intimate and integrated relationship between the logical and emotional parts of the mood system.

Drug therapy will work by normalising the ventral system first, with subsequent improvements in the dorsal system. CBT/IPT works first on the dorsal system, with the ventral-system improvements following later.

In relation to bipolar mood disorder, the depression phase changes seen in this dis-order are similar to those in unipolar depression. The mania phase involves over-activ-ty of the dopamine, noradrenalin and serotonin cables. Of note, many of the same structural changes in the mood departments seen in unipolar depression (with some differences, like an increase in the size of the amygdala) are found in this illness. There are also many similarities in neuro-imaging functioning in bipolar depression – but also important differences in some areas.

The simplest way to view these models is to look again at the ventral/dorsal model described above for unipolar depression. Once again, the ventral system is generally overactive due to structural difficulties. In particular, the amygdala is actually enlarged in size, in comparison to unipolar depression. The dorsal system is under-active, so cog-nitive control of emotion is diminished. The final result is mood/emotional lability.

A great deal of work is also being done on the relationships between G protein cell membrane proteins, and their links with second messengers, like cyclic AMP, which, through complicated intercellular mechanisms, involving molecules like Creb and BDNF, influence neuronal plasticity and survival.

There are many structural difficulties and other biological findings in this disorder. To go into them all is beyond the scope of this book. A full review of all these changes and how they differ from unipolar depression can be found in both the Philips/Drevets and Manji articles and, in particular, in an excellent summary on the subject by Kapczinki et al (see Bibliography).

Another interesting question is how the various treatments for this illness work. We dealt with this to some extent in the Red Flag section, but it is useful to review some of the treatments in more detail:

§ *Exercise* Increased activity of endorphins released during exercise can raise the mood. Exercise also boosts the dopamine system and increases activity in the hip-pocampus. It also helps to dampen down over-activity in the amygdala. This latter may also help to elevate our mood if we are down.

§ *Diet and supplements* A good diet produces nutrients for all neurons and support cells. B vitamins supply the raw material for production of neurotransmitters. Fish oils (and oily fish) increase the activity of the mood cables.

Apart from the fact that the cell membrane of every cell in the body depends on the presence of these essential fatty acids, these acids also improve the quality of the myelin sheaths which are wrapped around the neurons which make up these cables. These sheaths in turn are manufactured by the glial support cells (oligodendrocytes), which are in close proximity to their 'bosses', the neurons. The function of this protective layer is to speed up the conduction of electrical impulses from one neuron to another. This sheath is mainly composed of fatty tissues, with fatty acids like EPA in particular playing an important role in the structure and function of the myelin sheath. Some researchers feel that the anti-inflammatory effects of EPA may also play a role in the treatment of this illness. How, we do not as yet know. As our diet is usually quite poor in providing these fatty acids, supplementation is often the best source. Mackerel, herring, tuna, salmon, flax seeds and nuts are the best dietary sources of Omega 3 oils.

My own opinion is that the use of supplements, in conjunction with other forms of therapy, is important. The brain needs at least the minimum daily requirement of 500 milligrams EPA in order to function properly. This has to be supplied by two portions of oily fish or flax-seed oils, or as a supplement. When one looks at the effects this illness has on the mood cables and departments, it cannot help if we are lacking these basic nutrients! I usually recommend 500 to 1,000 milligrams EPA as part of a total treatment package.

§ *Counselling and psychological therapies* Through the work of Mayberg, Goldapple and others, we have developed a much clearer idea of what happens to the brain in CBT. It seems as though ITP (and possibly counselling) behaves in a similar manner. We already know that the emotional brain is more powerful than the logical one, so it would make sense that the former would have to work very hard to overcome the negativity pouring out of the former; that is what happens in practice.

The experts demonstrated that the PFC initially was over-active in CBT therapy and then began to settle down as the person 'got the hang of' the approach and their negative thinking and mood lifted. Area 25, the ventral sub-genual cortex, eventually settled down if the therapy was successful, but at a much slower rate than with drug therapy.

Area 24, the rostral cingulate PFC, was shown to increase in activity. The result of all these changes is a secondary reduction in the activity of the amygdala. Another key finding was an increase in activity of the hippocampus, which was obviously activated to memorise the cognitive/behavioural mechanisms learned during therapy. As a result of all this, the mood circuit gradually returns to normal.

All of this demonstrated that CBT/ITP acted from the top of the brain downwards, the reverse of what happens in drug therapy. If we reflect back on the ventral/dorsal systems noted earlier, it seems as though the latter becomes more activated, with eventual dampening down of the negative emotions emanating from the former. Those who would like to examine these results in more detail should consult the Mayberg/Goldapple articles; see Bibliography.

§ *Drug treatments* The main action of these has also been thought to have been through the activation of our mood cables. This explains their ability to reduce most of the physical effects of depression, such as sleep, fatigue, drive, concentration and so on. This seems to be their target initially. But how do they reduce negative thinking and raise self-esteem and mood? Many now feel that they may have a more delayed secondary effect on the cells of the left PFC (possibly by stimulating the whole mood circuit), increasing their efficiency, and improving their ability to communicate. This may occur through their effects on glutamate neurotransmitters. By increasing activity in the left PFC, this may in turn help to switch off the powerful negative dominance of the amygdala. As a result of this, our mood lifts, our negative thinking improves, and our anxiety lessens. This, allied to the lifting of the above physical symptoms, explains how these drugs contribute to the increased well-being of the person.

Now, as promised in the Red Flag section, I include a more detailed explanation of how we think these drugs work (and why it takes up to two weeks for them to work), for those who are interested. We will deal here particularly with the SSRIs, but the same principles also apply to drugs affecting the noradrenalin cable.

Firstly, the antidepressant blocks the re-uptake of serotonin back into the neuron which initially released it. Then the level of serotonin in the synapse tries to rise. However, neurons have a healthy feedback system, where some serotonin receptors (such as 5HT1B and 5HT1D on the pre-synaptic neuron) act as 'auto receptors', sensing this sudden rise in levels of the neurotransmitter, and preventing the cell from releasing more serotonin into the synapse. The result is that no major rise in serotonin occurs. After two weeks, this inhibitory mechanism weakens; gradually, the level of serotonin begins to rise, and the initial improvement in symptoms begins.

As the serotonin receptors (particularly 5HT1A, which seems to be the most likely culprit in depression) begin to be more actively stimulated, they activate G proteins in the cell membrane to release messengers, which pass into the nucleus of the cell to stimulate the genes/DNA. The genes in turn promote the production of a molecule called BDNF (Brain Derived Neurotrophic Factor). This in turn promotes the building of new dendrites, improving connections between neurons, and thereby improves the functioning of key mood sections such as the PFC and the hippocampus.

The improvement in both the activity and functioning of the serotonin mood cable and the mood departments it serves re-stabilises the mood neural circuit, leading to a gradual and sustained improvement in the symptoms of depression. The functioning of the other cable improves accordingly, and the Red Flag turns green.

What about the effects of both SSRIs and mood stabilisers like Lithium on the structures of the mood system? The present feeling is that, although the former improve the functioning of the various departments, they are unable to reverse the structural changes. They seem to increase BDNF/dendrite regrowth but cannot reverse the glial-cell loss.

Lithium, which seems to be an exception to the above, is increasingly thought to work by increasing inter-cellular neuro-protective factors, with evidence of some regrowth of grey matter through this process. It also seems to increase intra-cellular proteins, which protect the neuron from cell death. In some cases of chronic use, neuronal growth has been noted. It is likely that this process affects the PFC, which stabilises bipolar sufferers and reduces self-harm in those with borderline personality disorder.

We mentioned in the Red Flag section potential new drugs which act on melatonin. One very promising one in the pipeline is called Agomelatonine. This acts by increasing the activity of the melatonin receptors MT1 and MT2 and by blocking the 5HT2C serotonin receptors in the mood system. The antidepressant effect of this drug is believed to be due to its effects on the serotonin receptor; and the improvement in sleep patterns due to its effects on the melatonin receptors. What makes this new drug prospect interesting is its effectiveness, combined with a very clean side-effect profile (particularly in relation to sexual side effects). We will have to see if it proves itself in clinical practice in the future.

Most complementary therapies, such as massage, reflexology, meditation and yoga, probably act by dampening down the stress system and in the process dampening down an over-active amygdala. Acupuncture may work by increasing endorphins. Herbs like St John's wort probably work by stimulating the serotonin mood cable, just like fish oils, but are probably less effective.

PART III: THE YELLOW FLAG

The main player in anxiety disorders is now thought to be the amygdala. This important part of the limbic mood department is the 'commander-in-chief' of the stress system. It also acts as a storage area for emotions related to negative memories and experiences, particularly unconscious ones.

We saw in the Red Flag how the amygdala is the main culprit in producing many of the emotional symptoms attached to negative thinking, poor self-esteem and anxiety seen in that illness. It comes as no surprise that over-activity of this little box is seen by many as the biological reason for most of the fears, and thoughts of worry, apprehension and doom, seen in anxiety disorders, both acute and chronic.

Before dealing with anxiety, it is worth looking at the biology of the 'fear response' and the role of the amygdala.

Suppose a leopard confronts you – something which has actually happened to me! The initial visual response, which takes 12 milliseconds, is processed by a key structure called the 'thalamus', and arrives in the amygdala, which sets in motion the acute stress response often called 'fight or flight'. (Personally, I froze, which is probably why I am still here to write this book!) We have already seen that this is caused by massive bursts of adrenalin and noradrenalin. Before we have a chance to think about the situation, our heart pounds, our breathing gets shallow, and our stomach churns.

At the same time, the thalamus is also sending the visual information by a more roundabout system to the PFC; this takes around 30 to 40 milliseconds. Now the brain logically evaluates the danger, which in this case is very real. It then agrees with the initial response of the amygdala and begins to plan evasive action. The stress response is now allowed to continue till the threat is gone. In my own case, luckily the leopard felt that I was too scrawny and moved on to more juicy titbits! It still took some time following the event for my stress symptoms to settle. The emotional response to the event is, however, firmly embedded in my brain (with the help of the hippocampus and the amygdala). To this day, a large cat springing out of the shadows activates the fear response before my logical PFC overrules it! If, however, it had turned out that the danger was false, and I had seen a shadow rather than a real leopard, the PFC would have sent instructions to the amygdala to switch off the stress response, and all would have returned to normal.

When we move on to examine the biology of anxiety, it is worth keeping this natural fear response in mind, for the former is simply a dysfunctional response of the internal stress system. It is also worth mentioning the way in which the PFC and the hippocampus are closely linked in with the amygdala, forming the so-called fear circuit. This is relevant to panic attacks.

The above example also verifies the concept promoted by the great research expert Joseph Le Doux, namely that the emotional brain communicates more efficiently and quickly with the logical one due to the structural disparities in neural connections between them.

It now seems that, in anxiety disorders, the amygdala, through a combination of genetic vulnerability and early childhood experience, becomes hypersensitive by the time we become adults. In anxiety disorders, the PFC may inappropriately set off the amygdala to trigger the whole stress system into action. Thus, bursts of stress peptides pour forth, our noradrenalin cables buzz into life, and our adrenal gland starts to pour out adrenalin, noradrenalin and glucocortisol. We have already dealt with the symptoms of extreme anxiety in the Yellow Flag section of this book.

The hippocampus plays an important role in anxiety as well. Like the PFC, it has the potential to modulate or switch off the amygdala/stress-response activity. In anxiety, however, it struggles to do so, as does the PFC; those who doubt the latter should try talking to a person who is having a severe panic attack. It is difficult to convince such a person logically that their symptoms are not due to a serious illness. This is because the increased activity of their amygdala is overruling the normal, sensible control and reason that the PFC normally exerts. Thankfully, CBT can help to reverse this process.

The hippocampus also contributes to the 'fear of fears' seen in panic attacks by keeping the memory of previous attacks firmly in the consciousness of the victim. Once again, CBT is helpful in reversing this.

Many people who suffer from general anxiety disorder (GAD) may wonder where their background feelings of worry, doom and apprehension come from. Once again, our amygdala is the most likely source. The more stressful episodes that those with GAD experience in their lives, the more their feelings of worry increase. This is because the neurons in the amygdala strengthen their connections, as a result of constant over-stimulation, which consolidates the negative feelings of worry and apprehension. This explains why many people with this illness feel that their condition deteriorates as they get older and the momentum of life's many and varied problems begin to build.

In those with long-standing GAD, the hippocampus is subjected to a constant barrage of stress peptides and glucocortisol in particular. This has the opposite effect to what happens in the amygdala. New neuron production is reduced, and the communication between the neurons in this section is damaged. This leads to a symptom commonly experienced by people suffering from this condition: that they feel 'scattered' when it comes to coping with day-to-day activities.

Symptoms such as fatigue and poor concentration in GAD are probably caused by the noradrenalin cable being depleted due to chronic over-stimulation of the whole stress system.

Obsessive compulsive disorder (OCD) has proven to be a very difficult illness to explain biologically. Advances in functional neuro-imaging have helped partially to increase our understanding of this illness. Once again, the frontal mood department (the orbito-frontal PFC) is involved, along with other areas of the brain close to the limbic system (for those who are interested, the main area involved is the thalamus). It seems that over-activity of the former may lead to obsessive thoughts, and abnormal activity in the latter, to compulsive actions. Other research suggests that abnormalities in our serotonin and dopamine cables may also play a part. It will take some time before the whole story is revealed.

By comparison, in acute anxiety states such as panic attacks, the noradrenalin cable is over-stimulated by a hypersensitive amygdala, and this, together with over-production of adrenalin and noradrenalin by the adrenal gland, leads to the symptoms usually experienced during these episodes.

The secret to treating all anxiety disorders is to use various mechanisms to try to calm down or switch off the over-active amygdala. CBT is a very powerful tool for this purpose: it seems to put the thinking part of the mood system (the PFC) back in control. This in turn dampens down the part of the brain that deals with emotions (the limbic system), particularly the amygdala, which in turn reduces the physical and psychological symptoms of acute and chronic anxiety. Relaxation exercises are also very helpful. These work by encouraging the amygdala to calm down. Breathing exercises lie at the heart of this form of treatment.

Drug therapy can sometimes be of help. Tranquillizers work by increasing the activity of the GABA 'chill out' receptors but have a great potential for abuse and should only be used with caution. Drugs, such as SSRIs and Buspar, which increase the activity in the serotonin cable, seem to help in some cases of chronic anxiety. In general, their use is best combined with CBT and relaxation exercises.

Omega 3 fish oils and exercise can also play a role. The latter helps to reduce symptoms of anxiety and worry, increasing feelings of well-being, and encouraging activity in the hippocampus. Fish oils in particular work on the serotonin mood cable.

Once again, a holistic approach is the answer. Proper diet, supplements like fish oils, exercise, relaxation exercises, and meditation, together with psychological therapies like CBT, can put us back firmly in control of our own lives. Sometimes drug therapy may help in this process.

The real tragedy is that so many will go through their lives with so many symptoms of the Yellow Flag, unaware that help is available.

PART IV: THE PURPLE FLAG

For years, it has been clear to both doctors and other health professionals involved in the area of addiction that there are many traits and patterns present in all addicts. The mechanisms to explain these traits and patterns were poorly understood until very recently. However, due to exciting new research, we are starting to develop a much clearer understanding of the mechanisms behind addiction.

It is useful, before we go into some of these mechanisms, to refresh our memories of the normal pathways by which all of us experience normal pleasures. We may remember from Chapter One how our dopamine control box sends its cables through the limbic system and up into the PFC. On the way, we talked about a very important structure called the pleasure box: the *nucleus accumbens*. The dopamine control box is called the ventral tegmental area (VTA). When we are enjoying the good things in life, such as good meals, alcohol, sex, and other activities which give us a sense of enjoyment, this is the pathway which is activated. Information is passed from the ventral tegmental area (dopamine control box) via axons to the *nucleus accumbens* (the pleasure box). This box then lights up. It is in the process of this happening that we feel a great sense of pleasure and enjoyment.

It is interesting to note that, when the axons coming from our dopamine control box arrive in the *nucleus accumbens*, the main molecular development is that dopamine is released into the synapse of the cell, travels across the synapse, and attaches itself to the dopamine receptors on the neuron of the *nucleus accumbens*. It activates the cell and then travels back, to be reabsorbed back into the cell of origin. This is the typical way in which one neuron talks to another. It is this release of dopamine which stimulates the cell of the *nucleus accumbens* (pleasure box) and causes the changes within the cell that give us feelings of pleasure.

Let's move on now to the molecular biology of addiction itself. Most addictive substances end up having their effect at the level of the synapse, between the neurons of the dopamine system and their connections with the neurons of the *nucleus accumbens* or pleasure box. Nicotine, for example, encourages the cells of the VTA, or dopamine system, to release large amounts of dopamine into the *nucleus accumbens* synapses. Drugs such as cocaine end up blocking dopamine re-uptake at these synapses, increasing the amount of dopamine available to stimulate the *nucleus accumbens* neurons. Alcohol and opiates enhance dopamine release into these synapses. The final result of all these addictive substances is that we get a build-up of dopamine within the synapses.

It seems, however, as though it is the effects that this dopamine has on the cells of the *nucleus accumbens* itself which actually produces addiction. Other activities, such as gambling and food addiction, probably work by stimulating the VTA (pleasure system) and encouraging the dopamine control box to produce more dopamine to be released into the synapses between its neurons and the neurons of the *nucleus accumbens*.

Two terms that we have already dealt with in the chapter on the Purple Flag were 'tolerance' and 'dependency'. As stated before, tolerance means that the more a person uses a drug or an activity to which they are becoming dependent, the less 'buzz' they get from it, and the more of the substance they have to use to get the same effect. Dependency relates to the physical and psychological effects that appear when the drug or activity is withdrawn.

It now seems that the reasons for both of these states occurring relate to changes within the cells of the pleasure box or *nucleus accumbens* itself. The high dopamine levels in the synapses seem to encourage the release of secondary messengers from the cell membrane of the cell, which travel into the cell to interact with the genes. This apparently happens through the formation of an interesting molecule called Creb1. This molecule acts by dampening down the 'buzz' produced by these addictive substances. This is the reason for the development of tolerance. If the person then abstains from the addictive substance or activity, the level of this molecule falls, and the person starts to get an intense physical and psychological craving for the substance or activity.

Longer-term use of these addictive substances or activities leads to the formation of a second molecule from within these cells, called 'Fos p'. As the level of this molecule rises, its capacity to act upon the genes in the cell seems to last for a much longer period of time, and in some cases up to many years. It seems that the longer the exposure to these addictive substances, the greater the levels of this build-up, and the longer the person remains at risk of developing these cravings for the substance or activity.

It also seems obvious that memory plays a large role in addictive processes. Our hippocampus and amygdala are closely inter-connected. Our limbic system plays an important role in our feelings in relation to addiction, and our PFC in relation to our behaviour. The latter seems to become increasingly important in older chronic addicts.

All of these key structures are connected to the nucleus accumbens, and play their part in this illness. Some experts regard the nucleus accumbens, the amygdala and the PFC as being part of a 'reward circuit'. Stress, for example, seems to be a crucial trigger, through the amygdala connections, to the nucleus accumbens. The experts are beginning to focus more and more on this circuit, and the importance of both the serotonin and glutamate systems. We now know, for example, that chronic alcoholics suffer from under activity of the serotonin system in the brain; this may explain the links between alcohol addiction and depression. (For those who would like more detailed information on this subject, please consult the Bibliography.) But the core of the addictive forces seems to lie in the excess production of dopamine being released from the cells of the dopamine cable into the pleasure box, and the changes that subsequently occur.

One can justifiably ask what role our genes play in this process? Clearly, they must play an important role, as there is such variation in relation to people and their potential for addiction. The simplest example of this is alcohol. While many people misuse alcohol on a regular and constant basis, the majority do not become addicted. This would seem to suggest that there are genetic predispositions (either through personality development or possibly within the *nucleus accumbens*/dopamine system) which make it more likely for some people to become addicted. In the area of smoking, while it is clear that nicotine is highly addictive, some people have much greater difficulty in giving up smoking than others.

From years of experience, it seems to me that people who have a generally addictive nature will have much greater difficulty coming off cigarettes than those who do not. It is also clear that drugs such as cocaine, particularly when taken in the form of crack, seem to be highly addictive in themselves. Once again, however, some people seem to be able to misuse this drug and not become completely addicted to it. It seems likely that at least 50 percent of people who become addicted to drugs probably have underlying genetic predispositions to addiction to begin with. Gambling, for instance, seems to be an extremely addictive activity, but once again not everybody who gambles becomes addicted to it. One would have to assume that there are also some genetic predispositions in this addiction (most likely personality-related) that we do not as yet fully understand.

The above biological mechanisms explain the phenomenon that family doctors have known about for so many years: cross-addiction. It is quite common for one addiction to be interwoven with one or more other addictions. Good examples of this are combinations of gambling and alcohol, and cigarettes and drug abuse. When we understand that the same pathway (i.e. the dopamine system/*nucleus accumbens*) are involved in all of these addictions, it becomes much simpler to explain cross-addiction. If cocaine, nicotine, alcohol, opium and gambling are all responsible for the release of excess dopamine to feed into the pleasure box, it becomes clear that it is very likely that an addict will move from one addiction to another quite freely. The common denominator is that the addict experiences a 'buzz' in his or her *nucleus accumbens*.

For many years, the excuse was that the above pathways, which are obviously very biological in nature, could not be helped by the addict. However, our PFC behaviour box does have the capacity to make a decision to override all other factors. Although the biological changes noted above cause the intense cravings and psychological dependence associated with addiction, it is therefore possible for an addict, with the help of fellow addicts, to overrule the feelings that these molecular changes are producing.

We now have a greater understanding of the illness of addiction, from which so many people suffer. The biological mechanism outlined above explains the incredible cravings that sometimes lead alcoholics to binge-drink. The long-term changes occurring within the cells explain why people, after quite a long period of abstinence from these addictive substances, cave in and return to their addictions of choice. For many, counteracting these internal changes is a lifelong battle.

This biological mechanism also explains why so many smokers have so much difficulty in quitting. At the end of the day, it is a battle between our feelings and our behaviour: in addiction, the pleasurable feelings desperately try to overrule our behaviour and control mechanisms. Unfortunately, in the majority of cases, the pleasure box wins. It is only when the consequences of giving in to these addictive substances and activities becomes so great that many addicts are forced to change their behaviour and try to deal with these internal biological cravings. The intensity of the cravings also explains the incredible selfishness of many addicts, where they will feed their addiction to the exclusion of everything – and everyone – around them.

Addiction, therefore, is an illness, but we have a responsibility in how we manage our own illnesses.

PART V: THE WHITE FLAG

In the chapter on the White Flag of suicide, we dealt with the biological and social causes of suicide. I would like in this section to deal in more detail with the biology of suicide.

The difficulty in studying the changes in the brain of those who have taken their own lives through suicide is that we have to readjust the way we look at things, and in many cases work in reverse. This is what a pathologist does in a post mortem: he studies the changes seen in the organs of the deceased, and works out what illnesses they had when they were alive and what led to their death.

Suicide is no different, but study of the brain is more difficult. However, some excellent post-mortem research, allied to modern neuro-imaging of those who have made serious attempts on their own lives, has started to lift the veil on what is going on biologically in the mood systems of those who are at risk of suicide or have succumbed to this deadly illness.

Post-mortem studies of those who have committed suicide have identified some key common denominators. The key seems to be serotonin levels. We cannot measure the serotonin levels in those who have died, but we can learn a lot by studying slides of brain tissues. These show an increase in 5HT1A serotonin receptors and a reduction in pre-synaptic serotonin transporter sites in the ventral (ventromedial) PFC behaviour box, a sure sign that this section was starved of serotonin.

When this section of the brain cannot produce enough serotonin, it compensates by manufacturing extra 5HT1A receptors to make maximum use of the amounts of serotonin that are available. It also tries to achieve the same purpose by reducing the transport back into the pre-synaptic neuron.

As this part of the PFC, which we described earlier as the 'impulse control box', is the control mechanism inhibiting aggressive or impulsive thoughts and behaviour, starving it of serotonin inevitably increases the likelihood of suicide. Of interest, reduced activity in this part of the PFC may also explain the poor decision-making that so often precedes suicide.

We know that serotonin is manufactured under the careful eye of our serotonin control box, i.e. the *raphe nucleus*, and stored in small vesicles in terminal buttons of the axons of our serotonin mood cable which supplies the frontal cortex, in particular the PFC behaviour box. In suicide, there seems to be a particular under-activity of this cable, irrespective of the illness underlying it.

Post-mortem studies of some suicides show evidence of the *raphe nucleus* trying desperately to make more serotonin. Other findings supporting this theory relating to the importance of the lowered activity of the serotonin system is the constant finding of lower levels of the breakdown product 5HIIA in the spinal fluid of those who died by suicide, irrespective of the illness underlying it. Increased numbers of 5HT2A receptors (implying a shortage of serotonin) on platelets circulating in the bloodstream have also been noted. This is of interest because it mimics the situation in the brain. Some wonder whether this might help to screen out those who are more at risk of self-harm J. J. Mann, in an excellent review, noted that genetic factors, childhood neglect and abuse, substance abuse, cigarette smoking, and low cholesterol were all factors which could cause under-activity of the serotonin system.

The key to suicide probably lies in the starvation of the serotonin mood cable of serotonin itself, and the resulting reduction in activity of the impulse-controlling centre in the PFC. Other key post-mortem studies revealed higher levels of stress peptides like CRH, with corresponding reductions in receptors in the frontal cortex and limbic mood departments. Other studies have shown enlargement of the adrenal gland in some who have committed suicide. There is also evidence of noradrenalin-cable depletion in the PFC from constant over-activity as a result of stress prior to the event. Some feel that the depletion of this cable leads to the feelings of hopelessness and helplessness that are associated with suicide.

These findings, when put together, suggest the following possibilities:

1   That huge inner stress turmoil may have been going on in the lives of those with the White Flag for some time before the event.

2   That their mood system internally was in severe distress due to major disruption of their serotonin mood cable and control box. This leads to the strong possibility that depression (either on its own or associated with schizophrenia, alcohol and substance abuse, and personality disorder), often undiagnosed, lies at the heart of the condition.

3   That decreased activity of the ventral PFC behavioural box, supplied by the serotonin cable, provides the key to the impulsive nature of this illness.

4   That reduction in the regulatory activity of the ventromedial PFC over the amygdala, leading to over-activity of the latter, together with noradrenalin-cable under-activity, creates the symptoms of hopelessness, negative thinking and helplessness that are at the core of this illness.

5   That alcohol, by disrupting glutamate receptors and switching off the PFC, further increases chances of impulsive violent suicidal behaviour.

Neuro-imaging of those who have survived major suicide attempts supports this hypothesis, as it has shown a reduction in activity of the PFC behaviour box. It has also been shown that those who are regarded as being at higher risk of impulsive suicidal behaviour seem to have lower activity in the ventral, medial and lateral PFC. Interesting PET (positron emission tomography, a form of three-dimensional neuro-imaging) studies by Oquendo comparing high-lethality versus low-lethality suicide survivors confirmed the above; she actually earmarked two key sites of the brain, one involving Areas 8 and 32, and the other Areas 6 and 24.

Other key research findings relating to suicide include a reduction in total cholesterol associated with suicidal behaviour. This is probably due to the importance of cholesterol in the maintenance of the neuron cell membrane. As a result, cholesterol seems to play a role in the serotonin system.

In relation to suicide, there is definite evidence that, independent of the mental illness underlying it, there seems to be a genetic basis for suicidal behaviour in certain families. A great deal of research in such cases has been done into the genetics of the serotonin system. One particular set of genetic alleles (alternative forms of a gene) studied are responsible for the manufacture of TPH (tryptophan hydroxylase), an enzyme involved in the manufacture of serotonin. Those with the LL allele seem to have a greater risk of suicide. Many other genes involved have been studied, but so far no clear candidate has emerged. We are only at an early stage, however, in our understanding of the myriad of genes which may be involved.

Many of us know of cases of young males who have committed suicide where there is no obvious genetic basis or family history of mental illness. In the absence of other illnesses such as schizophrenia and addiction, it is likely that hidden depression (or at least a vulnerability to it), perhaps with the presence of this serotonin vulnerability, may be the explanation, often triggered by environmental factors.

Good examples of the latter are cases where the individual is experiencing severe bullying or loss of a significant personal relationship. The stress barrage of such triggers in those who are at risk causes depletion of the serotonin box and cable, a subsequent drop in activity in the left side of the PFC and an increase in activity of the amygdala, gradual depletion of noradrenalin in the noradrenalin cable, and the arrival of hopelessness, helplessness and, through the mechanisms already discussed, impulsive suicidal thoughts and actions.

In the case of schizophrenia (in particular where alcohol substance abuse is a factor), and in addiction itself, the combination of the illness plus the addictive substances themselves may cause both depression and depletion of the serotonin box and cable.

As these substances also reduce the control of the left side of the PFC, it is not surprising that suicide is a major risk in these cases.

We must continue to learn from all this biological post-mortem and other research, just as we have learned so much about coronary heart disease from such studies. This is where the key to the future prevention of suicides will lie.

One final point of note is the importance of brain development in this discussion. Our limbic mood system rules the roost from the ages of twelve to eighteen in particular, and the controlling influence of the PFC behaviour box is slowly maturing from the ages of eighteen to twenty-five, so there is an obvious risk of suicide in young males, in particular between the ages of fifteen to twenty-five. Emotions are ruling their lives, despite attempts by the behaviour box to put a break on impulsive activities. If we are feeling down during this period, we may experience an even greater intensity of emotion. This may make everything seem more hopeless, further reducing self-esteem. It is hard for the rational mind to rationalise these feelings.

Alcohol is particularly dangerous within this age group in particular. First, it and other substances have the capacity to alter the neurochemistry of the immature brain, increasing the risks of developing depression in those who are at risk. Second, in those who are suffering from (usually undiagnosed) depression, particularly if the at-risk trait is present, and who may be experiencing suicidal thoughts, alcohol removes any remaining control from the ventral PFC, which is already probably starved of serotonin by low mood. Control is quickly lost, and impulsive actions may occur. How many wonderful young people have been lost in this way? How many more will be? It is up to all of us to take a serious look at this question.

In summary, biological research is slowly unmasking the inner pain and turmoil, and the feelings of hopelessness, being endured by many of those who take their own lives. It is also beginning to explain why many people with mental illness do not experience major suicidal thoughts or actions; rather, that there is a specific subgroup of people who are primarily at risk of suicide. Biological research is also revealing in such people the presence of unrecognised stress which may have been present for some time. This combination, often in conjunction with alcohol, may lead eventually to the brain's normal control of impulsive thoughts and actions breaking down, and the White Flag of suicide unfurling.

Appendix 2

Suicide Tables

MALE SUICIDE DEATHS BY TEN-YEAR AGE GROUP, 1980–2004, REPUBLIC OF IRELAND

	0-14	15-24	25-34	35-44	45-54	55-64	65-74	75+
1980	3	27	39	36	44	30	21	4
1981	0	35	45	37	40	29	16	7
1982	1	38	52	48	28	30	22	9
1983	2	53	52	33	36	37	31	5
1984	3	29	51	33	28	36	24	6
1985	1	56	55	36	23	51	34	5
1986	2	51	54	49	41	42	28	7
1987	1	40	50	47	29	40	27	6
1988	0	51	61	29	22	42	21	18
1989	2	47	53	57	44	33	29	12
1990	5	50	58	52	46	44	20	9
1991	0	68	75	70	33	38	20	10
1992	3	73	86	43	43	35	28	12
1993	9	47	61	62	30	35	23	8
1994	2	72	78	54	49	31	17	13
1995	5	76	67	74	41	24	25	15
1996	4	83	91	75	44	32	13	15
1997	4	114	85	86	54	38	15	12
1998	1	118	114	88	72	34	26	15
1999	3	99	98	65	61	49	23	12
2000	1	97	115	86	70	45	20	7
2001	3	98	122	97	80	49	27	11
2002	1	104	127	75	64	45	29	9
2003	2	101	92	77	50	49	19	11
2004	1	87	91	86	60	49	16	9

2 FEMALE SUICIDE DEATHS BY TEN-YEAR AGE GROUP, 1980–2004, REPUBLIC OF IRELAND

	0-14	15-24	25-34	35-44	45-54	55-64	65-74	75+
1980	1	13	18	13	16	19	12	4
1981	0	6	13	19	22	19	6	1
1982	0	9	7	16	12	21	10	5
1983	0	10	15	15	15	29	9	2
1984	1	10	10	20	17	19	11	1
1985	1	5	14	16	15	14	14	1
1986	1	13	11	13	21	19	13	1
1987	1	10	9	18	12	13	7	6
1988	1	8	14	19	17	17	11	3
1989	1	10	10	15	12	16	20	9
1990	0	14	22	18	15	15	9	5
1991	0	4	15	12	15	11	9	4
1992	0	7	12	7	9	13	10	4
1993	0	9	13	15	14	11	5	4
1994	2	13	9	17	21	12	17	3
1995	2	11	20	19	18	11	3	3
1996	0	14	15	13	14	7	1	2
1997	0	20	12	16	17	10	15	3
1998	1	15	15	25	20	14	5	4
1999	1	20	18	20	23	18	10	6
2000	3	24	13	27	20	9	13	5
2001	0	18	18	22	26	20	3	3
2002	2	16	26	19	24	14	6	5
2003	2	16	22	12	23	14	2	4
2004	2	12	20	24	30	18	8	3

3   TOTAL SUICIDE DEATHS BY TEN-YEAR AGE GROUP, 1980–2004,
     REPUBLIC OF IRELAND

	0-14	15-24	25-34	35-44	45-54	55-64	65-74	75+
1980	4	40	57	49	60	49	33	8
1981	0	41	58	56	62	48	22	8
1982	1	47	59	64	40	51	32	14
1983	2	63	67	48	51	66	40	7
1984	4	39	61	53	45	55	35	7
1985	2	61	69	52	38	65	48	6
1986	3	64	65	62	62	61	41	8
1987	2	50	59	65	41	53	34	12
1988	1	59	75	48	39	59	32	21
1989	3	57	63	72	56	49	49	21
1990	5	64	80	70	61	59	29	14
1991	0	72	90	82	48	49	29	14
1992	3	80	98	50	52	48	38	16
1993	9	56	74	77	44	46	28	12
1994	4	85	87	71	70	43	34	16
1995	7	87	87	93	59	35	28	18
1996	4	97	106	88	58	39	14	17
1997	4	134	97	102	71	48	30	15
1998	2	133	129	113	92	48	31	19
1999	4	119	116	85	84	67	33	18
2000	4	121	128	113	90	54	33	12
2001	3	116	140	119	106	69	30	14
2002	3	120	153	94	88	59	35	14
2003	4	117	114	89	73	63	21	15
2004	3	99	111	110	90	67	24	12

4   DEATHS FROM SUICIDE CLASSIFIED BY COUNTY OF RESIDENCE OF
      DECEASED AND SEX, 2004

PROVINCE	COUNTY OF RESIDENCE	ALL	MALE	FEMALE
LEINSTER	CARLOW	6	5	1
	DUBLIN BELGARD	31	21	10
	DUBLIN CITY	50	42	8
	DUBLIN FINGAL	12	11	1
	DUN LAOGHAIRE RATHDOWN	11	7	4
	KILDARE	13	13	0
	KILKENNY	10	9	1
	LAOIS	3	2	1
	LONGFORD	5	3	2
	LOUTH	12	8	4
	MEATH	24	20	4
	OFFALY	12	8	4
	WESTMEATH	7	6	1
	WEXFORD	11	10	1
	WICKLOW	12	10	2
MUNSTER	CLARE	14	8	6
	CORK CITY	18	13	5
	CORK COUNTY	51	38	13
	KERRY	21	17	4
	LIMERICK CITY	9	9	0
	LIMERICK COUNTY	16	11	5
	TIPPERARY NORTH	11	9	2
	TIPPERARY SOUTH	6	3	3
	WATERFORD CITY	10	6	4
	WATERFORD COUNTY	6	6	0
CONNACHT	GALWAY CITY	4	3	1
	GALWAY COUNTY	11	9	2
	LEITRIM	4	3	1
	MAYO	11	8	3
	ROSCOMMON	1	1	0
	SLIGO	10	8	2
ULSTER (PART OF)	CAVAN	9	7	2
	DONEGAL	18	15	3
	MONAGHAN	8	7	1
ALL		457	356	101

Appendix 3

Drugs Commonly Used for the 'Flag' Illnesses

Common Antidepressant Drugs in Use

Drugs which affect the Serotonin Cable
1. Fluoxetine (Prozac, Prozamel, Gerozac)
2. Citalopram (Cipramil, Citrol, Ciprager)
3. Escitalopram (Lexapro)
4. Paroxetine (Seroxat, Meloxat Parox)
5. Sertaline (Lustral) – this has minor effects on the dopamine cable as well

Possible main side effects of these drugs
1. Initial nausea in first week in some cases
2. Reduced libido and delayed orgasm in some cases
3. Slightly heavier periods in some women
4. Occasional mild tremors
5. Initial fatigue and anxiety in certain cases

Drugs which affect the Noradrenalin Cable
Reboxetine (Edronax)

Possible main side effects of this drug
1. Sweating, headaches and nausea
2. Sleep difficulties
3. Dry mouth
4. Impotence in some cases

Drugs which affect the Serotonin and Noradrenalin Cables
1. Venlafaxine (Efexor XL)
2. Cymbalta (Duloxetine)
3. Zispin (Mirtazapine)

Possible main side effects of these drugs
1. A mixture of both of the above groups of symptoms!
2. In the case of the latter: weight gain

4   OLDER ANTIDEPRESSANTS IN USE
      1   Amitriptyline
      2   Trazodone (Molipaxin)
      3   Tofranil (Imipramine)
      4   Trimipramine (Surmontil)
      5   Lofepramine (Gamanil)
      6   Dothepin (Prothiaden)

Main side effects of these drugs
      1   Drowsiness (apart from Imipramine)
      2   Higher risk of serious consequences if taken in overdose
      3   Dry mouth, constipation and blurred vision are quite common

5   THE MOOD STABILIZERS
      1   Lithium (Priadel or Camcolit)
      2   Lamotrigine (Lamictal)
      3   Sodium Valproate (Epilim)
      4   Carbamazepine (Tegretol)

Main side effects of these drugs
      1   Weight gain (particularly Lithium and sodium Valproate)
      2   Skin rashes (particularly Lamotrigine)
      3   Teratogenic (all bar Lamotrigine)
      4   Dangerous in overdoses (particularly Lithium)

COMMON ANTI-ANXIETY DRUGS IN USE

THE BENZODIAZEPAMS: LONG-ACTING
      1   Diazepam (Valium)
      2   Chlordiazepoxide (Librium)
      3   Clonazepam (Rivotril).

THE BENZODIAZEPAMS: SHORT- TO MEDIUM-ACTING
      1   Bromazepam (Lexotane)
      2   Alprazolam (Xanax, Gerax)

Possible main side effects of benzodiazepams
      1   Drowsiness
      2   Impairment of concentration
      3   High risk of becoming dependent if used for long periods
      4   High risk of developing tolerance to these drugs

Appendix 4

Help Groups and Contact Details

Aware

Aware is a voluntary organisation established in 1985 to support those experiencing depression and their families. Aware endeavors to create a society where people with mood disorders and their families are understood and supported, and obtain the resources to enable them to defeat depression. Weekly support group meetings at approximately fifty locations nationwide, including Northern Ireland, offer peer support and provide factual information, and enable people to gain the skills they need to help them cope with depression, and the 'Beat the Blues' educational programme is run in secondary schools.

72 Lower Leeson Street, Dublin 2 | (01) 661 7211 | info@aware.ie | www.aware.ie | Helpline: 1890 303 302

Samaritans

Samaritans was started in 1953 in London by a young vicar called Chad Varah; the first branch to be opened in the Republic of Ireland was opened in 1970, in Dublin. Samaritans is available twenty-four hours a day to provide confidential emotional support for people who are experiencing feelings of distress or despair, including those which may lead to suicide.

jo@samaritans.org | www.samaritans.org | Texts: 0872 60 90 90 | Helpline: 1850 60 90 90

Grow

Established in Ireland in 1969, GROW is Ireland's largest mutual help organisation in the area of mental health. It is anonymous, non-denominational, confidential and free. No referrals are necessary. Grow aims to achieve self-activation through mutual help. Its members are enabled, over time, to craft a step by step recovery or personal growth plan and along the way to develop leadership skills that will help others.

Barrack Street, Kikenny | 056 61624 | grownational@grow.ie | www.grow.ie | Helpline: 1890 474 474

Irish Suicidology Association

The Irish Association of Suicidology, an all-Ireland association, was established in 1996 in response to the tragedy of suicide in Ireland at a time when suicide rates were increasing rapidly. The aims and objectives of the IAS are to facilitate communication between clinicians, volunteers, survivors and researchers in all matters relating to suicide and suicidal behaviour; to promote awareness of the problems of suicide and suicidal behaviour in the general public by holding conferences and workshops and by communication of relevant materials through the media; to ensure that the public is better informed about suicide prevention; to support and encourage relevant research; and to encourage and support the formation of groups to help those bereaved by suicide.

16 New Antrim Street, Castlebar, County Mayo | 094 925 0858 | office@ias.ie | www.ias.ie

Console

Console is a registered charity supporting and helping people bereaved through suicide. We respect each individual's unique journey through the grieving process following their tragic loss. Console promotes positive mental health within the community in an effort to reduce the high number of attempted suicides and deaths through suicide.

Console Dublin: All Hallows College, Gracepark Rd, Drumcondra, Dublin 9 01 857 4300| info@console.ie | www.console.ie | Helpline: 1800 201 890

Rainbows Ireland

Rainbows was founded in America by Suzy Yehl Marta to help children and adults who have been bereaved through parental death, separation or divorce to work through the grieving process which follows any significant loss. The charity provides a safe setting in which children can talk through their feelings with other children who are experiencing similar situations.

Loreto Centre, Crumlin Road, Dublin 12 | 01 473 4175

Childline

Childline, a service run by the ISPCC, seeks to empower and support children using the medium of telecommunications and information technologies. The service is designed for all children and young people up to the age of eighteen years in Ireland.

Helpline: 1890 66 66 66

Cuan Mhuire

This is a charitable organisation founded by Sister Consilio Fitzgerald in 1965. It provides a comprehensive structured, abstinence-based residential program dealing with alcohol, gambling and drug addiction in the north and south of Ireland, with centres in Athy, Athenry, Newry, Limerick and Cork.

063 00555 | cuanmhuire@gmail.com

Gamblers Anonymous Ireland and GamAnon

Self-help meetings for gamblers and those close to them.

Dublin 01 872 1133 | Cork 087 349 4450 | Galway 087 349 4450 | nfo@gamblersanonymous.ie

Alanon/Alateen

Self-help meetings for spouses and teenagers (aged twelve to seventeen) affected by those addicted to alcohol.

5 Capel Street, Dublin 1 | 01 873 2699 | info@al-anon-ireland.org | Peace House, 224 Lisburn Road, Belfast | 028 9068 2368

Narcotics Anonymous

Self help groups for those addicted to drugs.

4–5 Eustace Street, Dublin 2 | 01 672 8000 | na@ireland.org

The Irish Council for Psychotherapy

Offer a guide to and directory of psychotherapists who work in Ireland.

73 Quinns Road, Shankhill, County Dublin | 01 272 2105 | info@icpty.ie

Schizophrenia Ireland

Schizophrenia Ireland is the national organisation dedicated to upholding the rights and addressing the needs of all those affected by enduring mental illness, including, but not exclusively, schizophrenia, schizo-affective disorder and bipolar disorder, through the promotion and provision of high-quality services and working to ensure the continual enhancement of the quality of life of the people it serves.

38 Blessington Street, Dublin 7 | 01 860 1620 | info@sirl.ie

BIBLIOGRAPHY

Altman, J. (1996), 'A biological view of drug abuse', *Molecular Medicine Today*, 2 (6), 237–41

Anderson, R. (2003), 'Alcohol abuse', forum, Dublin: Newmedia.

Arango, V., M. D. Underwood and J. J. Mann (2002), 'Serotonin brain circuits in major depression', *Progress in Brain Research*, 136, 443–53

Ballamier, M., A. W. Toga, R. E. Blanton, E. R. Sowell et al. (2004), 'Anterior cingulate, *gyrus rectus*, and orbito-frontal abnormalities in elderly depressed patients: An MRI-based parcellation of the prefrontal cortex', *American Journal of Psychiatry*, 161, 99–108.

Bates, T. (1999), *Depression: The Commonsense Approach*, Dublin: Newleaf

———— (2004), 'Conversations that keep us alive', 3TS Conference, Dublin

Benedetti, F., H. S. Mayberg, T. D. Wager, C. S. Stohler and J. Zubieta (2005), 'Neurobiological mechanisms of the placebo effect', *Journal of Neuroscience*, 25 (45), 10390–402

Brendel, G. R., E. Stern and D. A. Silbersweig (2005), 'Defining the neurocircuitry of borderline personality disorder: Functional neuro-imaging approaches', *Development and Psychopathology*, 17, 1197–2206

Brody, A. L., S. Saxena, L. Matthew et al. (2001), 'Neuroimaging profiles and the differential therapies of depression', *Archives of General Psychiatry*, 58, 651–53

Brophy, J. (2006), 'Bipolar disorder', forum, Dublin: Medmedia

Butcher, J. N., S. Mineka, J. M. Hooley and R. C.Carson (2004), *Abnormal Psychology*, Boston: Pearson Education.

Cahill, L. (2005), 'His brain, her brain', *Scientific American*

Carlson, N. R. (2004), *Physiology of Behaviour*, Boston: Pearson Education

Chao, J. and E. Nestler (2004), 'Molecular neurobiology of addiction', *Annual Review of Medicine*, 55, 113–32

Cloningerm, C. R., S. Sigvardsson, S. B. Gilligan, A. L. Von Knorring, T. Reich and M. Bohman, 'Genetic heterogeneity and the classification of alcoholism', *Advances in Alcohol and Substance Abuse*, 7 (34), 3–16

Cotter, D., D. McKay, S. Landau, R. Kerwin and I. Everall (2001), 'Reduced glial-cell density and neuronal size in the anterior-cingulate cortex in major depressive disorder', *Archives of General Psychiatry*, 58, 545–53

Coyle J. T. and R. Schwarcz (2000), 'Mind glue: implications of glial-cell biology for psychiatry', *Archives of General Psychiatry*, 59, 90–93

Davison, G. C., J. M. Neale and A. M. Kring (2004), *Abnormal Psychology*, New Jersey: John Wiley & Sons

De Paulo, J. R. and L. A. Horvitz (2002), *Understanding Depression*, New Jersey: John Wiley & Sons

Dinan, T. G. (1994), 'Glucocorticoids and the genesis of depressive illness. A psycho-biological model', *British Journal of Psychiatry*, 164, 365–71

———— (1999), 'Psychiatry-physical consequences of depressive illness', *Irish Medical Times*

Dineen, S. (1999), 'Advances in psychiatry: The genetics of alcoholism', *Irish Medical Times*

Dobbs, D. (2006), 'Mastery of emotions', *Scientific American Mind*

———— (2006), 'Turning off depression', *Scientific American Mind*

:evets, W. C. (1999), 'Pre-frontal cortical-amygdalar metabolism in major depression', *Annals of Academy of Sciences*, 877, 614–37

—— (2000), 'Neuroimaging of mood disorders', *Biological Psychiatry*, 48, 813–29

—— (2001), 'Neuroimaging and neuropathological studies of depression: Implications for the cognitive-emotional features of mood disorders', *Current Opinion in Neurobiology*, 11, 240–49

:yden, W. (2003), *Handbook of Individual Therapy*, London: Sage

uman, R. S., G. R. Heniger and E. J. Nestler (1997), 'A molecular and cellular theory of depression', *Archives of General Psychiatry*, 54 (7), 607–8

umser, T., A. Barocka and E. Schubert (1998), 'Weight of adrenal glands may be increased in persons who commit suicide', *American Journal of Forensic Medicine and Pathology*, 19 (1), 72–76

kin, A., C. Pittenger, J. Polan and R. Kandal (2005), 'Towards a neurobiology of psychotherapy: Basic science and clinical applications', *Journal of Neuropsychiatry–Clinical Neuroscience*, 17, 145–58

:zell, C. (2003), 'Why? The neuroscience of suicide', *Scientific American*

:zpatrick, C. (2001), 'Suicide and mental health: What's new in childhood and adolescence?', *Irish Medical Times*

age, F. H. (2003), 'Brain repair yourself', *Scientific American*

eaney, C. (2003), 'The true picture of parasuicide in Ireland', forum, Dublin: Medmedia

eorge, M. S. (2003), 'Stimulating the brain', *Scientific American*

oldapple, K. (2004), 'Modulation of cortical-limbic pathways in major depression: Treatment-specific effects of cognitive behaviour therapy', *Archives of General Psychiatry*, 61, 34–41

oldberg, E. (2001), *The Executive Brain*, New York: Oxford University Press

:eenwald, B. S., E. K. Ginsberg, K. R. R. Krishnan, M. Ashtari, C. Auerbacch, M. Patel (1998), 'Neuroanatomic localization of MRI signal hyperintensities in geriatric depression', *Stroke*, 29, 613–617

:oss, R. (2001), *Psychology. The Science Behind Mind and Behaviour*, London: Hodder and Stoughton

arrison, P. J. (2002), 'The neuropathology of primary mood disorder', *Brain* 125 (7), 1428–49

emby, S. E. (1999), 'Recent advances in the biology of addiction', *Current Psychiatry Reports*, 1 (2), 159–65

ilty, D. M., K. T. Brady and R. E. Hales (1999), 'A review of bipolar disorder among adults', *Psychiatric Services*, 50, 201–3

olford, P. (2003), *Optimum Nutrition for the Mind*, London: Judy Piaktus Ltd

ollaway, M. (2003), 'The mutable brain', *Scientific American*

awton, K and K. Van Heeringen (2002), *The International Handbook of Suicide and Attempted Suicide*, West Sussex: John Wiley and Sons

yman, S. E. (2003), 'Diagnosing disorders', *Scientific American*

mieson, K. and T. G. Dinan (2001), 'Glucocorticoids and cognitive function: from physiology to pathophysiology', *Human Psychopharmacology, Clinical and Experimental*, 16 (4), 293–302

lian, R. M. (2001), *A Primer of Drug Action*, New York: Henry Holt and Company, LLC

amali, M., M. A. Oquendo and J. J. Mann (2001), 'Understanding the neurobiology of suicidal behaviour', *Depression and Anxiety* 14, 164–176

Kapczinski, F., B. N. Frey and V. Zannatto (2004), 'Physiopathology of bipolar disorders: What h
changed in the last ten years?', *Revista Braileira de Psiquiatria*, 26 (3)

Kennedy, S. H., M. Javanmard and F. J. Vaccarino (1997), 'A review of functional neuro-imaging in mo‹
disorders: Positron emission tomography and depression', *Canadian Journal of Psychiatry*, 42, 467–7!

Khan, A., H. A. Warner and W. A. Browne (2000), 'Symptom reduction and suicide risk in patients tre
ed with placebo in antidepressant clinical trials: An analysis of the FDA database', *Archives of Gene
Psychiatry*, 57, 311–17

Kolb, B and I. Q. Whishaw (2002), *An Introduction to Brain and Behaviour*, New York: Worth

Koob, G. F. (2006), 'The neurobiology of addiction: A neuroadaptive view relevant for diagnos‹
Addiction, 101, 23–30

Kramer, P. D. (1994), *Listening to Prozac*, London: Fourth Estate

Lam, R. W. and R. D. Levitan (2002), 'Pathophysiology of seasonal affective disorder: A review', *Journa.
Psychiatry and Neuroscience*, 25 (5), 469–80

LeDoux, J. E. (2002), 'Emotion, memory and the brain', *Scientific American*

Leonard, B. E. (2007), 'Melatonin receptors and antidepressant strategies', *Irish Psychiatrist*, 8 (1), 37–40

Lingford-Hughes, A. and D. Nutt (2003), 'Neurobiology of addiction and implications for treatmer
British Journal of Psychiatry, 182, 97–100

Logan, A. C. (2004), 'Omega-3 fatty acids and major depression: A primer for the mental-health profe
sional', *Lipids in Health and Disease*, 3 (25)

——— (2003), 'Neurobehavioral aspects of Omega-3 fatty acids: Possible mechanisms and therapeu
value in major depression', *Alternative Medical Review*, 8 (4), 410–25

Lucey, J. V. (1999), 'Obsessive compulsive disorder', *Irish Medical Times*

——— (2004), 'Generalised anxiety disorder', forum, Dublin: Medmedia

Lynch, T. (2001), *Beyond Prozac*, Dublin: Marino Books

Manji, H. K., W. C. Drevets and D. S. Charney (2001), 'The cellular neurobiology of depression', *Nat.
Medicine*, 7 (5)

Manji, H. K., J.A. Quiroz, J. L.Payne, J. Singh, B. P. Lopes, J. L. Viegas and C. A. Zarate (October 200.
'The underlying neurobiology of bipolar disorder', *World Psychiatry*, 2 (3), 136–46

Mann, J. J. (2003), 'Neurobiology of suicidal behaviour', *Nature Review/Neuroscience*, 4

——— (2004), 'National strategies for suicide prevention', 3TS Conference, Dublin

Marano, H. E. (1999), 'Depression beyond serotonin', *Psychology Today*

——— (2002), 'The many faces of depression', *Psychology Today*

Marchand, W. R., D. V. Dilda, C. R. Jensen (2005), 'Neurobiology of mood disorders', *Hospital Physicie*
September, 17–26, 43

Mayberg, H. S., J. A. Silva, S. K. Brannan, J. L. Tekell, R. K. Malhurin, S. McGinnis and P. A. Jerabek (200:
'The functional neuroanatomy of the placebo effect', *American Journal of Psychiatry*

——— (2003), 'Modulating dysfunctional limbic-cortical circuits in depression: Towards development ‹
brain-based algorithms for diagnosis and optimised treatment', *British Medical Bulletin*, 65, 193–207

——— (2005), 'Deep-brain stimulation for treatment-resistant depression', *Neuron*, 45 (5), 651–60

McGaugh, J. L. (2002), 'Memory consolidation and the amygdala: A systems perspective', *Trends in Neurosciences*, 25 (9), 456–80

McGauran, A. T., D. Barry and S. Commins (2006), 'Disruption of consolidation of long-term spatial memories: A role for protein synthesis and glutaminergic (NMDA/AMPA) receptors', *FENS Abstracts*, 3, 68

McKeown, P. (1995), *Coping With Depression and Elation*, London: Sheldon Press

——— (1998), 'Suicide in Ireland: A global perspective and a national strategy', Aware Publications

——— (1999). 'Depression and suicide', forum, Dublin: Medmedia

McKeown, P., J. Healy, G. Bailey and G. Ward (2000), 'Depression: Keeping hope alive', Aware Publications

Mirza, K. A. H., A. Michael and T. G. Dinan, 'Recent advances in paediatric psychopharmacology: A brief overview', *Human Psychopharmacology: Clinical and Experimental*, 9 (1), 13–24

Murck, H. (2003), 'Atypical depression spectrum disorder: Neurobiology and treatment', *Acta Neuropsychiatrica*, 15 (4), 227–41

Nemeroff, C. B. and W. W. Vale (2005), 'The neurobiology of depression: Inroads to treatments and new drug discovery', *Journal of Clinical Psychology*, 7, 5–13

Nestler, E. (2001), 'Molecular neurobiology of addiction', *American Journal of Addiction*, 10 (3), 201–17

Nestler, E. and R. C. Malenka (2004), 'The addicted brain', *Scientific American*

Obrien, S. M., L. V. Scott and T. G. Dinan (2004), 'Cytokines: Abnormalities in major depression and implications for pharmacological treatment', *Human Psychopharmacology: Clinical and Experimental*, 19 (6), 397–403

Öngur, D., W. C. Drevets and J. L. Price (1998), 'Glial reduction in the subgenual prefrontal cortex in mood disorders', *Proceedings of the National Academy of Sciences*, 95 (22), 13290–95

Oquendo, M. A., G. P. Placidi, K. M. Malone, C. Campbell, J. Keilp, B. Brodsky, L. S. Kegeles, T. B. Cooper, R. V. Parsey and R. L. Van Heertuum, (2003), 'Positron emission tomography of regional brain metabolic responses to a serotonergic challenge and lethality of suicide attempts in major depression', *Archives of General Psychiatry*, 60 (1), 14–22

——— (2003), 'Identifying neurobiological correlates of suicide risk in depression', *Psychiatric Times* (3)

Park, A. (2004), 'What makes teens tick?', *Time*

Philips, M. C., W. C. Drevets, S. L. Rauch and R. Lane (2003), 'Neurobiology of emotion in psychiatric disorders', *Biological Psychiatry*, 54, 515–28

Pinel, J. P. J. (2003), *Biopsychology*, Boston: Pearson Education

Plomin, R., J. C. DeFries, G. E. MacClearn and P. McGuffin (2001), *Behavioural Genetics*, New York: Worth Publishers

Puri, B. K. and H. Boyd (2005), *The Natural Way to Beat Depression*, London: Hodder and Stoughton

Quitkin, F. M., J. G. Rabkin, J. Gerald, J. M. Davis and D. F. Klein (2000), 'Validity of clinical trials of antidepressants', *American Journal of Psychiatry*, 157, 327–37

Quitkin, F. M. and D. F. Klein (2000), 'What conditions are necessary to assess antidepressant efficacy?', *Archives of General Psychiatry*, 57, 323–24

Raine, A., T. Lenz, S. Bihrle, L. LaCasses and P. Colletti (2000), 'Reduced prefrontal grey matter volume and reduced autonomic activity in antisocial personality disorder', *Archives of General Psychiatry*, 54 (7), 607–8

Ressler, K. J. and C. B. Nemeroff (2003), 'Depression', in Rosenberg, R. N., S. B. Prusiner, D. S. DiMauro, R. L. Barchi and E. J. Nestler (2003), *The Molecular and Genetic Basis of Neurologic and Psychiatric Disease*, third edition, Woburn, Massachusetts: Butterworth Heinemann

Reyna V. F. and F. Farley (2006), 'Is the teen brain too rational?', *Scientific American Mind*

Sabbagh, L. (2006), 'The teen brain', *Scientific American Mind*

Sapolsky, R. (2003), 'Taming Stress', *Scientific American*

Servan-Screiber, D. (2004), *Healing Without Freud or Prozac*, London: Rodale

Sheline, Y. I., P. W. Wang, M. H. Gado, J. G. Csernansky and M. W. Vannier (1996), 'Hippocampal atrophy in recurrent major depression', Proceedings of the National Academy of Sciences, USA, Vol. 93, 3908–13

Szigethy, E., Y. Cornwell, N. T. Forbes, C. Cox and E. D. Caine, 'Adrenal weight and morphology in victims of completed suicide', *Biological Psychiatry*, 36 (6), 374–80

Thomas, A. J., J. T. O'Brien, S. Davis, C. Ballard, R. Barber, R. Kalaria and R. H. Perry (2002), 'Ischemic basis for deep white matter hyperintensities in major depression: A neuro-pathological study', *Archives of General Psychiatry*, 59, 785–92

Ulian, E. M., S. K. Sapperstein, K. S. Christopherson and B. A. Barres (2001), 'Control of synapse number by glia', *Science*, 5504, 657–61

Vythilingam, M., C. Heim, J. Newport, A. Miller et al. (2002), 'Childhood trauma associated with smaller hippocampal volume in women with major depression', *American Journal of Psychiatry*, 159, 2072–80

Walsh, M. T., T. G. Dinan, R. M. Condron, M. Ryan and D. Kenny, 'Depression is associated with an increase in the expression of the platelet adhesion receptor glycoprotein Ib', *Life Sciences*, 70 (26), 31555–65

White, F. J. (2002), 'A behavioural/systems approach to the neuroscience of drug addiction', *Journal of Neuroscience*, 22 (9), 3303–5

Wickens, A. (2005), *Foundations of Biopsychology*, Essex: Pearson Education

Willenberg, H. S., S. R. Bornstein, T. Dumser, M. Ehrhart-Bornstein, A. Barocka, G. P. Chrousos and W. A. Scherbaum (1998), 'Morphological changes in adrenals from victims of suicide in relation to altered apoptosis', *Endocrine Research*, 24 (3–4), 963–67

Zubenko, G. S., H. B. Hughes, D. S. Maher, J. S. Stiffler, W. N. Zubenko and M. L. Marazita. (2002), 'Genetic linkage of region containing the Creb1 gene to depressive disorders in women from families with recurrent early-onset major depression', *American Journal of Medical Genetics*, 114 (8), 980–87

'Reach Out: National Strategy for Action on Suicide Prevention" (2005–14), HSE, the National Suicide Review Group and the Department of Health and Children

'Strategic Task Force on Alcohol: Interim Report' (May 2002), Department of Health and Children

'A Vision for Change: Report of the Expert Group on Mental Health Policy' (2006–), Department of Health and Children